THE BEST INTENTIONS

Unintended Pregnancy and the Well-Being of Children and Families

Committee on Unintended Pregnancy

Division of Health Promotion and Disease Prevention

INSTITUTE OF MEDICINE

Sarah S. Brown and Leon Eisenberg, Editors

NATIONAL ACADEMY PRESS
Washington, D.C. 1995

Institute of Medicine · 2101 Constitution Avenue, NW · Washington, DC 20418

NOTICE: The project that is the subject of this report was approved by the Governing Board of the National Research Council, whose members are drawn from the councils of the National Academy of Sciences, the National Academy of Engineering, and the Institute of Medicine. The members of the committee responsible for this report were chosen for their special competencies and with regard for appropriate balance.

This report has been reviewed by a group other than the authors according to procedures approved by a Report Review Committee consisting of members of the National Academy of Sciences, the National Academy of Engineering, and the Institute of Medicine.

The Institute of Medicine was chartered in 1970 by the National Academy of Sciences to enlist distinguished members of the appropriate professions in the examination of policy matters pertaining to the health of the public. In this, the Institute acts under both the Academy's 1863 congressional charter responsibility to be an adviser to the federal government and its own initiative in identifying issues of medical care, research, and education. Dr. Kenneth I. Shine is president of the Institute of Medicine.

This project was funded by the Carnegie Corporation of New York, which does not take responsibility for any statements or views expressed; the Robert Wood Johnson Foundation; and the U.S. Public Health Service (specifically the Maternal and Child Health Bureau, the Centers for Disease Control and Prevention, the National Institute of Child Health and Human Development, and the Office of Population Affairs).

Library of Congress Cataloging-in-Publication Data

The best intentions : unintended pregnancy and the well-being of children and families / Committee on Unintended Pregnancy, Institute of Medicine, National Academy of Sciences ; Sarah S. Brown and Leon Eisenberg, editors.
p. cm.
Includes bibliographical references and index.
ISBN 0-309-05230-0
1. Pregnancy, Unwanted—Government policy—United States. 2. Birth control—Government policy—United States. 3. Birth control clinics—Utilization—United States. I. Brown, Sarah S. II. Eisenberg, Leon, 1922- . III. Institute of Medicine (U.S.). Committee on Unintended Pregnancy.
HQ766.5.U5B47 1995 95-12064
304.6'66'0973—dc20 CIP

Printed in the United States of America

The serpent has been a symbol of long life, healing, and knowledge among almost all cultures and religions since the beginning of recorded history. The image adopted as a logotype by the Institute of Medicine is based on relief carving from ancient Greece, now held by the Staatlichemuseen in Berlin.

COMMITTEE ON UNINTENDED PREGNANCY

Leon Eisenberg,* *Chair,* Maude and Lillian Presley Professor of Social Medicine and Professor of Psychiatry Emeritus, Department of Social Medicine, Harvard Medical School, Boston, Massachusetts

Larry Bumpass, N.B. Ryder Professor of Sociology, Center for Demography and Ecology, University of Wisconsin at Madison *(liaison from the Board on Children and Families, jointly sponsored by the Commission on Behavioral and Social Sciences and Education and the Institute of Medicine)*

Sharon Lovick Edwards, President, The Cornerstone Consulting Group, Inc., Houston, Texas

Carol J.R. Hogue, Professor of Epidemiology and Jules and Deen Terry Professor of Maternal and Child Health, Rollins School of Public Health of Emory University, Atlanta, Georgia

Sylvia Drew Ivie, Executive Director, T.H.E. Clinic, Los Angeles, California

Robert L. Johnson, Professor of Clinical Pediatrics and Psychiatry, Director of Adolescent and Young Adult Medicine, New Jersey Medical School, Newark

Lorraine V. Klerman, Chair, Department of Maternal and Child Health, School of Public Health, University of Alabama at Birmingham

George A. Little, Professor of Pediatrics and Obstetrics and Gynecology, Dartmouth-Hitchcock Medical Center, Lebanon, New Hampshire

Marie C. McCormick, Chair, Department of Maternal and Child Health, Harvard School of Public Health, Boston, Massachusetts *(liaison from the Institute of Medicine Board on Health Promotion and Disease Prevention)*

Sara S. McLanahan, Professor of Sociology and Public Affairs, Office of Population Research, Princeton University, Princeton, New Jersey

Mark R. Montgomery, Associate Professor, Department of Economics, State University of New York at Stony Brook, Stony Brook, New York

Helen Rodriguez-Trias, Pediatrician-Consultant in Health Programming, Brookdale, California

Allan Rosenfield,* Dean, School of Public Health, Columbia University, New York, New York

---

*IOM Member

Study Staff

Sarah S. Brown, Senior Study Director
Dana Hotra, Research Associate
Alison E. Smith, Research Assistant
Michael A. Stoto, Director, Division of Health Promotion and Disease Prevention

Acknowledgments

This report on unintended pregnancy represents the collaborative efforts of many groups and individuals, particularly the supervising committee and staff whose names appear at the beginning of this document. The topic addressed by this study proved to be an unusually complicated one, and it required great dedication and effort by all concerned to complete the report that appears here.

Particularly helpful were the many papers developed for the committee; a full listing of them is in Appendix A. These papers assisted the committee in understanding and integrating many disparate sets of information. In addition, major portions of some papers were incorporated directly into the report itself. For example, material drafted by Kristin Moore and Dana Glei formed the backbone of Chapter 2; sections drafted by Jim Marks and Kristin Moore and by committee members Larry Bumpass, George Little, Sara McLanahan, and, in particular, Carol Hogue, were relied on heavily in Chapter 3; the work of committee member Allan Rosenfield and of Lisa Kaeser, Cory Richards, Jane Brown, and Jeanne Steele contributed to much of Chapter 5; a review article by Nancy Adler and Warren Miller assisted in the conceptualization of Chapter 6; and the work of committee members Lorraine Klerman and Marie McCormick and of Vanessa Gamble, Judith Houck, Mort Lebow, William D'Antonio, and Allan Carlson contributed substantially to Chapter 7. Rebecca Maynard and committee members Mark Montgomery and Lorraine Klerman also provided much helpful material for Chapter 8. Finally, it is important to acknowledge the particular contributions of committee members Carol Hogue, Larry Bumpass, and Mark Montgomery who developed important technical materials in Appendixes D, E, and G, respectively. All sections benefited enormously from the careful review of research on the determinants of contraceptive use developed by Koray Tanfer, as well as from the thoughtful paper on men and family planning by Freya Sonenstein and Joseph Pleck. To all of these scientists and others listed in Appendix A, the committee expresses its deep admiration and appreciation.

In addition, we extend special gratitude to a number of colleagues who provided much assistance along the way, especially Christine Bachrach, Wendy Baldwin, Marie Bass, Jerry Bennett, Doug Besharov, Virginia Cartoof, Jan Chapin, Henry David, Sara DePersio, Judith DeSarno, Joy Dryfoos, Erica Elvander, Shelly Gehshan, Rachel Gold, Debra Haffner, Carol Herman, Ruth Katz, Woodie Kessel, Doug Kirby, Rebecca Maynard, Arden Miller, Warren Miller, Kathy Morton, Sarah Samuels, James Trussell, and Laurie Zabin. Analysts with the National Center for Health Statistics were of enormous assistance as well—William Mosher, Kathryn London, Linda Peterson, and Linda Piccinino. Similarly, the leadership and staff of The Alan Guttmacher Institute (AGI) were unfailingly helpful, especially Jeannie Rosoff and Jacqueline Forrest, as were AGI's countless publications on many issues central to this report. Finally, Elena Nightingale and Lisbeth Schorr in particular offered much encouragement and assistance in the early stages of this study; their special contributions are gratefully acknowledged.

The Institute of Medicine staff who assured the completion of this document, Dana Hotra and Alison Smith, worked exceedingly hard on this project and have the deepest respect and appreciation of all concerned. Dana helped to draft much of Chapter 2 and completed virtually all of Chapters 4 and 8 and Appendix F. Alison drafted two key sections of Chapter 3 and also prepared the manuscript for publication. In doing so she improved the appearance and accuracy of the final product immeasurably. Finally, we acknowledge the many contributions of our editors, Mike Edington, Michael Hayes, and Elaine McGarragh.

This report was funded by the combined efforts of three groups: the Carnegie Corporation of New York, the Robert Wood Johnson Foundation, and the U.S. Public Health Service (specifically the Maternal and Child Health Bureau, the Centers for Disease Control and Prevention, the National Institute of Child Health and Human Development, and the Office of Population Affairs). Their willingness to finance a study on the causes, consequences, and prevention of unintended pregnancy took no small degree of commitment, inasmuch as this issue continues to be sensitive, even controversial, in some sectors. Their encouragement and funding are gratefully acknowledged.

Sarah Brown, Senior Study Director
Leon Eisenberg, Committee Chair
Washington, 1995

Contents

APPENDIXES

The Best Intentions

Summary

Unintended pregnancy is both frequent and widespread in the United States. The most recent estimate is that almost 60 percent of all pregnancies are unintended, either mistimed or unwanted altogether[1]—a percentage higher than that found in several other Western democracies. Unintended pregnancy is not just a problem of teenagers or unmarried women or of poor women or minorities; it affects all segments of society.

The consequences of unintended pregnancy are serious, imposing appreciable burdens on children, women, men, and families. A woman with an unintended pregnancy is less likely to seek early prenatal care and is more likely to expose the fetus to harmful substances (such as tobacco or alcohol). The child of an *unwanted* conception especially (as distinct from a *mistimed* one) is at greater risk of being born at low birthweight, of dying in its first year of life, of being abused, and of not receiving sufficient resources for healthy development. The mother may be at greater risk of depression and of physical abuse herself, and her relationship with her partner is at greater risk of dissolution. Both mother and father may suffer economic hardship and may fail to achieve their educational and career goals. Such consequences undoubtedly impede the formation and maintenance of strong families.

In addition, an unintended pregnancy is associated with a higher probability that the child will be born to a mother who is adolescent, unmarried, or over age 40—demographic attributes that themselves have important socioeconomic and

[1]These terms have precise demographic meanings and are defined carefully in the body of the report.

medical consequences for both children and parents. Pregnancy begun without planning and intent also means that individual women and couples are often not able to take full advantage of the growing field of preconception risk identification and management, nor of the rapidly expanding knowledge base regarding human genetics. Moreover, unintended pregnancy currently leads to approximately 1.5 million abortions in the United States annually, a ratio of about one abortion to every three live births. This ratio is two to four times higher than that in other Western democracies, in spite of the fact that access to abortion in those countries is often easier than in the United States. Reflecting the widespread occurrence of unintended pregnancy, abortions are obtained by women of all reproductive ages, by both married and unmarried women, and by women in all income categories.

Of the 5.4 million pregnancies that were estimated to have occurred in 1987, about 3.1 million were unintended at the time of conception. Within this pool of unintended pregnancies, some 1.6 million ended in abortion and 1.5 million resulted in a live birth. Only 2.3 million pregnancies in that year were intended at the time of conception and resulted in a live birth.

During the 1970s and early 1980s, the proportion of births that were unintended at the time of conception decreased. Between 1982 and 1988, however, this trend reversed and the proportion of births that were unintended at conception began *increasing*. This unfortunate trend appears to be continuing into the 1990s. In 1990, about 44 percent of all births were the result of unintended pregnancy;[2] the proportion is close to 60 percent among women in poverty, 62 percent among black women, 73 percent among never-married women, and 86 percent among unmarried teenagers.

Many factors help to explain the nation's high level of unintended pregnancy. Most obvious is the failure to use contraceptive methods carefully and consistently—or sometimes even at all—as well as actual technical failures of the methods themselves. Women and their partners relying on reversible means of contraception (about 21 million women) and those using no contraception at all, despite having no clear intent to become pregnant (about 4 million women), contribute roughly equally to the pool of unintended pregnancies. Many women and couples who are not seeking pregnancy move between these two groups, sometimes using contraception, sometimes not.

Contraceptive use and unintended pregnancy are influenced by numerous factors: knowledge about contraceptive methods and reproductive health generally, individual skill in using contraception properly, a wide range of personal feelings and attitudes, varying patterns of sexual behavior, access to

---

[2]The difference between the percentage of pregnancies that are unintended (close to 60 percent) and the percentage of births resulting from unintended pregnancies (about 44 percent) is due to the intervening occurrence of abortion.

contraceptive methods themselves, cultural values regarding sexuality, religious and political preferences, racism and violence, the sexual saturation of the media, and others as well. The sheer number and complexity of these forces mean that no single or simple remedy is likely to "solve" the unintended pregnancy problem, particularly because the interrelationships among all of these factors are not well understood. Nonetheless, the information reviewed in this report, past experience in the public health sector with addressing complex health and social problems, and common sense are all helpful in developing a plan of action to address this important national problem.

COMMITTEE RECOMMENDATIONS

The extent of unintended pregnancy and its serious consequences are poorly appreciated throughout the United States. Although considerable attention is now focused on teenage pregnancy and nonmarital childbearing, along with continuing controversy and even violence over abortion, the common link among all these issues—pregnancy that is unintended at the time of conception—is essentially invisible. The committee has concluded that reducing unintended pregnancy will require a new national understanding about this problem and a new consensus that pregnancy should be undertaken only with clear intent. Accordingly, the committee urges, first and foremost, that the nation adopt a new social norm:

- **All pregnancies should be intended—that is, they should be consciously and clearly desired at the time of conception.**

This goal has three important attributes. First, it is directed to all Americans and does not target only one group. Second, it emphasizes personal choice and intent. And third, it speaks as much to *planning for* pregnancy as to *avoiding* unintended pregnancy. Bearing children and forming families are among the most significant and satisfying tasks of adult life, and it is in that context that encouraging intended pregnancy is so central.

The U.S. Department of Health and Human Services, through its National Health Promotion and Disease Prevention Objectives, has urged that the proportion of all pregnancies that are unintended be reduced to 30 percent by the year 2000. The committee endorses this goal and stresses that it is a realistic one already reached by several other industrialized nations. Achieving this goal would mean, in absolute numbers, that there would be more than 200,000 fewer births each year that were unwanted at the time of conception, and about 800,000 fewer abortions annually as well.

· To begin the long process of building national consensus around this norm, the committee recommends a multifaceted, long-term campaign to (1) educate the public about the major social and public health burdens of unintended pregnancy and (2) stimulate a comprehensive set of activities at national, state, and local levels to reduce such pregnancies.

It is essential that the campaign direct its messages to national leaders and major U.S. institutions, as well as to individual men and women. The problem of unintended pregnancy is as much one of public policies and institutional practices as it is one of individual behavior, and therefore the campaign should not try to reduce unintended pregnancies only by actions focused on individuals or couples. Although individuals clearly need increased attention and services, reducing unintended pregnancy will require that influential organizations and their leaders—corporate officers, legislators, media owners, and others of similar stature—address this problem as well. The campaign should also draw on the successful experience of other major efforts to address complicated public health problems, such as the national campaigns to reduce smoking, limit drunk driving, and increase the use of seat belts.

The campaign should emphasize that reducing unintended pregnancy will ease many contemporary problems that are of such concern. Both teenage pregnancy and nonmarital childbearing would decline, and abortion in particular would be reduced dramatically. More generally, the lives of children, women, men, and their families, including those now mired in persistent poverty and welfare dependence, would be strengthened considerably by an increase in the proportion of pregnancies that are purposefully undertaken and consciously desired.

The Campaign to Reduce Unintended Pregnancy

The campaign to reduce unintended pregnancy should stress five core goals:

1. improve knowledge about contraception, unintended pregnancy, and reproductive health;

2. increase access to contraception;

3. explicitly address the major roles that feelings, attitudes, and motivation play in using contraception and avoiding unintended pregnancy;

4. develop and scrupulously evaluate a variety of local programs to reduce unintended pregnancy; and

5. stimulate research to (a) develop new contraceptive methods for both women *and* men, (b) answer important questions about how best to organize contraceptive services, and (c) understand more fully the determinants and antecedents of unintended pregnancy.

In the balance of this summary, each of these five campaign goals is outlined in more detail.

· *Campaign Goal 1:* **Improve knowledge about contraception, unintended pregnancy, and reproductive health.**

An important reason for inadequate contraceptive vigilance, and therefore unintended pregnancy, is that many Americans lack adequate knowledge about contraception and reproductive health generally. The fact that many people mistakenly believe that childbearing is less risky medically than using oral contraceptives is a sobering example of this problem. The resulting fears and misconceptions that stem from such erroneous beliefs can impede the careful, consistent use of contraception, which in turn contributes to the risk of unintended pregnancy.

Accordingly, the campaign should include a series of information and education activities directed to women of all ages, not just adolescent girls, describing available contraceptive methods and highlighting, in particular, the common occurrence of unintended pregnancy among women age 20 and over, especially those over age 40 for whom an unintended pregnancy may carry particular medical risks. Activities should target boys and men as well, emphasizing their stake in avoiding unintended pregnancy, the contraceptive methods available to them, and how to support their partners' use of contraception. And both men and women need balanced, accurate information about the benefits and risks attached to specific contraceptive methods.

Parents, families, and both religious and community institutions should be major sources of information and education about reproductive health and family planning, especially for young people, and they should be supported in serving this important function. In addition, U.S. school systems should continue developing comprehensive, age-appropriate programs of sex education that build on new research about effective content, timing, and teacher training for these courses. State laws and policies should be revised, where necessary, to allow and encourage such instruction.

Information and education about contraception should include abstinence as one of many methods available to prevent pregnancy. And particularly in programs directed to adolescents, it is important to encourage and help young people resist precocious sexual involvement. Sexual intercourse should occur in the context of a major interpersonal commitment based on mutual consent and caring and on the exercise of personal responsibility, which includes taking steps to avoid both unintended pregnancy and sexually transmitted diseases (STDs).

The electronic and print media should reinforce the material presented in schools and elsewhere, thereby helping to educate adults as well as school-aged children about contraception and reproductive health. The media should present accurate material on the benefits and risks of contraception and should broaden current messages about preventing STDs to include preventing unintended pregnancy as well. Media producers, advertisers, story writers, and others should also balance current entertainment programming so that, at a minimum, sexual activity is preceded by a mutual understanding of both partners regarding its possible consequences, and accompanied by contraception when appropriate. Similarly, advertising of contraceptive products and public service announcements regarding unintended pregnancy and contraception should be more plentiful.

· *Campaign Goal 2:* **Increase access to contraception.**

Through a combination of financial and structural factors, the health care system in the United States makes access to prescription-based methods of contraception a complicated, sometimes expensive proposition. Private health insurance often does not cover contraceptive costs; the various restrictions on Medicaid eligibility make it an unreliable source of steady financing for contraception except for very poor women who already have a child; and the net decline in public investment in family planning services (especially those services supported by Title X of the Public Health Service Act), in the face of higher costs and sicker patients, may have decreased access to care for those who depend on publicly financed services, particularly adolescents and low-income women. Condoms, the most accessible form of contraception, provide valuable protection against STDs but must be accompanied by other contraceptive methods to afford maximum protection against unintended pregnancy. Unfortunately, other accessible nonprescription methods, such as foam and other spermicides, neither prevent the transmission of STDs nor offer the best protection against unintended pregnancy.

The campaign to reduce unintended pregnancy should promote increased access to contraception generally, but especially to the more effective prescription-based methods that require contact with a health care professional. Financial barriers in particular should be reduced by (1) increasing the proportion of all health insurance policies that cover contraceptive services and supplies, including both male and female sterilization, with no copayments or other cost-sharing requirements, as for other selected preventive health services; (2) extending Medicaid coverage for all postpartum women for 2 years following childbirth for contraceptive services, including sterilization; and (3) continuing to provide public funding—federal, state, and local—for comprehensive contraceptive services, especially for those low-income women and adolescents who face major financial barriers in securing such care.

This last point speaks to the major role that such public financing programs as Title X and Medicaid have played in helping millions of people secure contraception. Although evaluation research has not yet defined the precise effects of these programs on unintended pregnancy, there is no question that they help to finance contraceptive services for many women (and some men), the principal means by which unintended pregnancy is prevented. Accordingly, it is essential that such public investment be maintained. In addition, foundations and government should fund high-quality evaluation studies of the impact that both Title X and Medicaid have on unintended pregnancy and related outcomes. Without better data on the effects of these and other publicly funded programs active in the area of reproductive health, such programs remain particularly vulnerable to attack, and it is difficult to know how best to strengthen them.

As another way to increase access to contraceptive services, the campaign should also broaden the range of health professionals and institutions that promote and provide methods of birth control. Campaign leaders, for example, should work with medical educators to revise the training curricula of a wide variety of health professionals (physicians, nurses, and others) to increase their competence in reproductive health and contraceptive counseling for both males and females and, where appropriate, in actually providing contraceptive methods. The campaign should also encourage those who provide social work, employment training, educational counseling, and other social services to talk with their clients about the benefits of pregnancy planning and how to do so.

· ***Campaign Goal 3:*** **Explicitly address the major roles that feelings, attitudes, and motivation play in using contraception and avoiding unintended pregnancy.**

Although increasing knowledge about and access to contraception (Campaign Goals 1 and 2) are important first steps, they are not enough. The campaign to reduce unintended pregnancy must also address the fact that the personal attitudes, motivation, and feelings of individuals and couples clearly affect contraceptive use and therefore the risk of unintended pregnancy. Similarly, partner preferences, and particularly the quality of a couple's relationship, are also important influences, as is overall comfort with sexuality; and feelings about specific contraceptives can affect an individual's choice of method and the success with which it is used as well.

In truth, avoiding unintended pregnancy can be hard to do, requiring specific skills and steady dedication over time, often from both partners. The strong, consistent motivation that many forms of reversible contraception require is typically fueled by a view of life in which pregnancy and childbearing are seen, at a given point in time, as less attractive than other alternatives. Being pregnant and bearing a child often bring significant psychological and social rewards, and there must be good reason to forego them.

In order to address feelings, attitudes, and motivation more directly, contraceptive services should be sufficiently well funded (through adequate reimbursement rates and/or public sector support) to include extensive counseling—of both partners, whenever possible—about the skills and commitment needed to use contraception successfully. Similarly, school curricula and programs that train health and social services professionals in reproductive health should include ample material about the skills that contraception requires and about the influence of personal factors on successful contraceptive use, along with more conventional information about reproductive physiology and contraceptive technology.

The influence of motivation in pregnancy prevention also underscores the importance of longer-acting, coitus-independent methods of contraception (e.g. hormonal implants and injectables and, when appropriate, intrauterine devices) because they require only minimal attention once the method is established. Although few women and couples rely on these methods, their long-term potential for reducing unintended pregnancy is great. When offered with careful counseling and meticulous attention to informed consent, these methods constitute an important component of the contraceptive choices available in this country. They do not, however, protect against the transmission of STDs, which requires that condoms be used also.

On a broader level, policy leaders need to confront the notion that, especially for those most impoverished, reducing unintended pregnancy may well require that more compelling alternatives than pregnancy and childbearing be available. Such alternatives include better schools, realistic expectations that a high school diploma will lead to an adequate income, and jobs that are available and satisfying. Increasing knowledge about contraception and improving access to it as well may not be enough to achieve major reductions in unintended pregnancy when the surrounding environment offers few incentives to postpone childbearing. This comment is not meant to suggest that unless poverty is eliminated unintended pregnancy cannot be reduced. The point is rather that, in the poorest communities especially, only modest reductions in unintended pregnancy will likely be achieved by the usual prescription of "more education, information, and services." In this context, it is important to note that research findings do not support the popular notion that welfare payments (i.e., AFDC) and other income transfer programs exert an important influence on non-marital childbearing.

· ***Campaign Goal 4:*** **Develop and scrupulously evaluate a variety of local programs to reduce unintended pregnancy.**

Little is known about effective programming at the local level to reduce unintended pregnancy. Accordingly, the campaign to reduce unintended pregnancy should encourage public and private funders to support a series of new research and demonstration programs in this field that are designed to answer a series of clearly articulated questions, evaluated very carefully, and replicated when promising results emerge.

The focus and design of these new programs should be based, at a minimum, on a careful assessment of 23 programs identified by the committee whose effects on specific fertility measures related to unintended pregnancy have been carefully assessed. Evaluation data from these programs support several broad conclusions: (1) even those few programs showing positive effects report only small gains, which demonstrates how difficult it can be to achieve major decreases in unintended pregnancy; (2) because most evaluated programs target adolescents, especially adolescent girls, knowledge about how to reduce unintended pregnancy among adult women and their partners is exceedingly limited; (3) there is insufficient evidence to determine if "abstinence-only" programs for young adolescents are effective, but encouraging results are being reported by programs with more complex messages stressing both abstinence and contraceptive use once sexual activity has begun; (4) few evaluated programs actually provide contraceptive supplies; and (5) only mixed success has been reported from programs trying to prevent rapid repeat pregnancies among adolescents and young women.

The new research and demonstration programs should reflect several additional themes as well. Unintended pregnancies derive in roughly equal proportions from couples who report some use of contraception, however imperfect, and from couples who report no use of contraception at all at the time of conception. Although many individuals move back and forth between these two states over time, it may nonetheless be useful to develop specific strategies for each group, especially for the very high-risk group of nonusers. Another theme that should shape these research and demonstration programs is the need to develop and test out new ways to involve men more deeply in the issue of pregnancy prevention and contraception. And finally, these programs should explore how to build community support for contraception. Although contraceptive use is ultimately a personal matter, community values and the surrounding culture clearly shape the actions of individuals and couples. Accordingly, at least some demonstration programs should target both the community and the individual, and some might also work exclusively at the community level.

· *Campaign Goal 5:* **Stimulate research to (a) develop new contraceptive methods for both women *and* men, (b) answer important questions about how best to organize contraceptive services, and (c) understand more fully the determinants and antecedents of unintended pregnancy.**

The need to develop new contraceptive methods for both men and women is compelling. One of the reasons that unintended pregnancy continues to occur is that the available contraceptive methods are not always well suited to personal preferences or to various ages and life stages. Particularly glaring is the lack of effective male methods of reversible contraception other than the condom.

There is also a clear need for more health services research in the field of pregnancy prevention. For example, little is known about how access to prescription-based methods of contraception is enhanced or restricted by the many managed care arrangements now shaping health services.

Finally, there is a pressing need for more interdisciplinary research to understand the complex relationships among the cultural, economic, social, biological, and psychological factors that lie behind widely varying patterns of contraceptive use and therefore unintended pregnancy. Research on personal feelings, attitudes, and beliefs as they affect contraceptive use, and especially several recent ethnographic investigations of motivation, offer particularly intriguing explanations for the observed phenomena. Careful work is needed to integrate these ideas with the more traditional explanations of unintended pregnancy, such as inaccessible contraceptive services or insufficient knowledge about how to prevent pregnancy. Research is also needed on factors outside of individuals (such as the impact of media messages on the contraceptive behavior of individuals), on factors within couples (such as the relative power and influence of women and men in decisions to use or not use particular methods of contraception), and on the combination of individual, couple, and environmental factors considered together. In all such multivariate research, it will be important to study the determinants of sexual behavior as well as contraceptive use, inasmuch as the two are often intimately connected and may jointly influence the risk of unintended pregnancy.

Campaign Leadership

Progress toward achieving the five campaign goals outlined above would be enhanced by the existence of a readily identifiable, public–private consortium whose mission is to lead the recommended campaign. Funding and leadership of the consortium should be provided by private foundations, given their proven capacity to draw many disparate groups together around a shared concern. Members of this consortium should be recruited from numerous sectors, both public and private, and especially from the groups that speak on behalf of children and their needs, such as the maternal and child health community.

1

Introduction

This report is about unintended pregnancy, a general term that includes pregnancies that a woman states were either mistimed or unwanted at the time of conception.[1] Unintended pregnancy in the United States is an important and complex problem that has significant consequences for the health and well-being of all Americans.

The study that culminated in this report was shaped and influenced by a wide variety of both demographic and social phenomena. Some of these phenomena were evident at the outset, and others emerged only as the project progressed. In the former category were the numbers. Data published in the 1980s indicated that rates of unintended pregnancy in the United States were higher than those in several other industrialized countries (Jones et al., 1989). Then, in 1990, analyses from the 1988 National Survey of Family Growth showed that declines in births derived from unintended pregnancies during the 1970s had reversed in the 1980s, with particular increases noted among poor women (Williams and Pratt, 1990). These figures indicated that progress on one of the most basic measures of women's autonomy—determining whether and when to bear children—had eroded, a development that could only undermine efforts to improve women's capacity for self-determination and full participation in their communities. Moreover, the increases in the number of births derived from unintended pregnancies were not confined to adolescents, which suggested that the nation's continuing focus on teenage pregnancy might well be missing

---

[1]A definition of these and other terms is found at the beginning of Chapter 2 and in Appendix C.

a larger issue: that adults as well as teenagers have difficulty planning and preventing pregnancy.

Another major force stimulating the Institute of Medicine's initial interest in studying unintended pregnancy was a concern that too little attention had been given to the relationship of pregnancy intendedness to the health and well-being of children. Throughout the late 1980s and early 1990s, there was an appreciable amount of advocacy on behalf of children. Even in the face of limited budgets and competing demands, many states and the federal government found numerous ways to direct money and attention to children: expanding eligibility for Medicaid in order to finance health care for more low-income children and pregnant women; increasing authorizations for the popular Head Start program; and stimulating programs in virtually every state to address infant mortality and early childhood immunization, improve the quality of education, offer early intervention services for at-risk families, reach pregnant women with prenatal care, and use school settings in new ways to provide a wide variety of human services.

But the world of education, counseling, and care that supports careful contraceptive use—often called family planning—has been starkly absent from the "children's agenda" as articulated over the past 10 to 15 years. In fact, pregnancy prevention and family planning have generally been treated as marginal or controversial activities, rarely discussed in a broad, comprehensive way that recognizes the important role that fertility control plays in the lives of men and women, in child and family well-being, and in the overall tenor of communities.[2] In particular, pregnancy planning has not been included as a central, routine component of human services, especially preventive health care and education; by contrast, a number of other countries have found many ways to incorporate family planning services into primary care, often as part of maternal and child health services. As evidence of this neglect, public investment in family planning services declined during the 1980s, perhaps by as much as a third. In particular, federal outlays for family planning through the Title X program (that portion of the Public Health Service Act that provides grants to various state and local entities to offer family planning services to low-income women and adolescents) dropped precipitously during the 1980s, although increased commitments from other public and private sources helped to fill a portion of the gap (Ku, 1993; Gold and Daley, 1991).

An additional influence on this project was the intense debate about health care reform during the 103rd Congress and the growth of managed care systems

---

[2]Exceptions to this exclusion were the March of Dimes' report, *Towards Improving the Outcome of Pregnancy* (1993), and the Carnegie Corporation of New York's report, *Starting Points* (1994), both of which highlighted the key role that pregnancy planning can play in the health and lives of children, women, and families.

throughout the nation. Both developments have revealed underlying disagreements about whether and how contraception should be financed and about the systems that should be in place to provide reproductive health services generally. As first the White House and then the Congress attempted to design a standard package of benefits that should be available to all insured Americans as part of health care reform, controversy arose over whether contraceptive services and supplies (as well as abortion) should be included and the extent to which copayments and deductibles should be applied to these and related services. And as managed care networks increasingly dominate health care financing in states and communities, new questions have arisen about the fate of the Title X program and other categorical grant programs now operating side-by-side with growing numbers of health maintenance organizations and other integrated systems. In some communities, categorical family planning programs have found ways to work smoothly with managed care networks, and in others, the relationship has been more difficult (Rosenbaum et al., 1994). Some have suggested that categorical family planning programs are no longer necessary in communities with broad insurance coverage; others claim that the need for such specialized, comprehensive services remains apparent, especially for low-income and adolescent women, many of whom are uninsured. This issue has taken on new importance given the increasing use of managed care networks by state Medicaid programs, which often have heavy caseloads of women in their childbearing years who need a wide variety of reproductive health services.

Intensifying discussions about welfare reform, and, in particular, the issue of childbearing by single women currently receiving cash assistance, also shaped the environment in which this project unfolded. Policymakers have suggested—and some states have actually legislated—that welfare payments not be increased if women bear additional children while on welfare, the notion being that welfare itself might provide an inappropriate incentive for childbearing and that job training and educational programs for mothers on welfare are hindered by repeated pregnancies.

One particularly interesting aspect of the welfare debate is its focus on both childbearing by women under age 20 as well as on nonmarital childbearing, two overlapping but distinct phenomena that are often treated as though they were one and the same. Data on births to adolescent women show that the birthrate in 1991 continued the rise that began in the latter years of the 1980s. Between 1986 and 1991, the rate of births to teens rose 24 percent, from 50 to 62 births per 1,000 females aged 15–19. This increase in the birthrate has occurred among both younger and older teens and in nearly all states (Moore, 1994). More recent data show a slight decline in the birthrate among teenagers between 1991 and 1992; even so, overall levels remain 21 percent higher than they were in 1986 (Moore, 1995). Births among unmarried women have also increased such that, by 1991, nearly one-third of all births were to unmarried women.[3] Although the rate of childbearing among unmarried women is higher among black than white women (DaVanzo and Rahman, 1993), much of the recent overall increase in childbearing among unmarried women has been fueled by a steep rise in births among unmarried white women (Ventura et al., 1994). These troubling data raise a critical, largely ignored question: To what extent are pregnancies among adolescent and unmarried women intended, especially those occurring among poor women? Are these pregnancies accidents? Or are they consciously planned and actively sought, derived from a clear desire to have a child, despite very young age, poverty, or the absence of marriage or even a committed partner (Dash, 1989)? Answers to these questions have obvious relevance to evolving welfare policy. If, for example, data suggest that most such pregnancies are unintended, it may be that finding ways to increase the use of contraception should be a major part of strategies to reduce welfare dependency. In various sections of this report, this connection between the welfare debate and unintended pregnancy is highlighted.

Another factor shaping the course of the project was the fact that men have largely been excluded from the research, programs, and policies designed to reduce unintended pregnancy in the United States. Although there have been scattered attempts around the nation to involve men in family planning services, for example, or to develop materials on contraception that are oriented to male concerns, much of this activity has been driven by efforts to control the spread of acquired immune deficiency syndrome (AIDS) and other sexually transmitted diseases (STDs), leaving pregnancy prevention largely a woman's concern. Despite the ostensible logic to this state of affairs (inasmuch as it is the female, not the male, who becomes pregnant), men obviously play a significant role in family formation. It became increasingly apparent to the committee over the course of this project that men must be involved in pregnancy prevention in a variety of ways beyond just encouraging condom use (Edwards, 1994). In the related area of childbirth, for example, men are now welcomed into what had for years been a process managed exclusively by women in labor and their doctors. Fathers now increasingly participate in classes that prepare couples for

---

[3]Despite recent increases, the U.S. level of nonmarital childbearing remains significantly lower than that found in many other countries, including several European ones (United Nations, 1991). At the same time, it is important to point out that in these European countries, especially the Scandinavian ones, up to three-quarters of these nonmarital births are to couples who are cohabitating, which may provide a family context for children that is similar to that provided by marital unions. By contrast, much of the nonmarital childbearing in the United States is not accompanied by cohabitation (Bumpass and Sweet, 1989), thereby providing less favorable family contexts for children, as discussed in more detail in Chapter 3.

labor and delivery, and they are often present in delivery rooms also. This development in childbirth highlights the interest of men in family formation, and lends added weight to the notion that men could be more deeply involved in pregnancy prevention and planning as well.

Federal and state legislation designed to strengthen child support enforcement and paternity establishment also focuses attention on males in that it provides new incentives for unmarried men in particular to take greater responsibility for preventing unintended pregnancy. The Family Support Act of 1988 requires states to establish paternity for all children born outside marriage and to require all unmarried fathers to pay child support until their child reaches 18 years of age; although it is too soon to gauge the impact of this law definitively, early reports are that there has been an increase in the percentage of children born outside of marriage who have paternity established and who have a child support award (Hanson et al., 1995). Current welfare reform proposals put even greater emphasis on establishing paternity. Whereas in the past an unmarried father could, in essence, walk away from a child born outside of marriage if he chose to do so, today both the law and public opinion make this a less available option.

The human immunodeficiency virus (HIV) and AIDS epidemic was also an important part of this project's genesis. Data now suggest that the incidence of HIV infection among women is accelerating at an alarming rate. Moreover, the epidemic has apparently increased the willingness of the public and some elected officials to address more candidly such issues as high-risk sexual behavior and at least one form of contraception—condoms. Topics that were once expressly forbidden in the electronic media are now common fare on talk shows and news specials, signaling that new opportunities have opened for communication and education. The present study was organized in part to take advantage of this new willingness to address sexual behavior, in the hope that pregnancy prevention, too, could be approached more directly.

Finally, it is important to acknowledge two particular issues that shaped this study: the controversies over abstinence-based education and over abortion. During the 1980s, there was a movement at the federal level, and among some communities as well, to promote abstinence instead of contraception as the major means of preventing pregnancies (as well as AIDS and STDs) among unmarried adolescents. This argument spawned impassioned debates about whether abstinence was an outmoded concept in the late twentieth century that ignored the realities of adolescent sexual activity and about whether discussing contraception with teenagers gave tacit approval to their sexual activity, or perhaps even encouraged it. Disagreements were especially intense over whether school-based sex education for adolescents should stress abstinence only, or should combine messages about abstinence with material on contraception as well. Although some federal health officials took the former position, other people, especially those in the family planning field, took the latter view, thereby often finding themselves at odds with federal policy leaders. The intensity of the debate had the unfortunate effect of polarizing many groups who share a common interest in reducing adolescent pregnancy. Thus, the time seemed right for a review of the knowledge base regarding the causes, consequences, and prevention of unintended pregnancy, including the effectiveness of abstinence-based education.

Abortion is perhaps the most divisive issue related to unintended pregnancy. As any observer of the American scene over the last 20 years could readily discern, the abortion controversy has dominated discussions of reproductive health and has led to painful divisions across many ideological, political, and religious lines. The heated debate over the acceptability of abortion itself has diverted attention from many other important and closely related issues, such as finding ways to encourage couples to prevent both unintended pregnancy and STDs simultaneously or learning how best to offer contraceptive services in communities whose health care systems are changing rapidly. Put another way, in arguing about how to *resolve* problem pregnancies, less attention has been given to *preventing* such pregnancies in the first place. The controversy has also obscured the very important differences between abortion and contraception and has led, in some instances, to contraception being treated as gingerly as abortion. Among other results, this unfortunate confusion between abortion and contraception has shifted attention away from the proposition that better use of contraception is a highly effective way to reduce the incidence of abortion.

This is not to suggest, however, that unintended pregnancy in the United States would have been eliminated by now were it not for the abstinence and abortion controversies. In fact, only 40 years ago the notion of carefully planned, controlled fertility in this country seemed an elusive, futuristic goal with little reasonable chance of actually occurring. Many of the most effective reversible methods of contraception—for example, intrauterine devices and oral contraceptives—have only been available since the early 1960s and have just recently been joined by hormonal implants and injections. Moreover, it was only in 1965 that it was clearly declared legal in the United States for married couples to secure and use contraception (*Griswold* v. *Connecticut*); similar protection was not granted to unmarried individuals until 1972 (*Eisenstadt* v. *Baird*). Thus, modern patterns of contraceptive use in the United States—and even the legality of many methods—are recent developments. It would be unrealistic to expect that in the mid-1990s contraception would be used universally and with no errors, failures, or missteps along the way (additional historical perspectives are presented in Appendix B). The use of many forms of reversible contraception carefully and successfully can be a complicated undertaking that requires a unique convergence of several factors including a supportive social environment, peer and personal values consistent with diligent contraceptive use, affordable and accessible methods of contraception, and partner agreement and, often, active partner cooperation. The continuing occurrence of unintended pregnancy in the United States suggests that it may well take many years to realize the full promise of modern contraception and fertility control.

FOCUS OF THIS REPORT

Within this broad context, the Institute of Medicine's Committee on Unintended Pregnancy was established to explore the relationship of unintended pregnancy in the United States to the health and well-being of children and families and to make recommendations for policy, practice, and research. In so doing, the committee was asked to:

- define what is meant by unintended pregnancy and related terms used in the relevant data and research;
- summarize evidence regarding the effects that unintended pregnancy (e.g., both mistimed and unwanted pregnancy) has on the health and well-being of children, youth, and adults (to include commentary on the role of abortion in resolving unintended pregnancies);
- analyze patterns of and trends in unintended pregnancy, noting the populations in whom unintended pregnancy is concentrated;
- outline the various reasons that might help to explain the observed patterns;
- describe the range of programs that have been organized in the last 10 years or so to reduce the incidence of unintended pregnancy and, to the extent possible, comment on the effectiveness of various approaches; and
- make conclusions and recommendations for policy, practice, and research based on the data assembled and reviewed.

The audience for this activity was defined to be policymakers at the federal, state, and local levels; administrators of relevant health and social service programs, including those who are active in the fields of child welfare, family planning, and reproductive health generally; opinion leaders in foundations, the business community, and the media; and scientists in a position to act on the committee's research recommendations.

STUDY METHODS AND REPORT ORGANIZATION

In meeting its charge, the committee and staff used several methods to gather the needed information. They reviewed published data and analyses; studied numerous commissioned and contributed papers on a variety of topics about which the group felt it needed more information (Appendix A); talked informally, during committee meetings and at other times, with experts on the various topics it was studying; requested one original piece of analytic work by The Alan Guttmacher Institute using the 1988 National Maternal and Infant Health Survey; conducted an analysis of what the childbearing population in the United States would look like if unintended pregnancies were eliminated; and held five meetings of the full committee over a 14-month period (from September 1993 through October 1994). Both committee members and staff participated in drafting the report. In addition, a careful effort was made to learn about programs in place around the country that address unintended pregnancy; the methods used in that portion of the committee's work are described in more detail in Chapter 8.

Following this introductory chapter, Chapter 2 presents data on rates of and trends in unintended pregnancy and on the populations in which unintended pregnancy is concentrated. Chapter 3 summarizes data on the health and social consequences of unintended pregnancy from the perspective of children and adults and discusses abortion as a major consequence of unintended pregnancy. It also addresses the socioeconomic consequences for children and their mothers of both adolescent parenthood and childbearing among unmarried women, because unintended pregnancy is particularly common among women who are teenaged, unmarried, or both.

Subsequent chapters address the fundamental question that unintended pregnancy poses: Why do Americans report such high levels of unintended pregnancy, even in the presence of numerous contraceptive methods? The most immediate and obvious answer, of course, is contraceptive nonuse, misuse, or failure. Thus, Chapter 4 is devoted to reviewing patterns of contraceptive use as they relate to unintended pregnancy.

The report then moves on to a discussion of factors that influence contraceptive use. Information on these factors—often called determinants—is scattered and often confusing and is peppered with as much opinion as data. On one point, however, there is clear consensus: many, many factors affect the use of contraception and thus unintended pregnancy. The committee found it helpful to group these factors into three sets: (1) knowledge about contraception, unintended pregnancy, and human reproduction in general, as well as access to contraception itself; (2) personal motivation, attitudes, beliefs, and feelings related to contraceptive use; and (3) the overall socioeconomic and cultural environment.

Chapter 5 addresses the first set of factors, asking whether unintended pregnancy may be explained in part by insufficient knowledge about contraception and related topics, as well as by limited access to the most effective methods of birth control. In the discussion of knowledge about contraception, schools and the media are highlighted; in the area of access to contraception, the emphasis is on financial and other barriers that limit an individual's ability to secure various methods of birth control.

Chapter 6 discusses the second set of factors affecting unintended pregnancy—the complex web of individual motivation, feeling, attitudes, and beliefs that shape contraceptive use as well as sexual activity. This section contains some of the most provocative and important material in the report, inasmuch as it touches on the more emotional, sometimes irrational, dimensions of human behavior and male–female relationships that are so closely connected to the occurrence of any pregnancy, intended or not.

Chapter 7 addresses numerous social forces that influence fertility and the effective use of contraception: political and religious diversity, views about sexuality, historical and ongoing racism, economic factors, cultural and ethnic diversity, gender bias, the far-reaching effects of the antiabortion movement, and the pervasive influence of violence in American life. The broad scope of this chapter is highly consistent with deliberations at the recent United Nations International Conference on Population and Development in Cairo, which addressed both men and women in fertility decisions, the integral part that socioeconomic and cultural environments play in reproductive behavior, the pervasive influence of gender bias and other women's issues in population trends, and the importance of addressing human sexuality as part of reproductive health services and policies (United Nations, 1994).

Chapter 8 reviews several pregnancy prevention programs to determine whether there is a strong knowledge base at the local level about how to reduce unintended pregnancy. Although there are literally hundreds of programs recently completed or currently under way in the United States that in some way address unintended pregnancy, this chapter focuses squarely on the few that have been evaluated. The chapter also comments on both Medicaid and the Title X program because they are major sources of public funding for family planning services nationwide.

The final chapter, Chapter 9, presents the committee's conclusions and recommendations. These are addressed to public policy, provision of services, and, in particular, research.

As the foregoing overview suggests, this report is confined to an analysis of unintended pregnancy in the United States. Nonetheless, the report does occasionally draw on international data in order to put certain U.S. numbers into perspective, to consider how other countries may have handled particular problems, or to ponder the feasibility of selected remedies.

REFERENCES

Bumpass L, Sweet J. Children's experience in single-parent families: Implications of cohabitation and marital transitions. Fam Plann Perspect. 1989; 21:256–260.

Carnegie Corporation of New York. Starting Points: Meeting the Needs of Our Youngest Children. New York, NY; 1994.

Dash L. When Children Want Children. New York, NY: Penguin Books; 1989.

DaVanzo J, Rahman MO. American Families: Trends and Policy Issues. Santa Monica, CA: RAND; 1993.

Edwards SR. The role of men in contraceptive decision-making: Current knowledge and future implications. Fam Plann Perspect. 1994;26:77–82.

Gold RB, Daley D. Public funding of contraceptive, sterilization and abortion services, fiscal year 1990. Fam Plann Perspect. 1991;23:204–211.

Hanson T, McLanahan S, Garfinckel I, Miller C. Trends in child support outcome. Unpublished manuscript. Princeton University. 1995.

Jones EF, Forrest JD, Henshaw SK, Silverman J, Torres A. Pregnancy, Contraception and Family Planning Services in Industrialized Countries. New Haven, CT: Yale University Press; 1989.

Ku L. Financing of family planning services. In Publicly Supported Family Planning in the United States. Washington, DC: The Urban Institute and Child Trends, Inc.; 1993.

March of Dimes Birth Defects Foundation. Towards Improving the Outcome of Pregnancy: The 90s and Beyond. New York, NY; 1993.

Moore KA. Facts at a Glance. Washington, DC: Child Trends, Inc.; February 1995.

Moore KA. Facts at a Glance. Washington, DC: Child Trends, Inc.; January 1994

Rosenbaum S, Shin P, Mauskopf A, Funk K, Stern G, Zuvekas A. Beyond the Freedom to Choose: Medicaid, Managed Care and Family Planning. Washington, DC: Center for Health Policy Research, The George Washington University; 1994.

United Nations. Program of Action: Report from the International Conference on Population and Development. New York, NY; 1994.

United Nations. The World's Women 1970–1990: Trends and Statistics. New York, NY: United Nations; 1991.

Ventura SJ, Martin JA, Taffel SM, Matthews TJ, Clarke SC. Advance Report of Final Natality Statistics, 1992. Mon Vital Stat Rep. 1994;43(5 Suppl).

Williams LB, Pratt WP. Wanted and unwanted childbearing in the United States: 1973–1988. Advance Data from Vital and Health Statistics, no. 189. Hyattsville, MD: National Center for Health Statistics; 1990.

2

Demography of Unintended Pregnancy

A majority of all pregnancies in the United States are unintended. About half of these unintended pregnancies result in live births and the other half are resolved by abortion. This chapter explores these two facts in detail after first defining *unintended*, *mistimed*, and *unwanted* pregnancies and commenting on the available data. Overall trends in births derived from unintended pregnancies are presented, along with the characteristics of women who experience such pregnancies and births. The chapter's penultimate section discusses the position of the United States in relationship to other developed countries on these measures.

TERMINOLOGY

Women often informally discuss their personal feelings about the timing of the pregnancies they have had—whether a baby came just a bit too early, whether a pregnancy occurred at a time when it interfered with future plans but would have been wanted at a later time, whether a baby had been desperately sought for several years and was the answer to heartfelt prayers, or whether a pregnancy was not wanted at any time. Some women feel ambivalent or may disagree with their partners, one wanting a pregnancy and the other preferring to wait. Books, movies, dormitory discussions, real-life arguments, pillow talk, and conversations over the back fence focus on the complexities of wanted, unwanted, and mistimed pregnancies. It is difficult, however, to quantify people's feelings and sort them into categories that hold comparable meaning over time and across varied social groups. When an unmarried high school sophomore reports that her pregnancy occurred too early, her assessment of "too early" probably means something different from the report of a married engineer who wanted a baby after working for several years but got pregnant her first year on the job.

Information on the demography of unintended pregnancy—the subject of this chapter—is dominated by data from the National Survey of Family Growth (NSFG), a federally-sponsored survey that has developed quite specific terminology and definitions to measure "unintended pregnancy." Over the past four decades, a series of questions has been regularly asked of women by this survey and its predecessors, the Growth of American Families surveys and the National Fertility Studies, in an effort to learn more about women's plans and intentions at the time they became pregnant. In these surveys, women are asked about pregnancies during the previous 5 years, including whether contraception was being used at the time the woman became pregnant. The relevant NSFG questions appear in Appendix C, along with additional material on the history and future plans of this survey.

On the basis of these questions, pregnancies in the NSFG are defined as

- *intended* at conception: wanted at the time, or sooner, irrespective of whether or not contraception was being used; or
- *unintended* at conception: if a pregnancy had not been wanted at the time conception occurred, irrespective of whether or not contraception was being used.

Among *unintended* pregnancies, a distinction is made between *mistimed* and *unwanted*:

- *mistimed* conceptions are those that were wanted by the woman at some time, but which occurred sooner than they were wanted; and
- *unwanted* conceptions are those that occurred when the woman did not want to have any more pregnancies at all.

The labels and terms from the NSFG have many limitations and ambiguities that should be mentioned. First, it is important to emphasize that the NSFG questions are designed to probe feelings *at the time of conception, not at the time of birth*. This distinction is important because a woman's feelings can change in many ways over the course of pregnancy (Miller, 1974). For example, Poole and colleagues (1994) report that among a sample of low-income women who were queried both early and late in their pregnancies, 12.5 percent reported a positive shift in attitude toward the pregnancy, and 10 percent reported a negative shift. In particular, an unintended pregnancy can result in a much anticipated birth and a cherished child. To emphasize this critical distinction, this report does not refer to *unwanted births*, for example, but rather to births resulting from unwanted pregnancies or conceptions; similar precision is used with the term *mistimed*.

The distinctions that the NSFG draws between intended and unintended and between mistimed and unwanted carry important implications. For example, unintended pregnancies are far more likely to end in abortion than intended pregnancies, and births resulting from unwanted conceptions appear to carry particular risks for both mother and child. In Chapter 3, these consequences of unintended pregnancy are discussed in detail.

It is also important to note that knowledge about pregnancy intentions derived from the NSFG comes entirely from women. Bumpass (1994) has reported data about partners' preferences, as provided by female respondents in the 1988 National Survey of Families and Households (see also Williams, 1994), noting that in more than one-fourth of the cases in which a woman described a birth as resulting from an unintended pregnancy, she reported that her spouse or partner had either wanted the birth at that time or was indifferent to the timing. Such disagreement may be a factor in the occurrence of pregnancies that women do not intend; this issue of partner interaction is taken up in more detail in Chapter 6.

It is also apparent that the NSFG survey questions, and similar ones used in other surveys, are often not able to measure the complicated mix of feelings that can surround pregnancy, as described by recent ethnographic research in particular (Musick, 1993). It is not uncommon to learn from a pregnant woman, for example, that she both did not "intend" to become pregnant but also was not using contraception, or that perhaps she wanted to be pregnant but was less enthusiastic about having a child (Luker, 1975). In Chapter 6, these complexities are explored in detail.

Other caveats with regard to the NSFG measures of pregnancy intention have been raised. For example, the questions about intendedness are retrospective, asking about all pregnancies in the preceding 5 years, which may make the answers offered subject to distortion and recall error. The questions do not distinguish how many months or years pregnancy timing was off, nor do they reflect the intensity of the woman's feelings about the timing of conception. In commenting on data sources other than the NSFG, Chapter 3 and Appendix G also address these generic problems in measuring the intention status of a given pregnancy, noting in particular that the difference between an intended and an unintended conception is often more complicated than these terms imply. Well aware of these nuances, the 1995 NSFG cycle will use an elaborate approach to establishing the intendedness of a given conception (see Appendix C), recognizing that the concept of intended versus unintended is more a continuum than an either/or matter. Consistent with the new approach being taken by the NSFG, one of this report's recommendations is that researchers develop more refined and differentiated measures of intention status that can accommodate important concepts like ambivalence, denial, and confusion and that can address the feelings of men and couples as well as individual women (Chapter 9).

These various caveats about the NSFG measures are not meant to suggest that this national survey and other similar ones fail to capture important information about intention at the time of conception. In fact, despite errors at the individual level, the general validity of the aggregate levels and trends in these measures has been repeatedly demonstrated. The same questions have been used with older and younger women as well as married and unmarried women and across a period of years, ranging from the time before legal abortion became widely available in the 1970s through to the 1990s. In addition, very few women are unable to answer the series of questions; less than 1 percent fall into a residual "undetermined" category. If there is any bias in the NSFG on the issue of intendedness, available evidence indicates that the direction of this bias would be in underreporting unintended pregnancy (Ryder, 1985). That is, the NSFG data may well provide overestimates of intended pregnancies and underestimates of unintended pregnancies.

Finally, three other important limitations in the data available from the NSFG should be noted. First, most research and analysis regarding pregnancy intention are based on the 1988 NSFG, which is by now somewhat dated, predating in particular the introduction and use of both injectable and implantable hormonal contraceptives. Nonetheless, the 1988 survey remains a highly credible source of information on intention status.[1] Although there was a telephone reinterview of the 1988 NSFG sample in 1990, it reported a less-than-optimal response rate, and thus its results are used sparingly in this report. The next NSFG survey, being completed in 1995, will provide more current data to extend the rich information already available.

Second, the marital status groupings used by the NSFG in its fertility questions have changed over the years. For example, the 1965 and 1970 National Fertility Studies were conducted only among currently married women. It was not until the 1973 NSFG that separated, divorced, and widowed women were also queried along with currently married women. From 1982 on, however, the NSFG has sampled *all* women aged 15–44, irrespective of marital status.

---

[1]The 1988 National Maternal and Infant Health Survey also collected data on intention status. Although these data are briefly referred to in this report, they were not relied on as heavily as the NSFG because they are not part of a long-standing series and therefore cannot provide the perspective of trends over time.

Third, it is widely recognized that the NSFG underreports abortion. Many unintended pregnancies are resolved by abortion, as discussed later in this chapter;[2] therefore, if one wants to know, for example, how many pregnancies were unintended in a given year, data on the number of both births unintended at conception *and* the number of abortions would be needed—data that the NSFG does not have in full measure. Jones and Forrest (1992) suggest that the number of abortions reported in the 1988 NSFG represents only 35 percent of the number actually obtained. Important attempts have been made to supplement the NSFG data with more complete abortion information in order to provide an understanding of the overall level of unintended pregnancy (Forrest and Singh, 1990). The NSFG remains the key data set, however, for tracking the intention status of births, providing comprehensive information on the families in which such births occur and on many other issues as well.

PERCENTAGE RATES OF UNINTENDED PREGNANCY

Figure 2-1 shows the best available estimate of the percentage of pregnancies that are unintended. These data are based on the 1988 NSFG, supplemented by abortion data from 1987 compiled by The Alan Guttmacher Institute and the Centers for Disease Control. As that figure shows, in 1987, 57 percent of all pregnancies were unintended at the time of conception. This figure of 57 percent includes pregnancies that were aborted as well as both mistimed and unwanted pregnancies that led to live births.[3] Only 43 percent of all pregnancies in that year were intended at conception and resulted in live births.[4]

---

[2]Much research in this field tacitly assumes that all pregnancies ending in abortion were unintended at the time of conception. Although this is accurate as a general finding, it is important to acknowledge that some very small portion of abortions are obtained for pregnancies that were intended at conception, but subsequently became problematic because of the diagnosis of a serious genetic defect in the fetus, for example, or some other troubling turn of events (Torres and Forrest, 1988). This dynamic, however, affects only a small percentage of abortions and does not change the overall estimates presented in this report.

[3]Miscarriages are excluded from this analysis and all others in this report because the number of pregnancies ending in miscarriage is not well established and because there is no information on the distribution of miscarriages by intention status.

[4]These data are generally consistent with information beginning to emerge from the 1988 National Maternal and Infant Health Survey, which also examined the intention status of births to both married and unmarried women (Kost and Forrest, 1995).

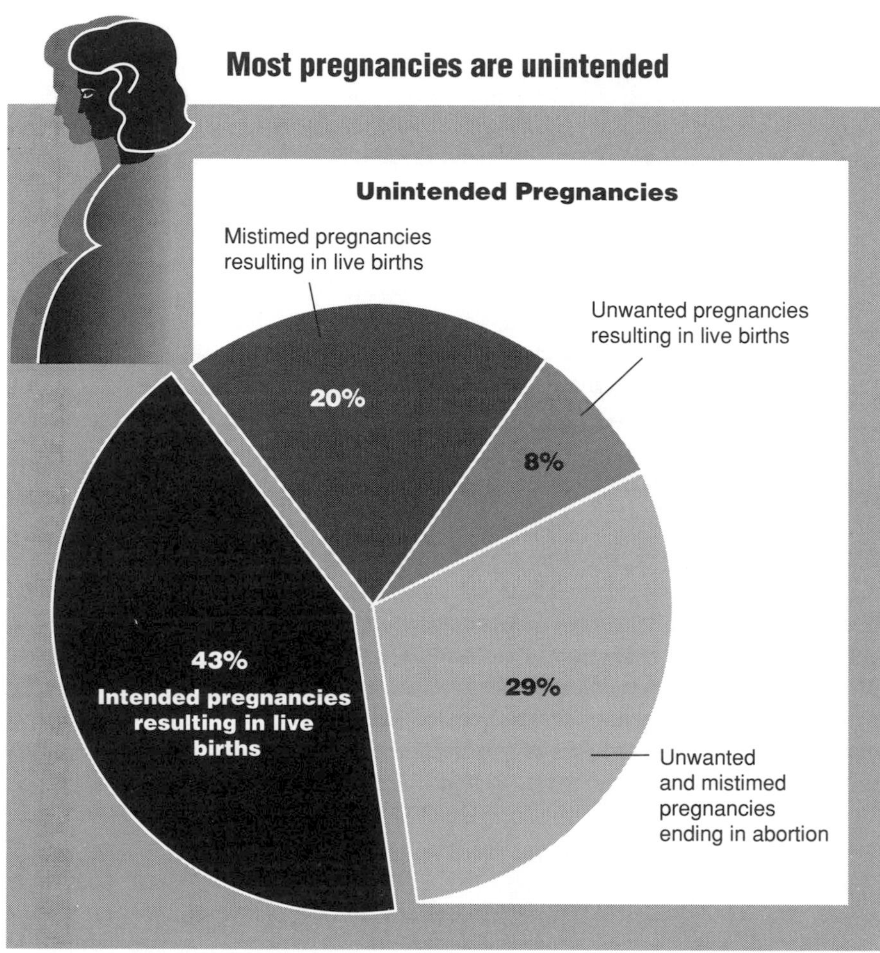

FIGURE 2-1 All pregnancies by outcome, 1987 (miscarriages excluded). Source: Forrest JD. Epidemiology of unintended pregnancy and contraceptive use. Am J Obstet Gynec. 1994;170:1485–1488.

Figure 2-2 is limited to unintended pregnancies only (i.e., intended pregnancies are not included), showing the outcomes of these pregnancies. One striking fact that this figure reveals is that more than half of all unintended pregnancies ended in abortion in 1987. The figure also shows that the majority of births from unintended pregnancies were from mistimed rather than unwanted pregnancies.

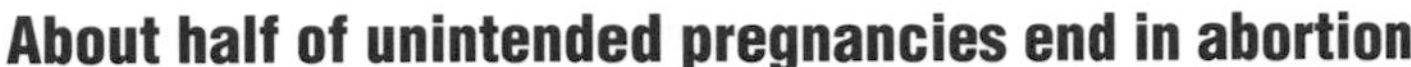

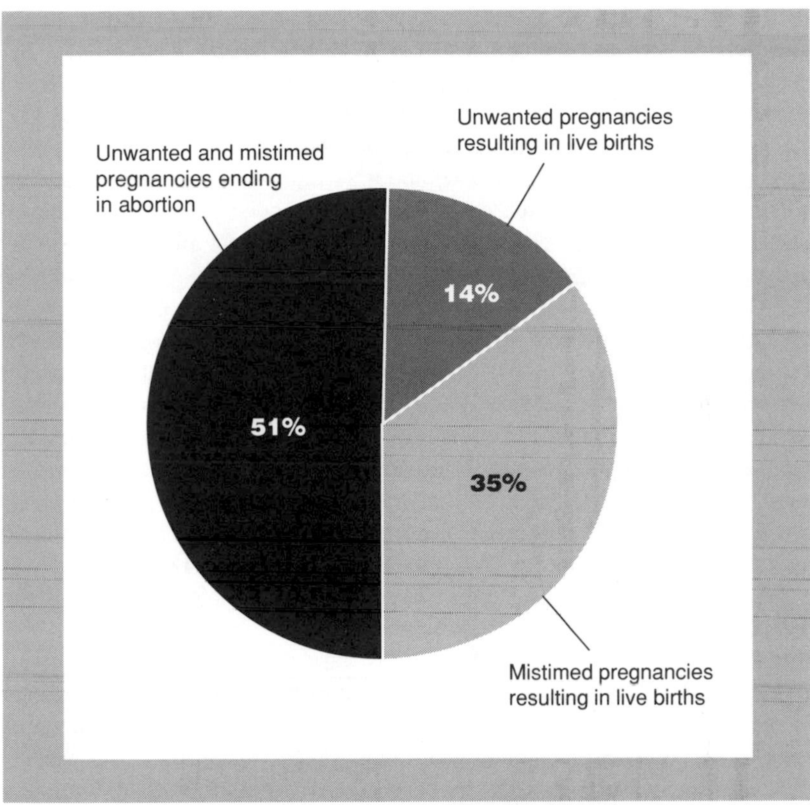

FIGURE 2-2 Unintended pregnancies by outcome, 1987 (miscarriages excluded). Source: Forrest JD. Epidemiology of unintended pregnancy and contraceptive use. Am J Obstet Gynec. 1994;170:1485–1488.

In absolute numbers, these proportions mean that in 1987, of the 5.4 million pregnancies that were estimated to have occurred, about 3.1 million were unintended at the time of conception. Within this pool of unintended pregnancies, some 1.6 million ended in abortion and 1.5 million resulted in a live birth. Only 2.3 million pregnancies in that year were intended at the time of conception and resulted in a live birth.

WOMEN AT RISK OF UNINTENDED PREGNANCY

In analyzing which women contribute to this pool of unintended pregnancies, it is helpful to begin with the profile of women "at risk" of such pregnancies. The definition of women at risk of unintended pregnancy is multifaceted. They are women who (1) have had sexual intercourse; (2) are fertile, that is, neither they nor their partners have been contraceptively sterilized and they do not believe that they are infertile for any other reason; and (3) are neither intentionally pregnant nor have they been trying to become pregnant during any part of the year.[5] In 1990, about 31 million women met these criteria and could therefore be considered at risk of unintended pregnancy (Table 2-1). These 31 million women represented about half of the 62 million women in the reproductive age range, defined as ages 13–44.

Not surprisingly, among women of reproductive age, the highest proportions at risk of unintended pregnancy are found at ages 18–29, the age range in which most women are fertile, have usually begun sexual activity but often prefer to delay pregnancy, and are generally too young to seek sterilization (Figure 2-3). Seventy percent of women in this age category are at risk of unintended pregnancy. This proportion drops dramatically among women age 30 and over, many of whom have been sterilized or have partners who have been sterilized. Nevertheless, nearly 12 million women aged 30–44 remain at risk of unintended pregnancy, compared with nearly 17 million women aged 18–29.

Within these various age categories, economic status clearly affects the level of risk (Table 2-1). The association between the proportion of women at risk of unintended pregnancy and economic status varies with the age of the woman. Among females aged 13–19, a higher proportion of teens from families in poverty are at risk, primarily because of earlier initiation of sexual activity among low-income teens. Among teens aged 15–17, for example, 46 percent of those with incomes below the poverty level were at risk of unintended pregnancy, compared with about a third of teens with family incomes 2.5 times the poverty level or above. On the other hand, among women in their 20s, slightly higher proportions of affluent women are at risk (three-fourths of women 2.5 times the poverty level or more versus two-thirds of women below the

---

[5]The concept of being "at risk" of unintended pregnancy is a complicated one with several definitions. For example, much of the research on contraceptive use summarized in Chapter 4 uses a definition in which only women who have been sexually active *in the last 3 months* are included in the pool of at risk, whereas the definition used here refers to sexual activity at *any* previous time. Moreover, other researchers suggest that even those women who have never had intercourse at all should sometimes be considered at risk. For example, young adults who have never had sexual intercourse but who are involved in increasingly intimate relationships may, in fact, be at risk of unintended pregnancy.

TABLE 2-1 Number of Women Aged 13–44 and Estimated Number and Percentage of Women at Risk[a] of Unintended Pregnancy, by Age, According to Poverty Status, 1990 (in 1,000s)

	No. of Women by Poverty Status[b]				
Age Group	Total	<100%	100–184%	185–249%	>249%
All women					
Total	61,808	9,242	8,841	7,638	36,087
13–14	3,226	551	561	457	1,657
15–17	4,875	819	753	611	2,692
18–19	3,777	8,854	585	431	1,907
20–29	19,963	3,689	3,213	2,620	10,441
30–44	29,967	3,329	3,729	3,519	19,390
Women at risk					
Total	30,508	4,897	4,300	3,593	17,719
13–14	271	63	47	38	123
15–17	1,734	374	273	221	866
18–19	2,644	646	411	301	1,286
20–29	14,099	2,440	2,153	1,743	7,763
30–44	11,762	1,374	1,417	1,290	7,681
Women at risk as percentage of all women					
Total	49.4	53.0	48.6	47.0	49.1
13–14	8.4	11.4	8.4	8.3	7.4
15–17	35.6	45.7	36.2	36.2	32.2
18–19	70.0	75.6	70.2	69.9	67.4
20–29	70.6	66.1	67.0	66.5	74.4
30–44	39.2	41.3	38.0	36.7	39.6

[a]Women "at risk" of unintended pregnancy are those who (1) have had sexual intercourse; (2) are fertile, that is, neither they nor their partners have been contraceptively sterilized and they do not believe that they are infertile for any other reason; and (3) are neither intentionally pregnant nor have they been trying to become pregnant during any part of the year.
[b]Poverty status as based on 1989 family income. Note: Numbers may differ slightly between tables because of rounding.

SOURCE: Henshaw SK, Forrest JD. Women at Risk of Unintended Pregnancy, 1990 Estimates: The Need for Family Planning Services, Each State and County. New York, NY: The Alan Guttmacher Institute; 1993.

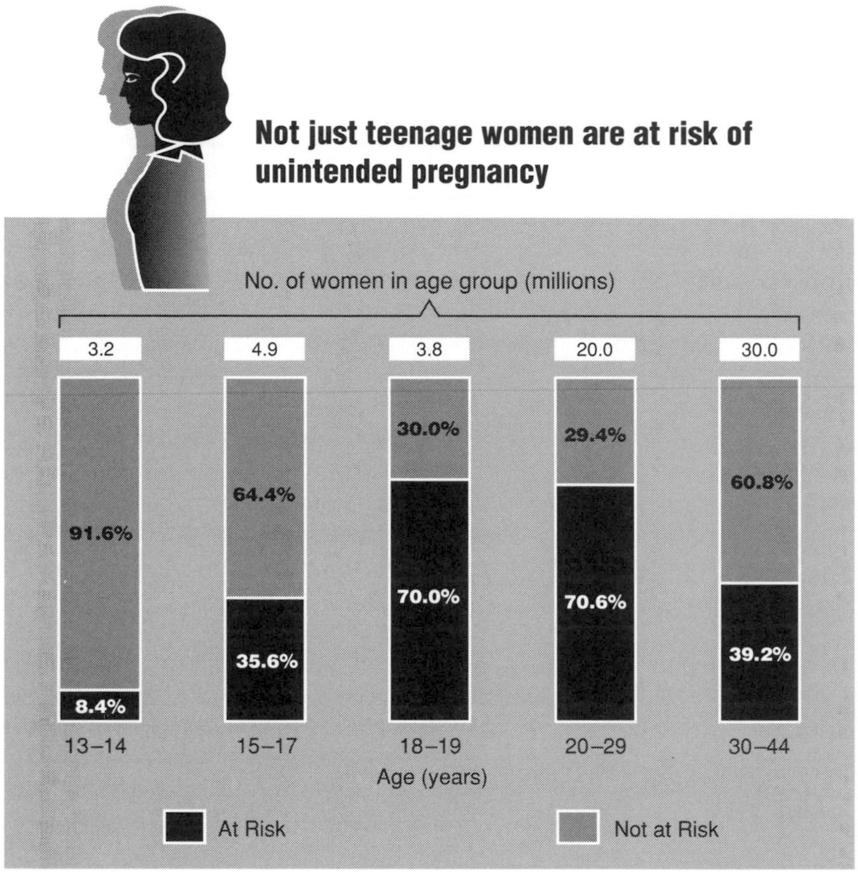

FIGURE 2-3 Proportion of women in age groups at risk of unintended pregnancy. Source: Henshaw SK, Forrest JD. Women at Risk of Unintended Pregnancy, 1990 Estimates: The Need for Family Planning Services, Each State and County. New York, NY: The Alan Guttmacher Institute; 1993.

poverty level). Among women aged 30–44 in all income groups about 4 in 10 are at risk of unintended pregnancy.

The proportion of women at risk of unintended pregnancy varies only slightly by race and ethnicity (data not shown). Non-Hispanic blacks and Hispanics are somewhat more likely to be at risk (52 percent for both groups) than non-Hispanic whites (49 percent). No similar data are available for Native or Asian Americans.

WOMEN WHO HAVE UNINTENDED PREGNANCIES

As noted above, the most recent data show that 57 percent of all pregnancies were unintended at the time of conception (Figure 2-1). This number includes pregnancies that were aborted, as well as both mistimed and unwanted pregnancies that led to live births. Only 43 percent of all pregnancies were intended at conception and resulted in live births.

Women of all socioeconomic, marital status, and age groups contribute to this pool of unintended pregnancies, as shown in Table 2-2. (This table displays pregnancies by both intention status and outcome for several demographic groupings, and also includes the actual number of pregnancies involved in each demographic category.) As this table shows, even among currently married women, 4 in 10 pregnancies were either mistimed or unwanted. However, the incidence of unintended pregnancy varies substantially by marital status, age, and economic group, being higher among unmarried and low-income women and among women at either end of the reproductive age span. (Variations in unintended pregnancy according to patterns of contraceptive use are discussed in Chapter 4.) Pregnancies during the teen years are particularly likely to be described as having been unintended. In 1987, for example, 82 percent of the pregnancies experienced by teenagers aged 15–19 were unintended, as were 61 percent of the pregnancies experienced by women aged 20–24.[6] Similarly, among women over age 40, 77 percent of the pregnancies experienced were unintended, as were 56 percent of the pregnancies to women aged 35–39. However, even among women between the ages of 25 and 34, between 42 and 45 percent of all pregnancies were described as having been unintended when they occurred.

Marital status, which is highly correlated with age, is also strongly related to whether a pregnancy is unintended. The vast majority of pregnancies to never-married women—88 percent—are unintended. Moreover, 69 percent of the pregnancies among formerly married women are unintended. Nonetheless, even among currently married women, 4 in 10 pregnancies are unintended, as noted earlier.

Economic status is also strongly correlated with pregnancy intention. Among women whose family incomes fell below the poverty level in the 1988 NSFG, 75 percent of pregnancies were described as unintended, compared with 64

---

[6]Part of the unintended pregnancy phenomenon in adolescence and the early 20s may reflect the decreasing age of menarche and the rising age of first marriage, both of which, taken together, have lengthened the period during which pregnancies are particularly likely to be considered unintended. In 1890, for example, the average number of years between menarche and marriage was 7.2 years (menarche at about 15.5 years of age and marriage at about 22 years of age); in 1988 the interval was almost 12 years (menarche at about 12.5 years and first marriage at about 24 years of age) (The Alan Guttmacher Institute, 1994:Figure 1).

TABLE 2-2 Estimated Proportions of Pregnancies (Excluding Miscarriages) by Outcome and Intention, Percentage of Pregnancies Unintended, and Percentage of Unintended Pregnancies Ending in Abortion, 1987, by Marital Status, Age at Outcome, and Poverty Status at Interview

	All Pregnancies (miscarriages excluded)					
Demographic Characteristics	Total Pregnancies	Intended Pregnancies Ending in Births	Unintended Pregnancies Ending in Births	Abortions	Percentage of Pregnancies Unintended	Percentage of Unintended Pregnancies Ending in Abortion
Total	100.1	42.8	28.4	28.9	57.3	50.4
Marital status						
Currently married	100.0	59.9	29.7	10.4	40.1	25.9
Formerly married	100.0	31.5	32.4	36.1	68.5	52.7
Never married	100.0	11.8	22.0	66.2	88.2	75.1
Age						
15–19	100.0	18.3	40.0	41.7	81.7	51.0
20–24	100.0	39.4	29.7	30.9	60.6	51.0
25–29	100.0	54.8	23.8	21.4	45.2	47.3
30–34	100.0	57.9	21.0	21.1	42.1	50.1
35–39	100.0	44.1	25.1	39.7	55.9	55.1
40–44	100.0	23.1	31.3	45.6	76.9	59.3
Poverty status						
<100%	100.0	24.6	35.6	39.8	75.4	52.8
100–199%	100.0	36.0	26.8	37.2	64.0	58.1
≥200%	100.0	55.0	25.7	19.3	45.0	42.9

SOURCE: Forrest JD. Epidemiology of unintended pregnancy and contraceptive use. Am J Obstet Gynec. 1994;170:1485–1488.

percent among women with incomes between 100 and 200 percent of the poverty level. Among women whose incomes exceeded 200 percent of the poverty level, 45 percent of all pregnancies were unintended.

Consistent with the higher rates of unintended pregnancy among women in poverty, unintended pregnancy is much more common among black than white women. Data from the 1990 NSFG show that the percentage of births reported as unintended at time of conception was 62 percent among black women; among white women, the comparable figure was 41 percent[7] (Piccinino, forthcoming).

Among some smaller subgroups, the proportions of pregnancies that are unintended may be appreciably higher than for the nation as a whole. Groups for whom this appears to be the case include, for example, women who are homeless, teenagers who have dropped out of school and engage in multiple high-risk behaviors, of which sexual intercourse without contraception is only one, and women who are heavy abusers of alcohol and illegal drugs (Centers for Disease Control and Prevention, 1994; Armstrong et al., 1991).

TRENDS IN UNINTENDED PREGNANCY

A key question is whether unintended pregnancy is becoming more or less prevalent. The data available to answer this question are limited because of the underreporting of abortion within the NSFG, as noted above. Forrest and Singh (1990) supplemented the 1982 and 1988 NSFG data on births with more complete information on abortions and found that the overall incidence of unintended pregnancy increased very slightly between 1982 and 1987, from 55.5 to 57.3 percent. Over those same years, however, there was a larger increase in the proportion of births resulting from unintended pregnancies, primarily because of a small decrease in the proportion of unintended pregnancies that were aborted.[8] Put another way, given an unintended pregnancy, slightly fewer women obtained abortions in 1987 than in 1982, resulting in more children being born who were unintended at the time of conception (Forrest and Singh, 1990). Similar data are not available after 1987 on this complex relationship among pregnancies, abortions, and births.

---

[7]Data are reported here on births rather than pregnancies because the research summarized in Table 2-2, which is the source for the narrative text in this section, did not include differential rates of unintended pregnancy by race, but only by marital status, age, and poverty level.

[8]Possible reasons for this phenomenon include the passage by states of restrictive abortion laws, decreased numbers of facilities performing abortions, changing views about the acceptability of abortion as a solution to unintended pregnancy, and increased social tolerance for nonmarital childbearing.

However, using data from the NSFG, it is possible to track trends in *births* derived from unintended pregnancies, both those that were mistimed and those that were unwanted at conception, as summarized in the next several sections. The first section briefly presents overall trends; subsequent, more detailed sections present trends by marital status because, as noted above, the marital status groupings used by the NSFG in its fertility questions have changed over the years.

Overall Trends for All Women

Data from the large pool of "ever-married women" show that, broadly speaking, the proportion of births resulting from unintended pregnancies decreased steadily in the 1970s through to 1982. Between 1982 and 1988, however, the picture changed. Looking at births to women aged 15–44 in all marital status groupings (Figure 2-4), the percentage of births unintended at conception increased (from 37 to 39 percent). Data from the 1990 NSFG telephone reinterview suggest that the increase continued through to 1990 (rising from 39 to 44 percent). That is, 44 percent of all births in 1990 were the result of unintended pregnancy. Preliminary data from the 1993 National Survey of Families and Households (Wave 2) indicate that the increase may extend into the early 1990s as well (Figure 2-5). Given the serious consequences that can burden births derived from unintended pregnancy (Chapter 3), this overall trend is troubling.

Trends Among Currently Married Women

Data on the intention status of pregnancies that result in live births to currently married women cover the longest time period—from 1965 to 1990—and are given in Figure 2-6. The overall proportion of births unintended at conception decreased steadily from 1965 to 1982 (from 55 to 30 percent). In particular, births unwanted at conception dropped dramatically over this period, decreasing from 24 percent in 1965 to 7 percent in 1982. Between 1982 and 1988, however, the percentage of births derived from unintended pregnancies among these currently married women increased, from 30 to 33 percent, largely because of an increase in births unwanted at conception. Between 1988 and 1990, the proportion of births unintended at conception increased again, to 37 percent, this time entirely because of an increase in births mistimed at conception. The broad trends displayed in Figure 2-6 appear to be statistically significant, at least at the extremes (e.g., 1982 versus both 1965 and 1990). Trends in unintended pregnancy among the slightly larger group of "ever-married" women (data not shown), which includes those who are separated,

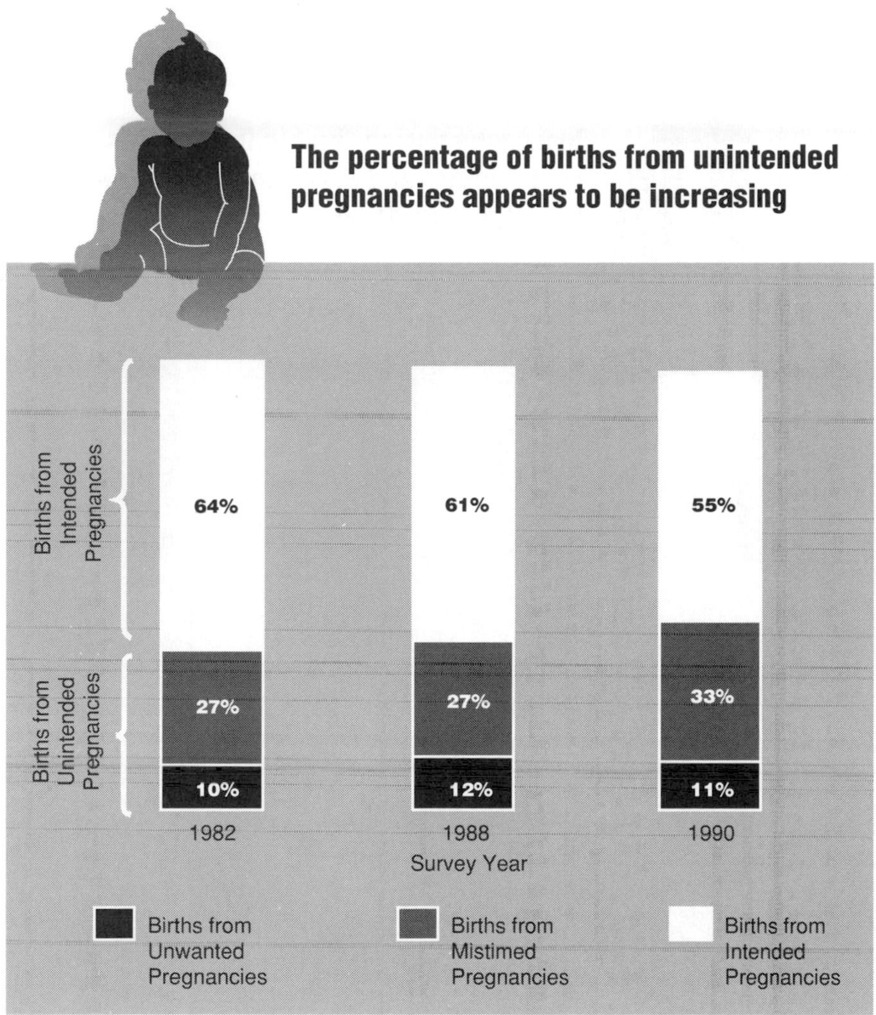

FIGURE 2-4 Intention status at conception of recent live births (births within exactly 5 years of interview date or within 2 years of interview date for 1990) to all women ages 15–44: United States, 1982 to 1990. Note: Because of rounding, totals may not add up to 100 percent. Source: Centers for Disease Control and Prevention, National Center for Health Statistics. National Survey of Family Growth 1982 and 1988. Telephone Reinterview; 1990 (preliminary data).

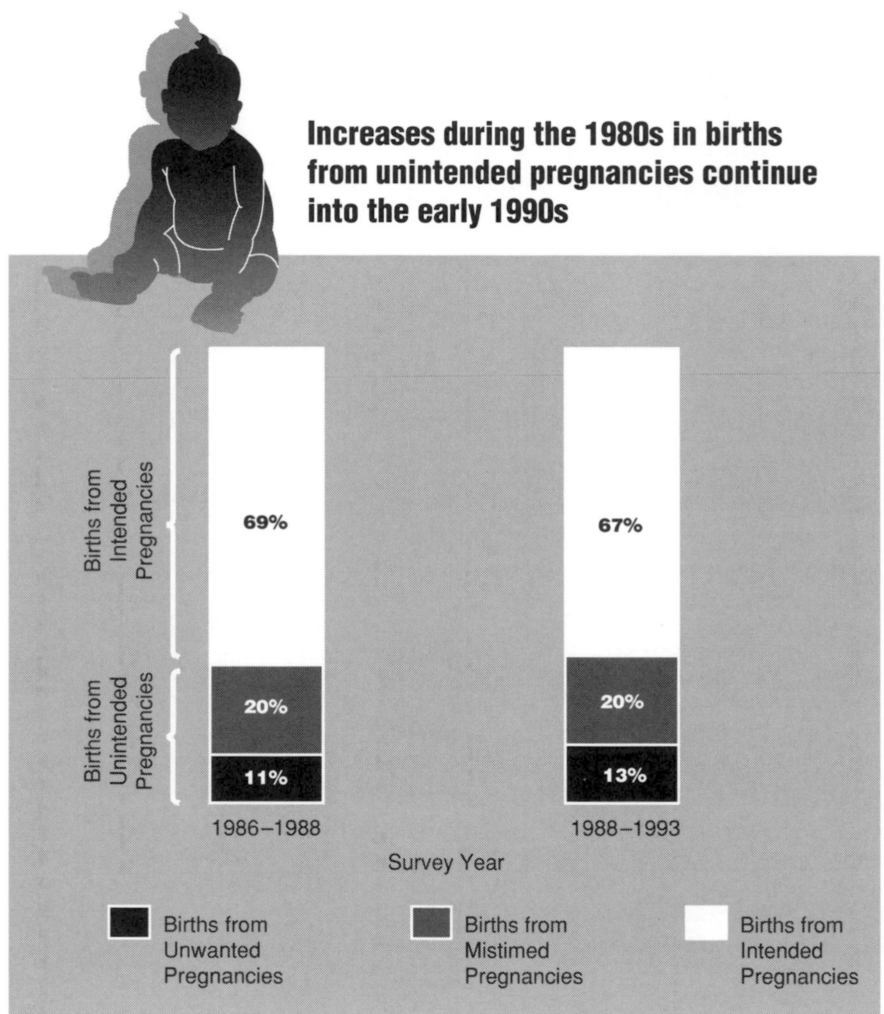

FIGURE 2-5 Intention status at conception among births in 1986–1988 (National Survey of Family Growth) and 1988–1993 (National Survey of Families and Households, Wave 2), among non-Hispanic white women ages 25–44. Source: Bumpass L. Unpublished data tabulated for the Institute of Medicine Committee on Unintended Pregnancy, October, 1994.

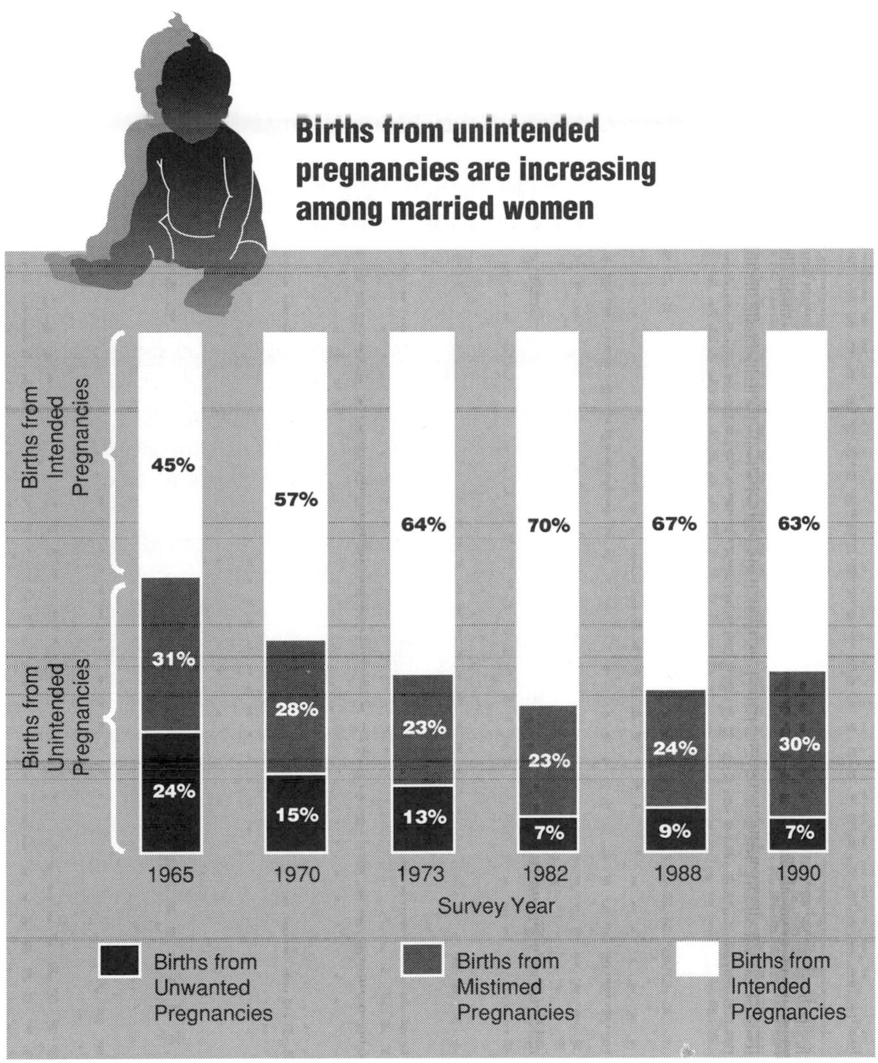

FIGURE 2-6 Births in the preceding 5 years among currently married women aged 15–44 at interview, by intention status at conception, 1965–1990. Note: In calculating percentages, it is assumed that missing data are distributed proportionately across intention groupings (missing data make up less than 1 percent of all data). Sources: Centers for Disease Control and Prevention, National Center for Health Statistics. National Survey of Family Growth 1982 and 1988. Telephone Reinterview; 1990 (preliminary data); Williams LB, Pratt WF. Wanted and unwanted childbearing in the United States: 1973–1988. Advance data from Vital and Health Statistics, no. 189. Hyattsville, MD: National Center for Health Statistics; 1990; Westoff CF. The decline of unplanned births in the United States. Science. 1976;191:38–41. (Calculations by Child Trends, Inc.)

divorced, or widowed, follow the same patterns seen among currently married women.

Trends Among Never-Married Women

As one might predict, a larger proportion of births to unmarried women (although certainly not all) are unintended at the time of conception than is the case for currently married and ever-married women; but interestingly, trends in births derived from unintended pregnancies among these women follow a different pattern. Between 1982 and 1990, both currently married and ever-married women experienced a steady *increase* in births unintended at conception, as noted above. By contrast, the percentage of births to never-married women derived from unintended pregnancy decreased between 1982 and 1988, and then appeared to increase between 1988 and 1990. Changing proportions of births derived from mistimed and unwanted pregnancies fueled these fluctuations (Figure 2-7).

Understanding the intention status of births to never-married women is particularly important given the increasing public policy focus on both nonmarital childbearing and childbearing among unmarried teenagers, as noted in Chapter 1.[9] One important question in this policy arena is whether births to these two groups are consciously undertaken (intended) or not. In fact, available data show that the overwhelming majority of births to both never-married women generally and to unmarried teenagers in particular were the result of unintended pregnancies: in 1990, 73 percent of births to never-married women were the result of unintended pregnancies (Figure 2-7; Williams and Pratt, 1990), and in 1988, 86 percent of births to unmarried teenagers (i.e., under 20 years of age) were unintended at conception (The Alan Guttmacher Institute, 1994:Figure 32). Clearly, most births to women who have never been married and the vast majority of births to unmarried teenagers are not the result of conscious intent.

Trends in Births Unwanted at Conception

The broad trends noted in the preceding sections mask some subgroup differences that are important to underscore, especially as regards births from

---

[9]These two phenomena—nonmarital childbearing and teen childbearing—are closely related but not synonymous; in fact, most births among unmarried women (70 percent) occur among women who are not teenagers.

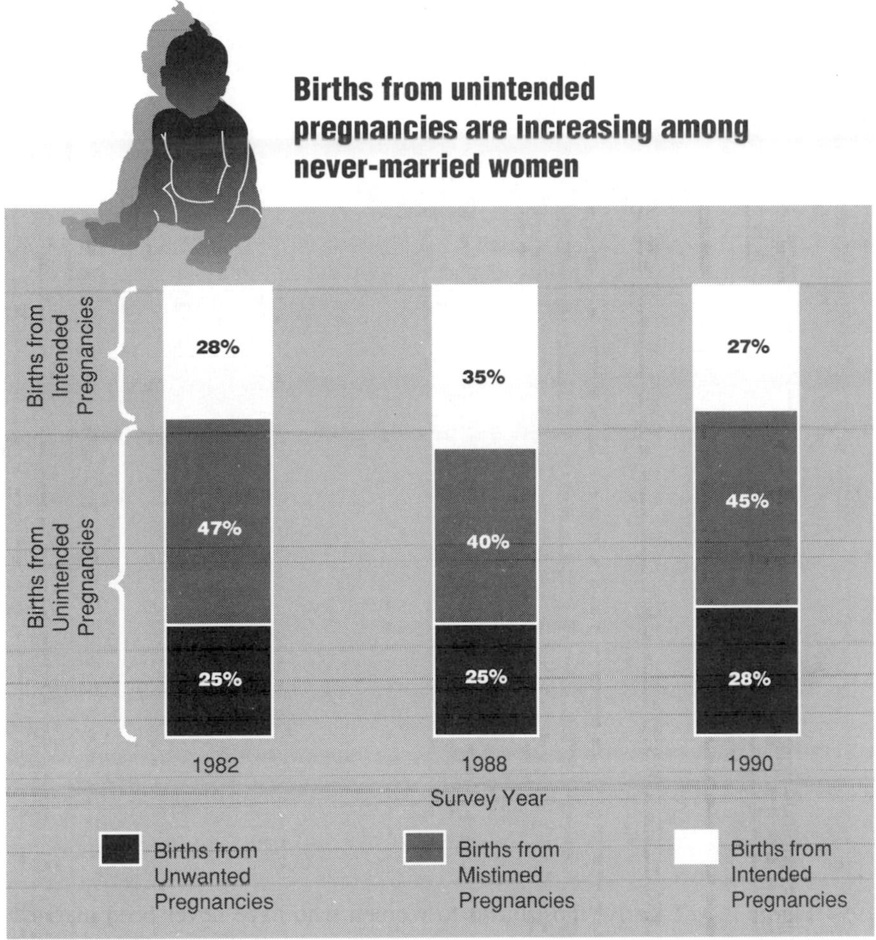

FIGURE 2-7 Percentage of births in the preceding 5 years to never-married women aged 15–44 by intention status at conception, 1982–1990. Source: Centers for Disease Control and Prevention, National Center for Health Statistics. National Survey of Family Growth 1982 and 1988. Telephone Reinterview; 1990 (preliminary data), unpublished tables.

unwanted pregnancies, which carry particularly serious risks (Chapter 3). Table 2-3 shows data on the intention status of births to ever-married women (which excludes the important group of never-married women) broken out by both income and by race (black, white) over the period 1973–1988. The intention status of births among ever-married women below the poverty level followed the same pattern as that of all ever-married women from 1973 to 1988; that is, the proportion of births derived from unintended pregnancies decreased from 1973

TABLE 2-3 Intention Status at Conception of Births in the Last 5 Years to Ever-Married Women and to Ever-Married Women with Incomes Below the Poverty Level, by Race, 1973–1988 (in Percent)

	Births Derived from Intended Pregnancies			Births Derived from Mistimed Pregnancies			Births Derived from Unwanted Pregnancies		
Group	1973	1982	1988	1973	1982	1988	1973	1982	1988
All ever-married women	61.7	68.3	64.7	24.0	24.0	25.0	14.3	7.7	10.3
Below poverty, ever-married women	48.6	56.6	45.0	25.3	31.5	34.3	26.1	11.9	20.7
Ever-married white women	64.3	69.7	65.6	23.4	23.6	25.6	12.3	6.7	8.8
Below poverty, ever-married white women	53.4	58.8	45.3	27.5	31.0	37.3	19.1	10.2	17.4
Ever-married black women	40.6	56.0	51.0	28.9	28.1	26.2	30.5	15.9	22.8
Below poverty, ever-married black women	35.9	47.5	37.6	20.3	31.5	27.1	43.8	21.0	35.3

SOURCE: Williams LB, Pratt WF. Wanted and unwanted childbearing in the United States: 1973–1988. Advance data from Vital and Health Statistics, no. 189. Hyattsville, MD: National Center for Health Statistics; 1990.

to 1982 and then increased in 1988.

Following trends in *unwanted* pregnancies, however, reveals more dramatic changes. Although births from unwanted pregnancies among all ever-married women showed a slight increase between 1982 and 1988 (increasing from about 8 to 10 percent), births among women below poverty in this group registered much steeper increases (rising from about 12 to 21 percent). This means that by 1988 one of every five births to ever-married women below the poverty level was the result of an unwanted pregnancy—a level approaching the 1973 level of one in four, with most of the progress in the interim having effectively been erased. For black women below poverty, the trend is more pronounced. In 1973, 44 percent of births among this group resulted from an unwanted pregnancy; by 1982, this percentage had dropped to 21 percent. By 1988, however, this number was sharply up again, to 35 percent; thus, in 1988, about one birth in three to ever-married black women below poverty was due to an unwanted pregnancy.

As noted above, these figures exclude data for never-married women, who are known to have very high proportions of births that were either mistimed or unwanted at conception (see Figure 2-7). Accordingly, it is reasonable to believe that the proportion of births unwanted at the time of conception among *all* women below poverty is probably even higher than the levels noted in the preceding paragraph, which is addressed only to those below poverty who have ever been married.

THE ROLE OF ABORTION

Reflecting the high proportion of pregnancies that are unintended, U.S. abortion rates are also high. That is, the nation's high abortion rate can be viewed as reflecting high levels of unintended pregnancies. More than a million and a half abortions occurred in the United States every year during the 1980s; in both 1991 and 1992, the total number was about 1.5 million (Figure 2-8). As already shown in Figure 2-2, over half of all unintended pregnancies end in abortion.

Factors That Affect Who Obtains an Abortion

Among women experiencing unintended pregnancies, marital status has a strong effect on the proportion obtaining an abortion (Table 2-2). Indeed, the proportion of unintended pregnancies terminated by abortion ranges from 75 percent among never-married women to 53 percent among formerly married women and 26 percent among currently married women. Whether the pregnancy was unwanted or mistimed does not affect the proportion of pregnancies ending

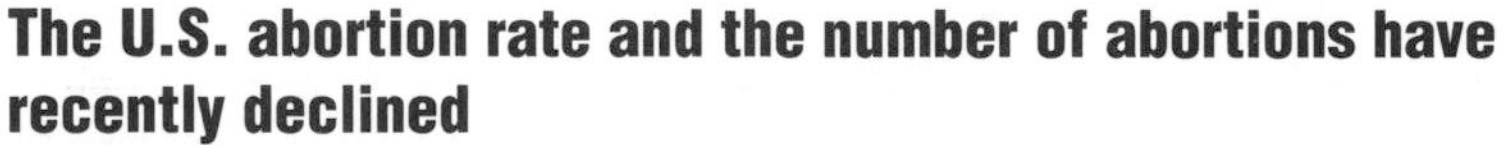

The U.S. abortion rate and the number of abortions have recently declined

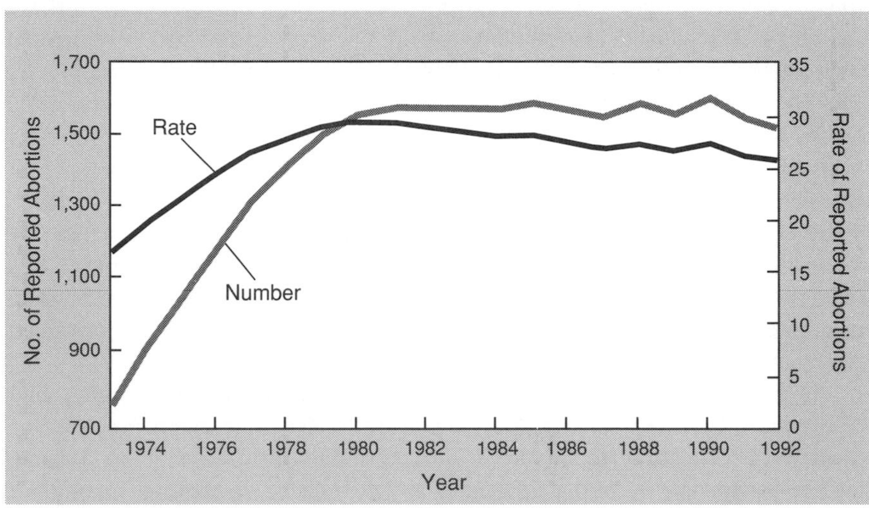

FIGURE 2-8 Number of reported abortions and rate of abortions per 1,000 women aged 15–44, United States, 1973–1992. Source: Henshaw SK, Van Vort J. Abortion services in the United States, 1991 and 1992. Fam Plann Perspect. 1993;26:100–106.

in abortion; 51 percent of mistimed pregnancies and 50 percent of unwanted pregnancies end in abortion (Forrest, 1994). The more critical factor is whether or not the woman is married.

Compared with marital status, age is a less powerful predictor of the propensity to abort an unintended pregnancy (Table 2-2). About half of women under age 35 who experience an unintended pregnancy obtain an abortion. The proportion rises among older women, with nearly 6 in 10 women ages 40–44 who experience an unintended pregnancy obtaining an abortion.

The proportion of women obtaining an abortion in the event of an unintended pregnancy is slightly lower among affluent women than low-income women. But, again, the effect of poverty status is weak and irregular compared with the very strong effect of marital status.

INTERNATIONAL COMPARISONS

International comparisons help to put many of these numbers into perspective. Data from other industrialized democracies demonstrate that the rate of unintended pregnancy experienced among teenagers in the United States is considerably higher than that in other countries and is often higher for adults as well (Jones et al., 1988, 1985). Figure 2-9 compares the level of intended and unintended pregnancies in the United States with the levels in a number of other industrialized nations.[10] It is apparent from Figure 2-9 that the rate of intended pregnancy[11] was fairly constant across countries, ranging only between 1.18 and 1.39 pregnancies per woman. However, there is substantial variation across nations in the unintended pregnancy rate, with only France having rates of unintended pregnancy comparable to those found in the United States. Levels of 0.28 in The Netherlands, 0.63 in Great Britain, 0.79 in Canada, and 0.80 in Sweden illustrate that a variety of nations have achieved rates of unintended pregnancy that are considerably less—some a great deal less—than the level of 1.31 in the United States. The information in Figure 2-9 is obviously dated; nonetheless, it clearly suggests that lower rates can be achieved in the United States.

U.S. Abortion Rates Versus Other Western Democracies

Although the U.S. abortion rate has declined slightly since the early 1980s (Figure 2-8), the rate remains high compared with that in other Western democracies.[12] Table 2-4 depicts the abortion rate (number of abortions per 1,000 women aged 15–44) for a number of developed industrialized nations. Compared with those nations, the U.S. abortion rate is two to four times higher. Few other Western democracies have abortion rates that even approach those of the United States; the U.S. rate is more than 50 percent higher than the

---

[10]If all unintended pregnancies were prevented, it is not the case that the total fertility rate would be as low as is implied by the intended pregnancy rate, because many unintended pregnancies are mistimed and would occur later as intended pregnancies.

[11]The intended pregnancy rate is derived from the total pregnancy rate. The total pregnancy rate is the average number of pregnancies (i.e., births plus abortions) that a woman would have, assuming a continuation of current age-specific rates over her reproductive lifetime. This rate can be broken down into the planned (or intended), unplanned (or unintended), and abortion rates by applying the distribution of births by planning and intention status to the levels of fertility and abortion that prevailed in the year following the survey.

[12]The term "Western democracies" is used in this section to clarify that the comparisons being made are between the United States and selected European countries, plus Canada. Other nations, such as China, the former Soviet Union, countries in Eastern Europe, and some developing countries report ratios of abortions to live births that are significantly higher than those in either the United States or in other Western democracies.

TABLE 2-4 Abortion Rates per 1,000 Women Ages 15–44 by Country, 1980, 1985–1991

Country	1980	1985	1986	1987	1988	1989	1990	1991	1992
Australia	13.9	15.6	16.4	16.3	16.6	—	—	—	—
Belgium	—	7.5	—	—	—	—	—	—	—
Canada	12.6	11.3	11.2	11.3	11.6	12.6	14.6	14.7	14.9
Denmark	21.4	17.6	17.7	18.3	—	—	18.2	—	—
Finland	—	12.4	—	11.7	—	—	11.5	—	—
France[a]	15.3	14.6	13.9	13.3	13.2	—	—	—	—
Federal Republic of Germany (former)[a]	6.6	6.1	6.3	6.6	6.3	5.6	5.8	—	—
Ireland[b]	4.8	5.2	5.2	4.8	5.0	4.9	5.4	—	—
Italy[a]	18.7	16.8	16.0	15.3	15.3		12.7	—	—
The Netherlands[c]	6.2	5.1	5.3	5.1	5.1	5.1	5.2	—	—
New Zealand	8.5	9.3	10.5	11.3	12.8	12.9	14.0	14.4	—
Norway	16.3	16.3	17.1	16.8	17.1	17.9	16.7	—	—

United States	29.3	28.0	27.4	26.9	27.3	26.8	27.4	26.3	25.9
United States, whites[d]	24.3	22.6	21.8	21.2	21.2	20.9	21.5	20.3	—

[a]Statistics for France, Germany, and Italy may be incomplete.
[b]Abortion is illegal in Ireland and the reported rate is based on abortions obtained in England and Wales by women reporting Irish addresses.
[c]Data from The Netherlands are for residents only.
[d]Data for whites in the United States include most hispanic women.

SOURCES: The Alan Guttmacher Institute. Unpublished data. 1994. Henshaw S, Morrow E. Induced Abortion: A World Review, 1990 Supplement. New York, NY: The Alan Guttmacher Institute; 1990. Henshaw S, Van Vort J. Abortion services in the United States, 1991 and 1992. Fam Plann Perspect. 1993;26:100–106: Table 1. Canadian Center for Health Information. Therapeutic Abortions, 1991. Ottawa, Ontario: Statistics Canada; 1993. United Nations. Abortion Polices: A Global Review, Vol. I. New York, NY: Department of Economic and Social Development, United Nations; 1992. United Nations. Abortion Policies: A Global Review. Vol. II. New York, NY: Department of Economic and Social Development, United Nations; 1993.

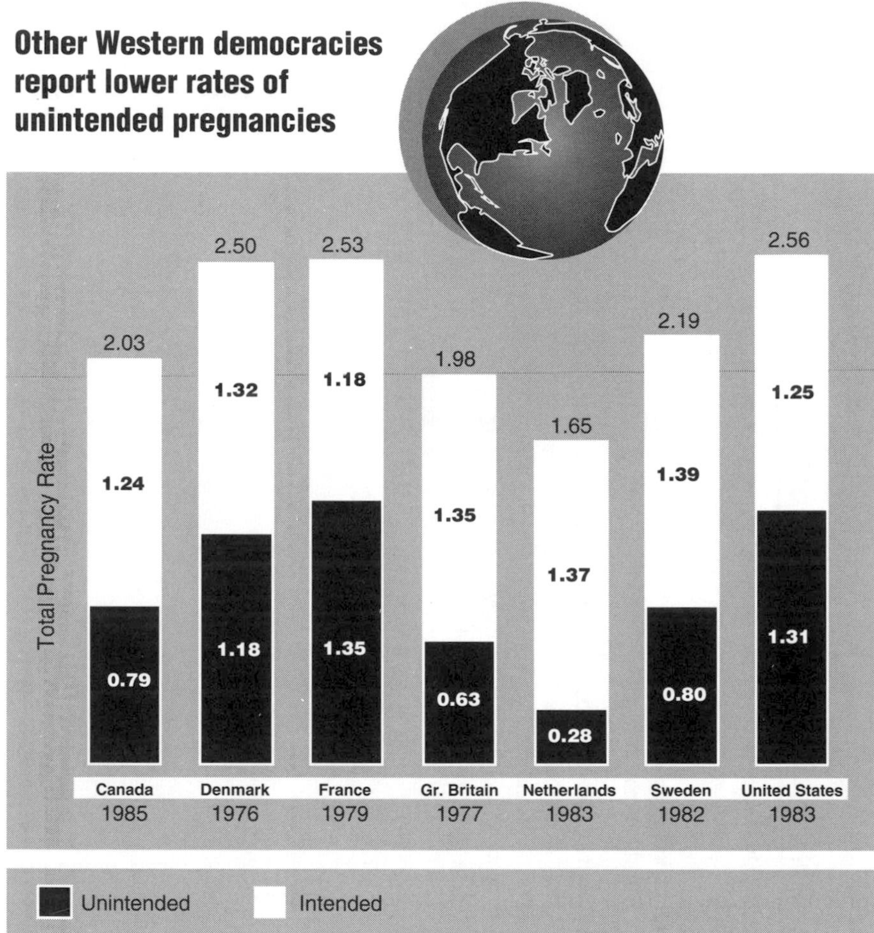

FIGURE 2-9 Total pregnancy rate and its components, the intended pregnancy rate and the unintended pregnancy rate, selected countries, selected years. Note: The total pregnancy rate is the average number of pregnancies (i.e. births plus abortions) that a woman would have, assuming a continuation of current age-specific rates over her reproductive lifetime. This rate can be broken down into the planned (or "intended"), unplanned (or "unintended") and abortion rates by applying the distribution of births by planning/intention status to the levels of fertility and abortion that prevailed in the year following the survey. Source: Henshaw SK, Van Vort J. Abortion services in the United States, 1991 and 1992. Fam Plann Perspect. 1993;26:100–106.

Norwegian rate, for example. The abortion rate for U.S. whites is also presented to confirm that the higher U.S. rate is not explained by the higher incidence of abortion among minority women in the United States. The data show that the U.S. abortion rate is higher than the rate found in other Western nations among whites as well as among all U.S. women.

A detailed study conducted by The Alan Guttmacher Institute comparing the United States with four other comparable areas illustrates the degree to which the U.S. abortion rate reflects the high proportion of pregnancies that are unintended. In the United States, women were estimated to have a total pregnancy rate (defined in Footnote 11) of 2.6—that is, an average of 2.6 pregnancies during their reproductive years. This represents a considerably higher total pregnancy rate than that found in the other study areas: 1.7 in The Netherlands, 1.7 in Quebec, 2.0 in Great Britain, and 2.1 in Ontario.

The higher total pregnancy rate in the United States is due entirely to the higher rate of unintended pregnancies (births resulting from unintended pregnancies plus abortions). And even though many unintended pregnancies are resolved by abortion, the rate of births derived from unintended pregnancy is still higher in the United States than in any of the other study areas. Moreover, compared with the four study countries, the U.S. abortion rate remains two to four times higher, as in the earlier comparison (Table 2-4).

CONCLUSION

Unintended pregnancy is common in the United States; the most recent estimate is that almost 60 percent of all pregnancies are unintended, either mistimed or unwanted altogether. Reflecting the high proportion of pregnancies that are unintended, abortion rates are also high; about half of these unintended pregnancies are aborted. Although unintended pregnancies occur among women of all socioeconomic, marital status, and age groups, unmarried and poor women as well as women at either end of the reproductive age span are especially likely to become pregnant unintentionally.

During the 1970s and early 1980s, a decreasing proportion of births (as distinct from pregnancies) were unintended at the time of conception; between 1982 and 1988, however, this trend reversed such that the proportion of births that were unintended at conception increased. These trends in the 1980s reflect both an overall increase in the proportion of unintended pregnancies and a decline in the proportion of unintended pregnancies that were resolved by abortion. Some data from the 1990s suggest that the proportion of births that were unintended at conception has continued to increase into this decade. In 1990, 44 percent of all births were the result of unintended pregnancy; among such subpopulations as women in poverty, black women, never-married women, and unmarried teenagers, the percentage of births resulting from unintended pregnancy was substantially higher (59, 62, 73, and 86 percent, respectively, in the late 1980s).

International comparisons show that U.S. women experience more unintended pregnancies—and therefore more abortions as well as births—than women in many other industrialized countries. Such data suggest that lower rates of unintended pregnancy could be achieved in the United States.

REFERENCES

The Alan Guttmacher Institute. Sex and America's Teenagers. New York, NY and Washington, DC; 1994.

The Alan Guttmacher Institute. Unpublished data. 1994.

Armstrong KA, Kenen R, Samost L. Barriers to family planning services among patients in drug treatment programs. Fam Plann Perspect. 1991;23:264–271.

Bumpass L. Unpublished data tabulated for the Institute of Medicine Committee on Unintended Pregnancy, October, 1994.

Canadian Center for Health Information. Therapeutic Abortions, 1991. Ottawa, Ontario: Statistics Canada;1993

Centers for Disease Control, National Center for Health Statistics. National Survey of Family Growth 1982 and 1988. Telephone Reinterview; 1990 (preliminary data).

Centers for Disease Control and Prevention. Health risk behaviors among adolescents who do and do not attend school—United States, 1992. MMWR. 1994;43:129–132.

Forrest JD. Epidemiology of unintended pregnancy and contraceptive use. Am J Obstet Gynec. 1994;170:1485–1488.

Forrest JD, Singh S. The sexual and reproductive behavior of American women, 1982–1988. Fam Plann Perspect. 1990;22:206–214.

Henshaw SK, Forrest JD. Women at Risk of Unintended Pregnancy, 1990 Estimates: The Need for Family Planning Services, Each State and County. New York, NY: The Alan Guttmacher Institute; 1993.

Henshaw S, Morrow E. Induced Abortion: A World Review, 1990 Supplement. New York, NY: The Alan Guttmacher Institute; 1990.

Henshaw SK, Van Vort J. Abortion services in the United States, 1991 and 1992. Fam Plann Perspect. 1993;26:100–106.

Jones EF, Forrest JD. Underreporting of abortion in surveys of U.S. women: 1976 to 1988. Demography. 1992;29:113–126.

Jones E, Forrest JD, Goldman N, Henshaw SK, Lincoln R, Rosoff J, Westoff CF, Wulf D. Teenage pregnancy in developed countries: Determinants and policy implications. Fam Plann Perspect. 1985;17:53–62.

Jones E, Forrest JD, Henshaw S, Silverman J, Torres A. Unintended pregnancy contraceptive practice and family planning services in developed countries. Fam Plann Perspect. 1988;20:53–67.

Kost K, Forrest, JD. Intention status of U.S. births in 1988: Differences by mother's socioeconomic and demographic characteristics. Fam Plann Perspect. 1995;27:11–17.

Luker K. Taking Chances: Abortion and the Decision Not to Contracept. Berkeley and Los Angeles, CA: University of California Press; 1975.

Miller WB. Relationships between the intendedness of conception and the wantedness of pregnancy. J Nerv Ment Dis. 1974;159:396–406.

Musick JS. Young, Poor and Pregnant: The Psychology of Teenage Motherhood. New Haven, CT: Yale University Press; 1993.

Piccinino L. Unintended pregnancy and childbearing in the United States: 1973–1990. Advance Data from Vital and Health Statistics. Hyattsville, MD: CDC, NCHS; Forthcoming.

Poole VL, Klerman LV, Goldenberg RL, Cliver SP. Pregnancy intendedness and maternal behaviors in a low-income high risk population. Unpublished manuscript. University of Alabama at Birmingham; 1994.

Ryder NB. The structure of pregnancy intervals by planning status. Popul Stud. 1985;39: 193–212.

Torres A, Forrest JD. Why do women have abortions? Fam Plann Perspect. 1988;20: 169–176.

United Nations. Abortion Polices: A Global Review, Vol. I. New York, NY: Department of Economic and Social Development, United Nations; 1992.

United Nations. Abortion Policies: A Global Review, Vol. II. New York, NY: Department of Economic and Social Development, United Nations; 1993.

Westoff CF. The decline of unplanned births in the United States. Science. 1976;191:38–41.

Williams LB. Determinants of couple agreement in US fertility decisions. Fam Plann Perspect. 1994;26:169–173.

Williams LB, Pratt WF. Wanted and unwanted childbearing in the United States: 1973–1988. Advance data from Vital and Health Statistics, no. 189. Hyattsville, MD: National Center for Health Statistics; 1990.

3

Consequences of Unintended Pregnancy

Does it matter whether a pregnancy is unintended at the time of conception—mistimed or unwanted altogether? There is a presumption that it does—that unintended pregnancy has a major impact on numerous social, economic, and cultural aspects of modern life. But it is important to define what these consequences might be. Accordingly, this chapter examines five sets of information that help to answer this important question. The first section addresses elective termination of pregnancy, because about half of all unintended pregnancies in the United States are resolved by abortion. As such, abortion can be seen as one of the primary consequences of unintended pregnancy. The second section considers the fact that unintended pregnancy is more common among unmarried women and women at either end of the reproductive age span (Chapter 2)—demographic attributes which themselves carry increased medical or social risks for children and/or their parents.

The final three sections address additional consequences of unintended pregnancy. The third section analyzes a complex set of studies in which the intendedness of pregnancy itself is related to a variety of outcomes for both the child (such as birthweight and cognitive development) and parents (such as educational achievement). These studies allow one to consider whether pregnancy intention itself affects various child and parental outcomes. The fourth consequence explored is that opportunities for preconception health assessment and care are often missed when pregnancy occurs unintentionally. Preconception care is still a developing field of clinical practice, but its potential impact is important. The fifth section of the chapter analyzes how some dimensions of the childbearing population in the United States would change if unwanted pregnancies were eliminated altogether and mistimed ones were redistributed (typically, postponed). This statistical exercise helps provide an understanding of the consequences of current demographic patterns of unintended pregnancy and subsequent childbearing.

ABORTION AS A CONSEQUENCE OF UNINTENDED PREGNANCY

As the Chapter 2 discussed, about half of all unintended pregnancies end in abortion. Accordingly, the occurrence of abortion can be seen as one of the primary consequences of unintended pregnancy. Voluntary interruption of pregnancy is an ancient and enduring intervention that occurs globally whether it is legal or not. The legalization of abortion in all of the United States, accomplished through the 1973 Supreme Court ruling *Roe* v. *Wade*, served in large part to replace illegal abortion (as well as abortion obtained outside of the United States) with legal abortion in this country. It is estimated that before the legalization of abortion, about 1 million abortions were being performed annually, few of them legally, and somewhere between 1,000 and 10,000 women died annually from complications following these often poorly performed procedures. Before the Supreme Court ruling, abortion was probably the most common criminal activity in this country, surpassed only by gambling and narcotics violations (Luker, 1984; Jaffe et al., 1981).

A 1975 report by the Institute of Medicine documented the benefits to public health by the legalization of abortion. The Supreme Court decision was followed not only by a decline in the number of pregnancy-related deaths in young women (Cates et al., 1978) but also by a decline in hospital emergency room admissions because of incomplete or septic abortions, conditions that are more common with illegally induced abortions (Institute of Medicine, 1975).

Given the long-standing reliance on abortion to resolve many unintended pregnancies, it is important to consider available information about the major medical and psychological risks that this procedure may pose (Centers for Disease Control and Prevention, Reproductive Epidemiology Unit, 1994; Frye et al., 1994; Lawson et al., 1994). From the voluminous data available for review, two important findings stand out that are often overlooked in the controversy over this procedure. First, whatever the risks associated with legal abortion in the United States, it remains a far less risky medical procedure for the woman than childbirth; over the 1979–1985 interval, for example, the mortality associated with childbirth was more than 10 times that of induced abortion (Council on Scientific Affairs, American Medical Association, 1992). Second, abortion in the first trimester of pregnancy carries fewer risks to health than abortion in the second trimester of pregnancy and beyond.

Medical Complications

As with any surgical procedure, abortion carries an inherent risk of medical complications, including death. Complications known to be directly related to the procedure include hemorrhage, uterine perforation, cervical injury, and infection, which is often due to incomplete abortion. Later complications that have been investigated include possible negative effects on subsequent pregnancy outcomes, particularly low birthweight, midtrimester spontaneous abortion, and premature delivery. The vast majority of abortions performed in this country are first-trimester vacuum aspiration procedures. Pregnancy outcomes among women who have had one vacuum aspiration abortion are no different than those among women who have not had an abortion. Results are mixed, however, as regards the influence on subsequent pregnancy outcomes of having had more than one abortion or having second-trimester abortions by vacuum extraction. At present, investigators are studying a possible relationship between abortion and an increased risk of developing premenopausal breast cancer (Daling et al., 1994).

Rates of Complications

To assess the frequency with which the well-documented complications of abortion occur, between 1970 and 1978 the Centers for Disease Control and the Population Council conducted the Joint Program for the Study of Abortion in three waves: 1970–1971, 1971–1974, and 1975–1978. These surveys showed that the risk of developing major complications[1] from legal abortion decreased greatly during the 1970s: from 1.0 percent in the first wave to 0.29 percent in the last (Buehler et al., 1985; Cates and Grimes, 1981; Grimes et al., 1977; Tietze and Lewit, 1972). Although the total complication rate[2] increased from 9.0 to 14.8 percent over the three waves, this probably reflected an increased follow-up rate, a change in the distribution of first- and second-trimester abortions among the study populations, and an increase in reports of minor complications. Alternatively, the change may have been due to an actual increase in complications. More recent data show a total complication rate of induced abortion of less than 1 percent (Gold, 1990; Hakim-Elahi et al., 1990).

---

[1]The major complications rate denotes the percentage of women sustaining 1 or more of 15 complications that include cardiac arrest, convulsion, fever for 3 or more days, hemorrhage necessitating blood transfusion, pneumonia, psychiatric hospitalization for 11 or more days, and death.

[2]The total complication rate refers to the percentage of women who sustained one or more complications of any variety or severity.

In all waves, the risk of all complications increased steadily with increasing gestational age, being lowest for women obtaining abortions at ≤ 8 weeks of gestation and increasing 2 to 10 times for procedures after 12 weeks of gestation. Complication rates were lowest among women whose abortions were performed using suction curettage and increased with more invasive procedures (those often used for more advanced pregnancies).

Trend data are also available on mortality. The annual number of legal-abortion-related deaths decreased from 24 deaths in 1972 to 6 in 1987, and the mortality rate decreased from 4.1 per 100,000 abortions in 1972 to 0.4 in 1987. As with overall complication rates, the risk of mortality is lower for abortions performed by suction or sharp curettage during the first trimester and for pregnancies of lower gestational age (Lawson et al., 1994). The risk of mortality is higher, however, for nonwhite women, women 35 years of age and older, and for women of higher parity.

The increased risk of both morbidity and mortality with increasing gestational age underscores the health risks averted by early rather than late abortion. At present, 11 percent of abortions are obtained after 12 weeks of pregnancy; these later abortions are obtained disproportionately by adolescents: for girls under age 15, 22 percent of abortions are done in the second trimester, whereas the comparable figure for women over age 20 is 9 percent (Rosenfield, 1994). Although late abortion may be due to delay in recognizing a pregnancy, in deciding what to do if the pregnancy is unwanted, or may be a consequence of a genetic defect not detected until the second trimester, public policies can also increase the chance that an abortion will be performed in the second rather than the first trimester. Policies that may discourage first-trimester abortions include mandatory waiting periods (now required in 13 states), parental involvement/judicial bypass laws (35 states), and various informed consent laws, many of which require that women be given antiabortion lectures and materials intended to discourage them from having an abortion (31 states) (National Abortion and Reproductive Rights Action League, 1994). Chapter 7 notes the important and related issues of insufficient training of providers in abortion techniques and of declining numbers of abortion providers.

Psychological Issues

Although the medical risks of abortion appear to be very small, the procedure may pose troubling moral and ethical problems to some women and providers as well. In addition, women (and those close to them) may find that confronting an unintended pregnancy and weighing the option of abortion are emotionally difficult experiences, and the procedure itself may involve appreciable pain and expense.

Accordingly, numerous researchers have attempted to determine the extent to which abortion results in psychological problems in the weeks and months following the procedure. Some have investigated what has been called "post-abortion syndrome," hypothesizing that abortion may lead to a form of post-traumatic stress disorder, even though abortion does not meet the American Psychiatric Association's definition of trauma (Gold, 1990). Most of the 250 studies dealing with the psychological effects of induced abortion suffer from substantial methodological shortcomings and limitations (Council on Scientific Affairs, 1992; Adler et al., 1990; Gold, 1990; Koop, 1989). In light of these problems, former Surgeon General C. Everett Koop concluded in 1989 that data "were insufficient . . . to support the premise that abortion does or does not produce a post-abortion syndrome." He also concluded that emotional problems resulting from abortion are "minuscule from a public health perspective" (Koop, 1989). Similarly, Adler et al. (1990:42) concluded that "studies [of the psychological impact of abortion] are consistent in their findings of relatively rare instances of negative responses after abortion and of decreases in psychological distress after abortion compared to before abortion."

Political Issues

It is important to add that even though the medical and psychological consequences of abortion for individual women are largely minor, the consequences for the nation's political and social life are less benign. The legality and availability of abortion have been associated with important and painful divisions throughout the country, even overt hostility and violence, including several murders of health care personnel working for clinics that provide abortions. Controversy over abortion has affected public discourse on a wide range of issues—health care reform, fetal tissue research, and public funding for contraceptive services and research, among other topics. Views about abortion have colored state and local elections, Supreme Court nominations, political conventions, presidential politics, and many other issues as well. Polling data show that although a majority of Americans continue to support the basic legality of abortion, there remain many differences of opinion about the extent to which abortion should be available without restrictions, the acceptability of using government funds to pay for abortions, whether parental consent should be required when a minor seeks an abortion, and other issues as well (Blendon et al., 1993). It appears that social and political controversy over abortion will likely remain a divisive force in the United States—a reality that underscores the importance of reducing unintended pregnancy, which is the principal antecedent to abortion.

MATERNAL DEMOGRAPHIC STATUS

As noted in Chapter 2, unintended pregnancy occurs among all populations of women. But the experience is relatively more common in several specific groups: women at either end of the reproductive age span and women who are unmarried. Although many of these unintended pregnancies are resolved by abortion, an appreciable number result in live births (see Table 2-2). Therefore, in assessing the consequences of unintended pregnancy, it is useful to review the available data on the extent to which these demographic attributes themselves carry increased risks for children and their parents. Information on both socioeconomic and medical risks are reviewed below; because poverty is intertwined with the issues of both age and marital status, as subsequent text reveals, it is not discussed as a separate issue. Data from selected developing countries on many of these issues have recently been reviewed but are not presented here (National Research Council, 1989a,b).

This focus on selected groups is not meant to obscure a major point made in Chapter 2: although it is true that women who are unmarried or at either end of the reproductive age span are disproportionately represented among those having births that were unintended at conception, the majority of such births are to women without these attributes. Unintended pregnancy remains a widespread problem, whatever its pockets of concentration.

Adolescent Childbearing: Socioeconomic Issues

The negative associations between early childbearing and a host of economic, social, and health outcomes have been found in a variety of data sets over time. The association is strong, consistent, and persistent. The critical question has been that of causality. Births during the teenage years are concentrated among disadvantaged groups, whose members are likely to experience multiple disadvantages as adults whether or not they have children as teenagers. Thus, it has been argued that the association between early childbearing may reflect the disadvantaged backgrounds of those adolescents who become parents rather than any negative effects due to the timing of the birth itself (Geronimus, 1992; Luker, 1991).

Before addressing the causality issue, it is important to note the strong association of teenage childbearing with various problems. The link to diminished socioeconomic well-being, for example, for both children and their mothers has been recognized for several decades (Bacon, 1974). Adolescents who have children are substantially less likely to complete high school than those who delay childbearing. In recent years, the proportion of teenage mothers with high school degrees has increased, in large part because many are able to complete requirements for the general equivalency diploma (Moore, 1992; Mott and Maxwell, 1981). However, few teenage mothers attend college, and less than 1 percent have been found to complete college by age 27 (Moore, 1992).

Moreover, teenage mothers are more likely to be single parents or, if they are married, to experience marital dissolution (Hayes, 1987). Indeed, the proportion of teenagers who are single parents has increased substantially over the years. For example, in 1970, 30 percent of all births to teenage girls occurred outside of marriage, whereas 67 percent of births occurred outside of marriage in 1991 (National Center for Health Statistics, 1994).

Larger families place greater demands on a family's economic assets. Although family sizes among younger as well as older mothers have declined over time, younger mothers continue to have more children than delayed childbearers (Moore, 1992). Because of their fewer years of schooling, larger families, and lower likelihood of being married, teenage mothers acquire less work experience, have lower wages and earnings, and are substantially more likely to live in poverty. Figure 3-1 illustrates the strong association between age at first birth and poverty. Although minority women generally face a higher probability of poverty regardless of their age at first birth, age at first birth is linked to lower economic well-being within each race/ethnicity group. A majority of Hispanic and black teenage mothers are poor; that is, the ratio of their family income to the poverty threshold is below 100 percent; less than one-fourth of women who delay childbearing into their 20s have such low incomes. Among whites, one-fourth of teenage mothers had family incomes below the poverty level, compared with less than 1 in 10 among delayed childbearers.

The lesser likelihood of marriage and lower earning capacity of teenage mothers are also related to more frequent welfare receipt. Figure 3-2 illustrates the very strong association between a mother's age at the birth of her first child and the probability that she will receive payments from Aid to Families with Dependent Children (AFDC) during her first-born's preschool years.

Again, though, there are important questions about whether these many associations are directly caused by the mother's young age. Untangling the question of causality is essential to understanding the impact of childbearing in adolescence on both the mother and her offspring and in designing remedial programs for the future. Specifically, if having a baby has no negative impact on socioeconomic status or health, then remedial efforts should focus less on delaying childbearing than on alleviating the disadvantages associated with and apparently contributing to teenage childbearing. Of course, for many service providers and policymakers confronted with the needs of young parents and their children, the causality issue is moot; teenage parents and their children represent a population with multiple and immediate needs who pose substantial public costs, and figuring out cause versus association has little urgency.

Selectivity into early parenthood has long been recognized (Waite and Moore, 1978), and researchers have employed a variety of strategies to control for the effects of socioeconomic background differences. For example, Moore

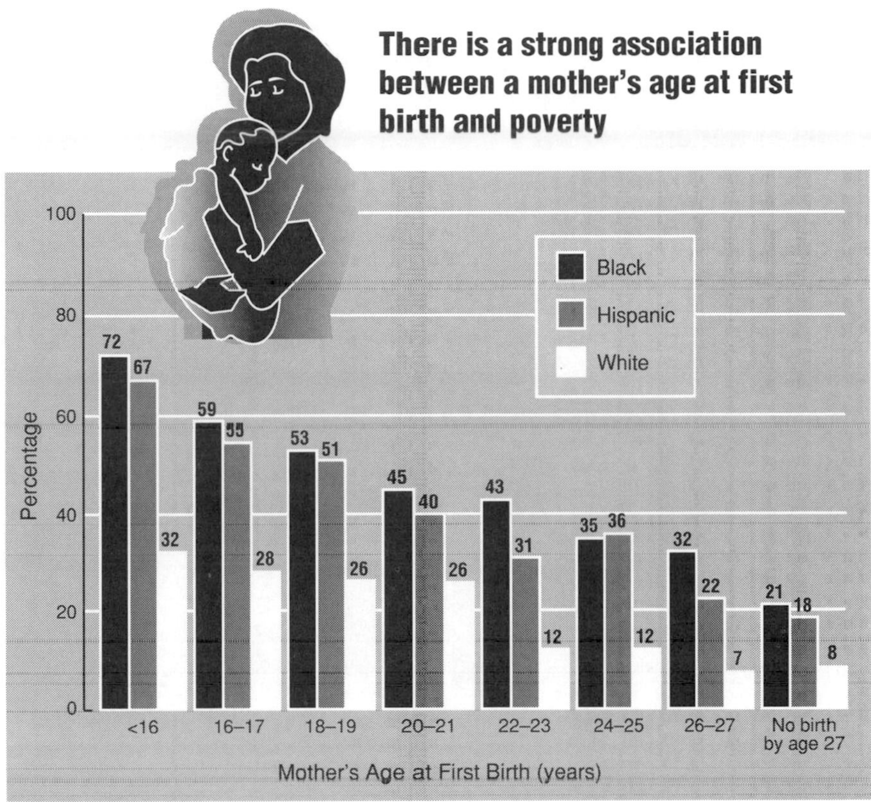

FIGURE 3-1 Percentage of mothers in poverty at age 27 by age at first birth. Source: Moore KA, Myers DE, Morrison DR, Nord CW, Brown B, Edmonston B. Age at first childbirth and later poverty. J Res Adol. 1993;3:393–422.

and colleagues (1993) estimated structural equation models including numerous background factors as controls; Hoffman et al. (1993) and Geronimus and Korenman (1992) compared outcomes for sisters, one of whom was a teenage mother and one of whom was not; Grogger and Bronars (1994, 1993) compared teenagers whose first birth was to twins with teens who had single births; and Hotz and colleagues are now comparing teens who have miscarriages with teens who deliver and raise their children (J. Hotz, pers. com., 1994).

Published results from these investigators find that the negative effects associated with teenage childbearing are much diminished when the mother's prepregnancy characteristics are accounted for. Nevertheless, virtually all researchers using varied approaches with varied data sets find that early childbearing is associated with negative outcomes over and above the effects of background. Put another way, there does appear to be a causal and adverse

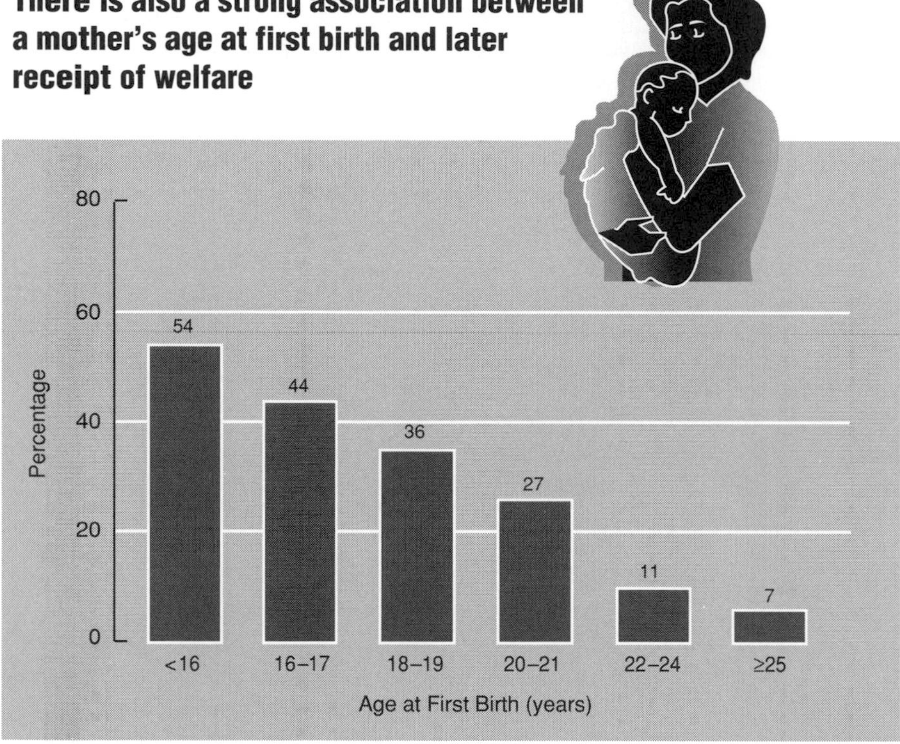

FIGURE 3-2 Percentage of mothers ever receiving Aid to Families with Dependent Children in the first 5 years after first birth by age at first birth, 1979 cohort National Longitudinal Survey of Youth. Source: Child Trends, Inc. based on public use files from the National Longitudinal Survey of Youth, 1979–1988 data, under Contract N01-HD-9-2919 from the National Institutes of Health.

effect of early childbearing on the health and social and economic well-being of children; this effect is over and above the important effects of background disadvantages.

Adolescent Childbearing: Medical Issues

In addition to the socioeconomic burdens accompanying childbearing by teenagers, adolescent pregnancy often poses serious health risks as well to both mothers and infants. Young adolescents (particularly those under age 15[3]) experience a maternal death rate 2.5 times greater than that of mothers aged 20–24 (Morris et al., 1993). Common medical problems among adolescent mothers include poor weight gain, pregnancy-induced hypertension, anemia, sexually transmitted diseases (STDs), and cephalopelvic disproportion (Stevens-Simon and White, 1991). It is also believed that teenagers are at greater risk of very long labor (American College of Obstetricians and Gynecologists, 1993), but whether this risk results in increased rates of labor abnormalities and cesarean deliveries has not been proven conclusively (Lubarsky et al., 1994). Less is known about the long-term physiological sequelae. Adolescent mothers tend to be at greater risk for obesity and hypertension in later life than older primiparas, but most studies have not clearly distinguished whether these conditions are linked to early childbearing or early maturation (Stevens-Simon and White, 1991).

Although potential risks to the adolescent mother are quite serious, the risks to the infant she delivers are even greater. Infants born to mothers less than 15 years of age are more than twice as likely to weigh less than 2,500 grams (about 5.5 pounds) at birth and three times more likely to die in the first 28 days of life than infants born to older mothers (McAnarney and Hendee, 1989). After controlling for birthweight, the postneonatal mortality rate is approximately twice as high for infants born to mothers under 17 years of age than for infants born to older women. The incidence of sudden infant death syndrome is higher among infants of adolescents, and these infants also experience higher rates of illness and injuries (Morris et al., 1993).

Many of these health risks derive from the demographic attributes of adolescents rather than from their physiological immaturity. For instance, pregnancy-induced hypertension appears to be connected more closely to low parity than to age. Several studies have indicated that very young adolescent mothers are underweight and give birth to smaller babies because of poor diets and inadequate or no prenatal care (Stevens-Simon and White, 1991). Similarly, the greater incidence of illness and injury in infants of adolescent mothers is more likely due to environmental factors such as poverty, poor health habits, and insufficient supervision than to the age of the mother per se (Stevens-Simon and White, 1991).

---

[3]The number of births to girls under age 15 is small. In 1992 there were only 12,220 live births to women under age 15, representing 0.3 percent of all live births that year (National Center for Health Statistics, 1994).

Childbearing at Older Ages: Socioeconomic and Medical Issues

Unfortunately, few data are available to help provide an understanding of the socioeconomic consequences to parents or children of childbearing late in life, and the consequences may well differ by parity. Older parents having a first or second child may be better educated, may be more likely to be married, and may have higher incomes than younger parents, especially those parents in their teens or early 20s. On the other hand, a birth occurring to an older mother can also be a higher-order birth—for example, a fourth or fifth child or more—whose addition to the family may add appreciable strain. Moreover, elderly parents may have less physical energy and perhaps less flexibility in outlook, despite the presumption of increased wisdom.

However, data are available to assess the important medical risks to the mother and her child that cluster at this end of the reproductive life span. In the aggregate, childbearing becomes riskier to both mother and infant as women get older. Maternal mortality rates are several times higher in women over age 40 than in younger women. From 1979 to 1986 the overall maternal mortality rate in the United States for women over age 40 was 56 deaths per 100,000 live births compared with only 9.1 deaths per 100,000 live births in the general population (Koonin et al., 1991). Maternal morbidity is also higher among women over 40 (Prysak at al., 1995). In a review of the literature on the effect that greater maternal age has on pregnancy outcome, Hansen (1986) found that the majority of studies show a two- to fourfold increase in the frequency of toxemia in older mothers compared with that in younger ones. Venous thrombosis, a serious condition usually occurring postpartum in 1 in 100 women, was reported in one study to occur in 1 in 12 women over age 40 (Lehmann and Chism, 1987). In addition, the incidence of chronic conditions that are aggravated by pregnancy, such as hypertension and diabetes mellitus, increase with maternal age. Unless these conditions are monitored closely, they can pose major maternal as well as perinatal health risks.

Risks to the fetus and infant of a woman over age 40 include spontaneous abortion, chromosomal defects, congenital malformations, fetal distress, and low birthweight. Although the chances of miscarriage for a woman under age 25 are only 1 in 400, after the age of 35 the rate jumps to 40 in 100 pregnancies (Hotchner, 1990). Down syndrome, a chromosome disorder commonly associated with advanced maternal age, occurs at an approximate rate of 1 in 1,167 in pregnancies to women age 20; by age 40 the rate is 1 in 106 (Scott et al., 1989). It is believed that Down syndrome and other chromosomal disorders occur more frequently in older women because of their longer exposure to such environmental risks as X-rays and certain drugs. Medical conditions more common to older women affect their infants as well. For example, diabetes, if not carefully monitored, can lead to congenital malformations among other problems, and high blood pressure can cause fetal distress. Older women appear to give birth more often to infants who weigh less than 2,500 grams and more than 4,000 grams, occurrences that are linked to biologic aging of maternal tissues and systems and/or the cumulative effects of disease (Lee et al., 1988). Low birthweight from growth retardation or prematurity is a risk factor for asphyxia, birth injuries, and susceptibility to infection (O'Reilly-Green and Cohen, 1993).

These various medical risks to the mother and infant are not always due to older age alone (Vercellini et al., 1993), although some may be, as noted above (Lee et al., 1988). It is more that as women age they have an increased chance of having a preexisting medical condition like diabetes or a long history of exposure to potentially harmful substances such as X-rays. And because these various conditions and factors can complicate pregnancy and childbearing, older women as a group are at increased risk of poor pregnancy outcome overall.

Childbearing by Single Women

Births resulting from unintended pregnancies are often conceived out of wedlock and the infants are born to unmarried women. More than 40 percent of infants born after unintended conception begin life with unmarried parents. Births to unmarried parents are twice as likely to be unintended as births to married parents (70.4 compared with 33.9 percent) (Kost et al., 1994). Moreover, couples who marry after conception—usually unintended—are more likely to divorce than couples who marry before conception (Bumpass and Sweet, 1989). Finally, unintended pregnancies within marriage are associated with a greater risk of divorce after the child's birth. For all these reasons, children born after unintended conceptions are very likely to live apart from one or both of their parents, usually their father, sometime during childhood.

A large body of research suggests that the absence of a father—either because of divorce or an out-of-wedlock birth—is associated with negative outcomes in children when they grow up. Although many children raised by single parents do very well and although many children raised in two-parent families develop serious problems, the absence of the father increases the risk of a number of negative outcomes. The increase in risk associated with father absence is about 1.5 to 2.5, depending on the outcome being studied (Grogger and Bronars, 1994; Haveman and Wolfe, 1994; McLanahan and Sandefur, 1994; Seltzer, 1994; Furstenberg and Cherlin, 1991).

Compared with children from the same social class background who grow up with both biological parents, children raised by only one parent, usually the mother, are more likely to drop out of high school, less likely to attend college, and less likely to graduate from college if they ever attend (Graham et al., 1994; Haveman and Wolfe, 1994; Knox and Bane, 1994; Wojtkiewicz, 1993; Sandefur et al., 1992; Haveman et al., 1991; McLanahan, 1985). According to one nationally representative sample of young adults—the National Longitudinal Survey of Youth (NLSY)—the high school dropout rate is 13 percent for children raised by two biological parents, compared with 29 percent for children raised by one or neither parent (McLanahan and Sandefur, 1994). Before leaving high school, children in one-parent households score lower on standardized achievement tests, have lower grade point averages, have more erratic attendance records, and have lower college expectations (Astone and McLanahan, 1991). These children also show more behavioral and emotional problems while growing up, as reported by parents and teachers (Thomson et al., 1994; Zill et al., 1993; Furstenberg et al., 1987).

Children raised by single mothers exhibit different patterns of home leaving and family formation. They leave home earlier than children in two-parent families (Kiernan, 1992; Thornton, 1991); they are more likely to become teenage parents and unmarried parents (Haveman and Wolfe, 1994; Wu and Martinson, 1993; McLanahan, 1988; McLanahan and Bumpass, 1988); and, if they are married, are more likely to divorce (McLanahan and Bumpass, 1988). Estimates from the NLSY show that the risk of becoming a teenage mother is 11 percent for children raised by both parents and 27 percent for children raised by single mothers (McLanahan and Sandefur, 1994).

Finally, children who live with only one parent have more problems finding and keeping a steady job after leaving school and are more likely to have encounters with the criminal justice system than children who live with both parents (Haveman and Wolfe, 1994; McLanahan and Sandefur, 1994; Powers, 1994). As noted above, these differences persist even after adjusting for differences in the parents' socioeconomic background.

The findings discussed above have been replicated with numerous data sets in the United States and by researchers in several other countries (McLanahan and Sandefur, 1994; Kiernan, 1992; Cherlin et al., 1991). They also have been examined by different statistical techniques to adjust for unobserved differences between families that break up and families that stay together (Haveman and Wolfe, 1994; Powers, 1994; Manski et al., 1992). Finally, the data have been replicated for children of different racial and ethnic groups and different social classes within the United States. The findings are quite robust across different samples, different countries, and different estimation techniques.

Although the risks associated with the absence of the father are similar for children from different backgrounds, the absolute effects are much larger for children from minority and economically disadvantaged families. This is because the underlying risk of dropping out of high school and becoming a teenage mother is much greater for these children than for children from white middle-class families. The average Hispanic child has a 25 percent chance of dropping out of high school if he or she lives with both parents and a 49 percent chance of dropping out if he or she lives with a single parent. For black children the percentages are 17 and 30 percent, respectively, and for non-Hispanic white children, they are 11 and 28 percent, respectively.

Although the absence of the father has become increasingly common among children of all racial and ethnic groups and among all social classes, Hispanic and black children and children from economically disadvantaged backgrounds are more likely than white children and children from economically advantaged families to live apart from their fathers. Thus, even though all children in families in which the father is absent face an increased risk, the consequences fall disproportionately on children from disadvantaged backgrounds.

Much of the research on children raised by a single parent does not distinguish between children born to unmarried parents and children whose parents experience a divorce or separation. In a few instances, however, researchers have been able to make this distinction and to compare children born outside marriage with children of divorced parents. Their findings show that once differences in parents' education and age are taken into account (on average never-married parents are younger and less educated than divorced parents), children born to unmarried parents are quite similar to children whose parents experience a divorce in terms of academic and social achievement (McLanahan and Sandefur, 1994; Thomson et al., 1994; McLanahan and Bumpass, 1988; McLanahan, 1985). Although some differences in outcomes among children with these two types of single parents have been observed, they are small compared with the differences between children raised by single parents and children raised by both of their biological parents.

THE EFFECTS OF INTENDEDNESS

A number of investigators have studied whether children born as a result of unintended pregnancies (both mistimed and unwanted) are at greater risk of various poor outcomes, such as low birthweight, than are children born as a result of intended pregnancies. This section of the report reviews a complex set of studies on this topic, after first presenting some introductory comments on the methodological problems faced in analyzing the effects of intention status as a single variable. A limited amount of material about the effects of unintended pregnancy on the parents is also included.[4]

---

[4]As noted earlier, additional material on some of these issues, drawn from developing countries, was recently compiled by the National Research Council's Committee on Population. Though not directed to unintended pregnancy per se, both the final report and its companion background papers provide international perspectives on the broader issue of how contraception and fertility control affect the health of women and children (National Research Council, 1989a,b).

Methodological Concerns

Studies on the consequences of unintended pregnancies for the health and well-being of children and families have used a wide variety of data sources, study methods, and sample populations. They have also used numerous terms and concepts to sort out and classify the complex feelings that often surround a given conception. One source of information on the effects of intention status is the National Survey of Family Growth (NSFG), which was discussed in detail in Chapter 2. There, some of that survey's strengths and limitations were discussed, especially as regards its terminology. In this section of the report, many more data sources and studies are reviewed that pose their own methodological challenges. In general, though, the problems are similar to those faced by the NSFG: accurately determining parental attitudes at the time of conception, and classifying those attitudes. Because studies have used different techniques to solve these two problems, it is sometimes difficult to synthesize results.

Researchers studying the effect of intention status on various outcomes have approached the problem of determining parental attitudes at conception in a variety of ways. One strategy, employed primarily in a series of European studies, is to use the request for an abortion as a marker of an unintended or, more particularly, an unwanted pregnancy. These studies have assessed outcomes for pregnancies in women denied abortions. One difficulty with such studies lies in disentangling the effects of factors that might have led to the denial of the abortion from the unwantedness of the pregnancy itself.

Another strategy is to inquire after the fact about the intention status of a given pregnancy. Theoretically, such retrospective measurement of parental attitudes should be made as soon after conception as possible, in order to increase the accuracy with which intention status is recalled. However, it is difficult to obtain a representative sample of the pregnant population shortly after conception. Most studies that ask pregnant women about intention at the time of conception rely on clinic-based, not population-based, samples of women. This means that a selection bias is built in from the outset—that is, the sample is composed entirely of women already in prenatal care; those who are not in care, for whatever reason, are excluded. Thus, results cannot be generalized to those with late prenatal care or none at all.

The most representative studies of the impact of parental intention at conception are such population-based surveys as the NSFG. But in this survey, as noted in Chapter 2, months or even years have sometimes passed between conception and the measurement of attitudes at the time of conception. The extended time between conception and measurement of parental attitudes increases the uncertainty that parents will accurately recall their pregnancy intentions at conception.

When parental attitudes toward the conception are measured at delivery or postpartum, the accuracy of parental recall may also be affected by the outcome of the pregnancy. Inaccuracies in recalling parental attitudes at conception are likely to bias studies toward a finding of no ill effect when there is a true effect. This is because people who did not originally intend the conception may be more likely to recall it as intended than are people who intended the conception to recall it as unintended (Ryder, 1979, 1976; Westoff and Ryder, 1977). Thus, when adverse effects are observed, they may be underestimates of the full impact of unintended pregnancy.

The second methodological problem faced in these studies is that classifications of intention status vary widely, which makes pooling their results particularly challenging. Different indicators of intendedness are often used across studies, and because many of them do not use questions identical or similar to those of the NSFG, it can be difficult to compare findings. Even small differences in methodology may create differences in estimates of mistimed and unwanted conceptions (see, for example, Kost and Forrest, 1995). In addition, some studies that assess the effects of intention status do not distinguish between *mistimed* and *unwanted* conceptions, the two types of pregnancies included under the umbrella term of *unintended*. When conceptions are lumped into a category of unintended conception, it cannot be determined whether there is a difference in pregnancy outcome between a mistimed or an unwanted conception.

This distinction is very important and bears once again on the issue of association versus causality that was noted above in the discussion of maternal demographic status. If it is clear that a negative effect is closely linked to *unwanted* pregnancy, it is not necessary to establish definitively whether the effect is *caused by* or merely *associated with* unwanted pregnancy. By preventing unwanted pregnancy (that is, helping couples to avoid pregnancies that they did not want at all), the ill effect will not occur, because no pregnancy or birth takes place. But with mistimed pregnancy, the distinction does matter. If it can be determined that the ill effect is caused by the pregnancy being mistimed, then there is some reason to hope that by helping couples to time their pregnancies better (which usually means postponing them), the incidence of the problem would decrease. If, on the other hand, the ill effect is merely associated with mistimed pregnancy, it is more likely that changing the timing of pregnancy would not affect the risk of the ill effect occurring. Thus, in reviewing studies on the effect of intention status on various outcomes, it is important (1) to distinguish mistimed from unwanted pregnancies, and (2) in the case of studies examining the effects of mistimed pregnancies on various outcomes, to consider whether the investigators have attempted to separate those effects that are associated with a timing failure from those that are caused by the timing failure. Because of this significant distinction, liberal use of italics is made in the balance of this section to distinguish between these two categories of unintended pregnancy. Also, where possible, comment is made on the causality/association issue.

Finally, it is important to note that the literature on the consequences of mistimed and unwanted conception spans three decades, during which time drastic changes occurred in couples' abilities to control their fertility. A cohort of parents in the early 1990s may look very different from a cohort in the 1960s, whose members were studied before the introduction of oral contraceptives, publicly funded family planning programs, or legalized abortion.

In summary, study results need to be interpreted in light of how well parental intentions were captured, that is, the degree to which the study may accurately reflect parental attitudes at conception, and the precision with which that measurement was made. Even with these inherent methodological problems and challenges, the literature in this area is nonetheless fairly coherent and compelling. It is summarized below by type of health behavior or condition examined (see also Appendix D).

Prenatal Care

In theory, there are many reasons why a woman faced with an unintended pregnancy might receive insufficient prenatal care. Ambivalence toward maintaining the pregnancy may lead to a delay in seeking prenatal care; time may be lost when women who are not intending to be pregnant do not recognize the symptoms of pregnancy. Or the youth and poverty that often accompany unintended pregnancy may make enrollment in prenatal care difficult. Regardless of the reasons for delaying care, the immediate costs to the woman and her developing fetus may be less vigilance in detecting problems such as pregnancy-induced hypertension, less support for practicing healthy behaviors such as smoking cessation, and less preparation for parenthood (Kogan et al., 1994).

A substantial literature documents a relationship between unintended pregnancy and insufficient participation in prenatal care. Women who have mistimed or unwanted conceptions tend to initiate prenatal care later in pregnancy and to receive less adequate care (Figure 3-3) than women who have intended the pregnancy. When compared with women who planned to conceive, women with an *unwanted* pregnancy are 1.8 to 2.9 times more likely to begin care after the first trimester (DePersio et al., 1994; Kost et al., 1994; Pamuk and Mosher, 1988; Watkins, 1968). Women with *mistimed* conceptions are between 1.4 and 2.6 times more likely to begin care after the first trimester as are women who intended the conception (DePersio et al., 1994; Kost et al., 1994; Pamuk and Mosher, 1988). Studies that combine these women into a group with *unintended* conceptions report intermediate odds ratios of 1.1 to 2.6 (Byrd, 1994; Cartwright, 1988; Marsiglio and Mott, 1988; McCormick et al., 1987; Wells et al., 1987). These studies show a persistent pattern over time (from 1968 through 1993) and across diverse medical care and cultural settings

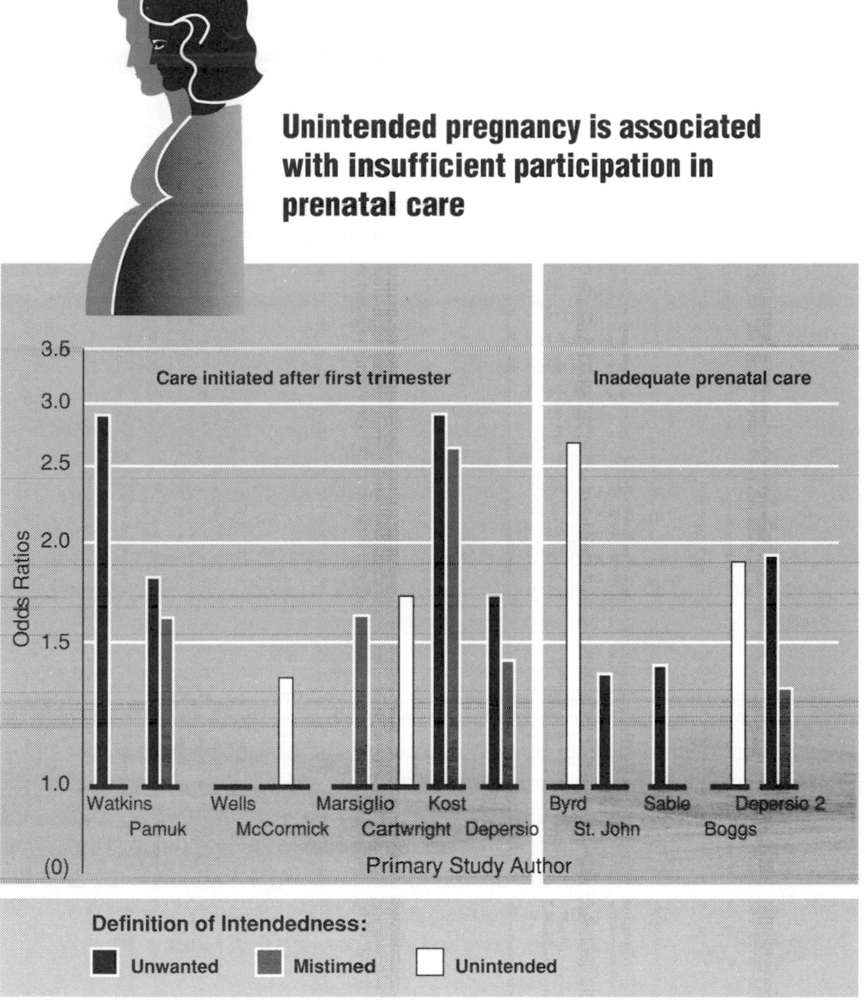

FIGURE 3-3 Studies of prenatal care attainment: odds ratios or relative risks of inadequate care by pregnancy intendedness. All rates displayed in this figure were developed by the Committee on Unintended Pregnancy from the published research except those for the DePersio study, which had already calculated the rates.

(e.g., women in England, black women in Harlem, Hispanic women in Houston, and representative samples of all U.S. women in the NSFG, the National Natality Survey, the NLSY, and the National Maternal and Infant Health Survey). When factors associated with both planning status and prenatal care initiation are controlled, the effect of mistimed or unwanted conception remains elevated, but its effect is reduced and sometimes no longer statistically significant (see tables in Appendix D). Thus, in most studies unintended pregnancy has been found to exert an additional barrier to the early initiation of prenatal care among women who are already at higher risk of later care.

The adequacy of prenatal care has been estimated by a combination of both early initiation and sufficient numbers of visits throughout pregnancy. In all of the relevant studies, a negative association between adequacy of prenatal care and desired or intended pregnancy is reported (Figure 3-3); the association may be more negative among *unwanted* than among *mistimed* conceptions. The association is attenuated when it is controlled for related factors. In particular, one study found that when the mother discussed her pregnancy with members of her support network or when she received support for the pregnancy from family members, the effect of *mistiming* on adequacy of prenatal care was no longer significant. Family support for obtaining care also reduced the effect of an *unwanted* conception on adequacy of care, but just discussing the pregnancy did not eliminate the effect (St. John and Winston, 1989). This suggests that a strong social support network may assist the pregnant woman in overcoming the barriers to obtaining care. Unfortunately, many women who find themselves with an unintended pregnancy lack such social resources.

Further evidence that intention to conceive is related to early access to prenatal care is provided in an examination of the impact of public funding of family planning services on the number of women seeking prenatal care after the first trimester. After controlling for the rate of publicly funded abortions, the ethnic and religious composition of the population, income, and female labor force participation, Meier and McFarlane (1994) found that for every additional dollar in state expenditures for family planning, there are significantly fewer births with late prenatal care. This study is discussed in more detail in Chapter 8.

Behavioral Risks in Pregnancy

Women with unwanted or mistimed conceptions may need additional, sometimes intense, care and supervision during pregnancy. They are more likely to smoke and to drink (Figure 3-4). The effect of pregnancy intention on other behaviors associated with pregnancy outcome, such as illicit drug use, weight gain during pregnancy, and use of multiple vitamins, is not as well studied.

Population-based studies (national as well as in selected states) linking smoking to intention status among pregnant women date from 1980 and show remarkable consistency. Women with mistimed or unwanted conceptions are

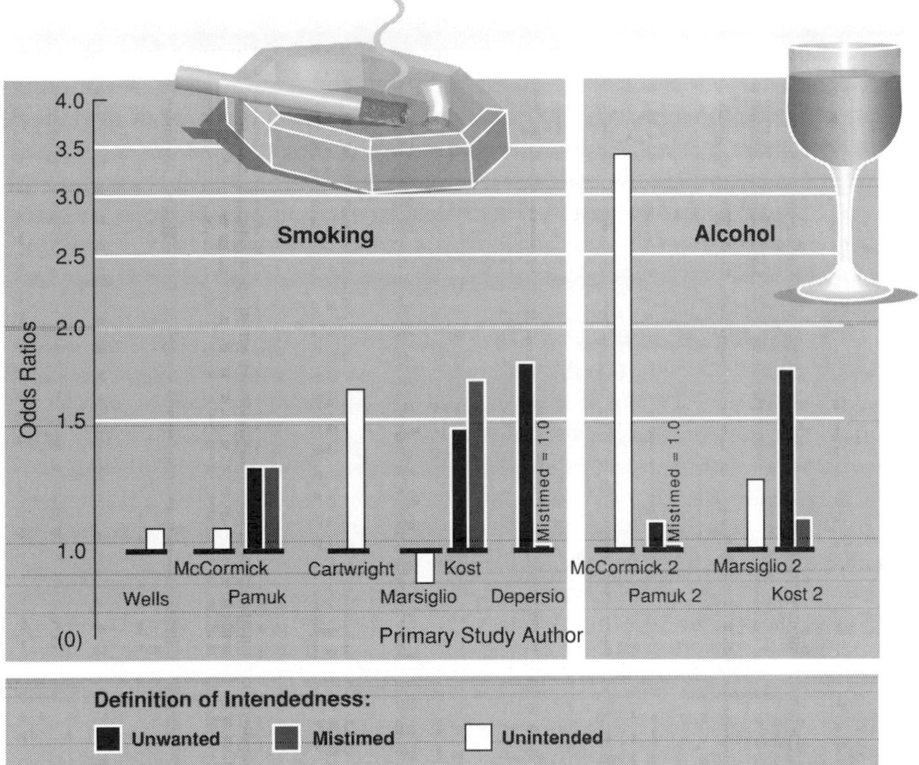

FIGURE 3-4 Studies of behavioral risk factors: odds ratios or relative risks of behavioral risks during pregnancy. All rates displayed in this figure were developed by the Committee on Unintended Pregnancy from the published research except those for the DePersio study, which had already calculated the rates.

about 30 percent more likely to smoke than are women with intended conceptions (DePersio et al., 1994; Kost et al., 1994; Cartwright, 1988; Marsiglio and Mott, 1988; Pamuk and Mosher, 1988; McCormick et al., 1987; Wells et al., 1987). The odds ratios are similar for both black and white women (Pamuk and Mosher, 1988). Adjustment for factors related to both pregnancy planning and smoking tend to reduce the estimates of effect, but planning status remains a significant factor in most studies. These are probably underestimates of the true effect, because of misclassification bias resulting from underreporting of smoking and alcohol consumption.

Beyond the health risks that many of these behaviors pose, it is important to consider this broad area of behavior for other reasons as well. In particular, to the extent that there is a connection between unintended pregnancy and drug or alcohol use especially, there are legal implications to consider. The issues of drug-exposed infants and fetal alcohol syndrome have attracted increasing attention in recent years. Much of the increased caseload of the child welfare system in the 1980s has been attributed to drug and alcohol related issues. Moreover, there has been an effort in many states to address the use and abuse of alcohol and other drugs by pregnant women through the legal system by application of both criminal laws and child welfare laws, approaches that have both financial costs and personal costs associated with them.

Low Birthweight

A number of researchers have examined the risk of delivering a low birthweight (<2,500 grams) infant following an unintended conception (Figure 3-5). Given the diversity of time and settings in which these studies took place, there is a surprising uniformity of results, with crude odds ratios for unwanted conceptions and for mistimed conceptions ranging from 1.2 to 1.4 (DePersio et al., 1994; Kost et al., 1994; Sable, 1992; Goldenberg et al., 1991; Cartwright, 1988; Marsiglio and Mott, 1988; Pamuk and Mosher, 1988; Morris et al., 1973). The data indicate that if all *unwanted* pregnancies were eliminated, there would be a 7 percent reduction in the low birthweight rate among black infants and a 4 percent reduction among white infants (Kendrick et al., 1990)—a change that would help to decrease the large disparity between rates of low birthweight among blacks and whites (Hogue and Yip, 1989). However, it is not clear that better *timing* would reduce the risk of low birthweight.

In the developing world, closely spaced births are associated with increased risk of infant mortality, and, less definitively, with increased risk of low birthweight (Haaga, 1989). In the United States and Norway, some studies have failed to find an increased risk of low birthweight for closely spaced births (Klebanoff M, 1988; Erickson and Bjerkedal, 1978). However, a recent prospective study suggests that white infants conceived within three months of a previous pregnancy and black infants conceived within nine months of a previous pregnancy are at greater risk of preterm delivery and low birthweight (Rawlings et al., 1995). To the extent that very closely spaced pregnancies are not planned (and clinicians have the strong impression that this is often the case), unintended pregnancy may increase the risk of low birthweight through this mechanism.

There have been a few studies of the components of low birthweight: preterm delivery (DePersio et al., 1994; DeMuylder et al., 1992; Goldenberg et al., 1991) and intrauterine growth retardation (Goldenberg et al., 1991). Although the data are sparse, they suggest that the association between pregnancy desire and low birthweight is through an increased risk of preterm delivery rather than through slowed fetal growth.

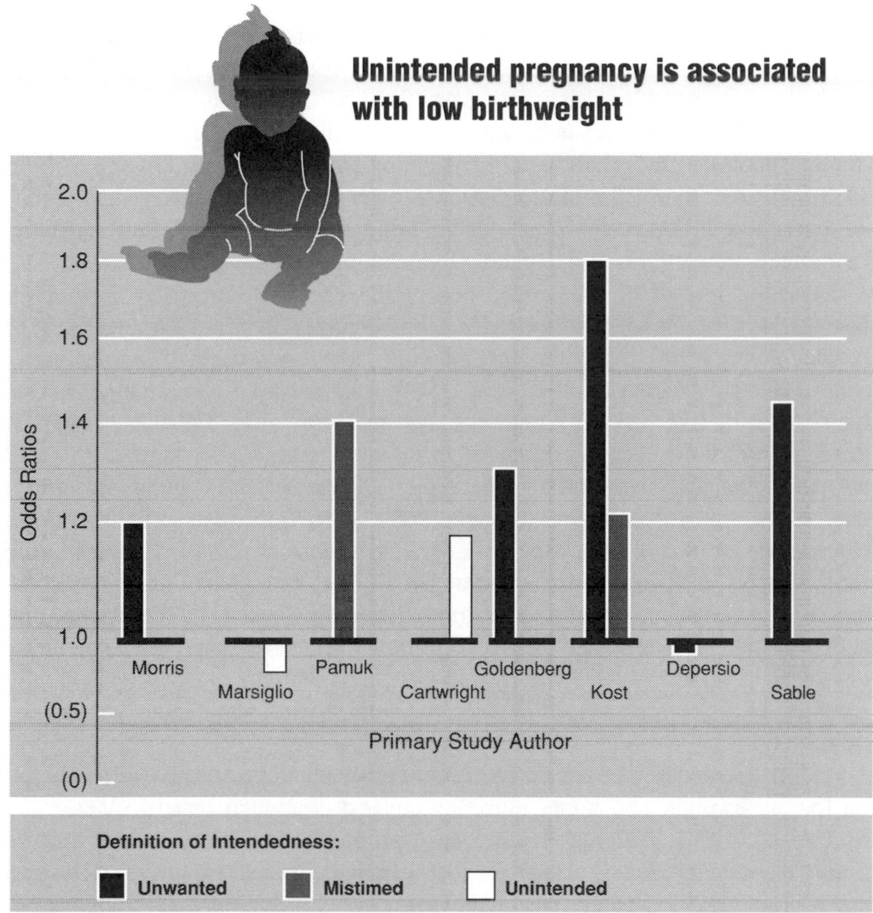

FIGURE 3-5 Studies of low birthweight: odds ratios or relative risks of low birthweight (<2,500 grams) by pregnancy intendedness. All rates displayed in this figure were developed by the Committee on Unintended Pregnancy from the published research except those for the DePersio study, which had already calculated the rates.

Infant Mortality

A link between unintended conception and infant mortality has been made using population-based data from a variety of sources and with a variety of methods. For example, using data from the NSFG and other surveys, it was estimated that if all sexually active couples had routinely used effective contraception in 1980, there would have been almost 1 million fewer abortions (533,000 rather than 1.5 million), 340,000 fewer live births that were unintended at conception, 5,000 fewer infant deaths, and a reduction in the infant mortality rate of 10 percent (World Health Organization, 1987). Another method to estimate the impact of unintended conception on infant mortality is to infer decreases in unintended pregnancies from changes in the characteristics of women giving birth. Using this methodology, about one-third of the decline in infant mortality between 1960 and 1968 was attributed to change in the distribution of live births by maternal age and birth order (Wright, 1975). A third method is to correlate changes in infant mortality over time with other temporal changes. Using this methodology, Grossman and Jacobowitz (1981) determined that between 1966 through 1968 and 1970 through 1972, the single most important factor associated with declining neonatal mortality (death in the first 28 days following birth) among both black and white infants was the increasing availability of induced abortion. Similarly, Joyce (1987) estimated that a decade later the reduced incidence of low birthweight and preterm births among black infants in 1977 was mostly associated with the availability of family planning clinics which helped women to avoid a birth unintended at conception.

More recent estimates of the impact of family planning and abortion services on low birthweight and infant mortality suggest continued benefit (Meier and McFarlane, 1994). Although the evidence of the public health value of current family planning programs argues for their continuation and expansion (Klerman and Klerman, 1994), the gap between existing services and the theoretical benefit of all conceptions being intended is enormous.

Poor Child Health and Development

To sustain normal health and development, children need a wide variety of resources that support cognitive stimulation and development, as well as affective and relational development. Baydar and Grady (1993) hypothesized that children born after mistimed or unwanted conceptions have fewer such resources. Using data from the NLSY, they tested this hypothesis for 1,545 children at two points in their development: at 0–2 and 3–5 years of age. The conceptions of approximately one-third of the children had been mistimed; about 5 percent of the conceptions had been unwanted. The study revealed significant deficits in the developmental resources available to these children; however, those deficits were associated with the sociodemographic differences among the families in which wanted, mistimed, and unwanted conceptions occurred. When background characteristics were controlled, a few developmental effects of planning status remained significant. Before 2 years of age, children whose conceptions had been mistimed or unwanted exhibited higher levels of fearfulness and lower levels of positive affect. When they were of preschool age, they had lower scores on verbal development tests, even though they had no deficit of verbal memory. The authors hypothesize that this critical developmental skill is lagging because "significant adults, particularly the mother may be less available" to the children (Baydar and Grady, 1993:14).

In the most extreme examples of unwanted conceptions—children born after women were denied abortions—various social development problems and relationship problems have been documented among children in Sweden (Forssman and Thuwe, 1981, 1966; Blomberg, 1980; Hook, 1975, 1963), Finland (Myhrman, 1988), and Czechoslovakia (Kubicka et al., 1994; David et al., 1988; Matejcek et al., 1978). All studies compared children born to women denied abortions (DA group) with children born to women with accepted pregnancies (AP group). Children in the first group were found to be less well adjusted socially, more frequently in psychiatric care, and more often found in criminal registers. In all but the Czechoslovakian study, the deficits of children born after their mothers had been denied abortion could have been due to the less favorable family environments in which they were raised. However, Matejcek and colleagues (1978) also compared the DA group with siblings in both AP and DA families when the original cohort was 35 years of age. They found that the siblings did share some of the less favorable characteristics within the DA group, but DA females were more frequently emotionally disturbed than their AP female controls whereas their female siblings did not exhibit emotional deficits. Girls were also at a greater disadvantage in the Finnish study by Myhrman (1988), but in the Czechoslovakian group earlier problems were more pronounced among male offspring. In all groups studied, differences attenuated with increasing age, but they did not disappear, even by the time the children were in their 30s.

In severe situations of financial and emotional deprivation, children whose conceptions had been mistimed or unwanted may be at higher risk of physical abuse or neglect (Zuravin, 1991). One controlled, prospective study of physical abuse supports this hypothesis (Altemeier et al., 1979), although three retrospective studies do not (Zuravin, 1991; Kotelchuck, 1982; Smith et al., 1974). Four other studies of children of parents reported for abuse or neglect found higher numbers of such families with children whose pregnancies had not been intended than among families with no reports of abuse or neglect (Murphy et al., 1985; Oates et al., 1980; Egeland and Brunnquell, 1979; Hunter et al., 1978). In a study that separated abused from neglected children and that included family size as a control variable, Zuravin (1991) found that unintended conception increased the risk of subsequent child abuse. Large family size, regardless of planning status, increased the risk of child neglect. On the basis of this and other analyses, Baumrind (1993:76), in a comprehensive study for the National Academy of Sciences, concluded that a child abuse prevention network should begin with "affordable contraceptive services." This echoes a previous analysis conducted for Surgeon General Koop, which stated that "the starting point for effective child abuse programming is pregnancy planning" (Cron, 1986:10). These research findings and perspectives also imply that by increasing the risk of child abuse and neglect, unintended pregnancy may increase the pressures on the child welfare system, including juvenile courts, the foster care system, and related social service agencies.

Consequences for the Parents

The birth of a child is a major event in parents' lives, regardless of whether the child was the result of an intended or unintended conception. When childbearing occurs without prior planning and preparation, it can cause severe disruption to other life plans, decreased resources for children already born, temporary or permanent lowering of educational and career aspirations, and a threat to present and future economic security. Its effects can be surprisingly far-reaching, contributing, for example, to the problem of insufficient child care in the United States. Child care is a major burden, largely for women, often beginning with teenagers who stay home from school to care for their infants and children (who are often the result of unintended pregnancies), but extending beyond that to older women, both married and single, who are unable to support themselves and their families because they cannot pay for or find adequate care for their children.

In particular, mistimed and unwanted pregnancies can place a strain on parental relationships. Marriages that begin after an unintended conception have a higher chance of failure, regardless of whether the marriage is a first or a second one (Wineberg, 1992, 1991; Teachman, 1983; Card and Wise, 1978; Furstenberg, 1976). The young age of the spouses does not entirely explain this observation, because it is found for second as well as first marriages.

Mothers

Worldwide, childbearing at very young or very old age, the bearing of many children, and the bearing of children who are closely spaced (less than two years apart) contribute to the high level of maternal deaths (about 500,000 per year) and to the reproductive complications that women suffer (National Research Council, 1989a,b; Zimicki, 1989). Even in the United States, where maternal mortality is low, pregnancy and childbirth carry risks, albeit small, of permanent disability and death (Franks at al., 1992; Atrash et al., 1990). A reduction in unintended pregnancies would reduce those risks, especially among women at highest risk of maternal morbidity and mortality, who are also the most likely to have an unintended pregnancy.

Current reports provide little systematic assessment of women's health following pregnancy and childbirth, but some data suggest that unintended pregnancy increases health risks for women. For example, unintended pregnancy can increase the likelihood of depression during pregnancy (Orr and Miller, 1995), and, regardless of marital status at birth, women who give birth following an unintended conception are more likely to suffer from postpartum depression as well (Salmon and Drew, 1992; Najman et al., 1991; Condon and Watson, 1987). They may also be at greater risk of experiencing domestic violence. For example, in a study done in New Zealand, 13.4 percent of women who experienced an unintended pregnancy also experienced physical violence from their partners over a 6-year period after conception; for those women who experienced intended pregnancies, the rate was 5.4 percent (Fergusson et al., 1986).

Data from the Pregnancy Risk Assessment Monitoring System (PRAMS)[5] are available on domestic violence during pregnancy and pregnancy planning for four states: Alaska, Maine, Oklahoma, and West Virginia (Gazmararian et al., 1994). Of the 12,612 women surveyed, physical abuse was reported among between 3.8 and 6.9 percent of them, depending on the state. Experience of violence was reported among between 5.6 and 10.7 percent of women with an unintended pregnancy.

Fathers

Very little is known about the impact of unintended childbearing on the fathers involved. The few studies of adolescent fathering and educational attainment have found an association between teenage fathering and dropping out of high school. However, those studies have not been able to determine whether problems in school lead to early parenting or whether early parenting increases the likelihood of dropping out of school (Parke and Neville, 1987; Marsiglio, 1986; Lerman, 1985; Card and Wise, 1978). Similarities in acting-out behavior among male students who had fathered, those who had caused a pregnancy that did not end in birth, and those who were unsure if they had caused a pregnancy suggest that educational and emotional problems precede rather than follow the

---

[5]PRAMS is an ongoing population-based survey of random samples of women giving birth in each participating state.

act of fathering (Resnick et al., 1993). These groups of young men were similar to each other but differed significantly from students who reported no involvement in causing a pregnancy.

Even less is known about the impact of unintended conception on the father's employment, but the scant available evidence suggests that there is less of an effect of early parenting on males than on females (Card and Wise, 1978). This is undoubtedly related to the greater responsibility that mothers assume in child rearing (Parke and Neville, 1987). "[T]o the extent that the adolescent father disassociates himself from the child and/or the mother, he may minimize the negative impact of early paternity on [his] own social or educational trajectories" (Parke and Neville, 1987:166).

An intriguing and important finding is that the ability of the father to provide "positive parenting" (i.e., positive involvement with one's child) may be strongly associated with whether the pregnancy was intended. Positive parenting is a benefit for the parent as well as the child. When the parents are unmarried, the father's involvement with his children may be limited by his own choice or by the mother's or her parents' functioning as gatekeepers to limit his contact (Parke and Neville, 1987; Parke and Beitel, 1986; Parke and Tinsley, 1984). Limited opportunities to learn about child development can affect a father's ability to parent effectively (Parke and Neville, 1987). Even married, adult fathers vary in their ability to achieve positive, significant involvement with their children (Cooney et al., 1993). When compared with younger fathers, men who became fathers after age 30 were more likely to be involved in a positive way with their children. Late parenting may more often reflect "intended parenting," with more time to prepare for the paternal role (Cooney et al., 1993:214).

PRECONCEPTION CARE

Another consequence of unintended pregnancy—the fourth reviewed in this chapter—is that opportunities for the mother and couple to engage in preconception risk assessment and intervention are often lost. The importance of preconception care derives from the notion that if a woman or couple is actively planning—or intending—a pregnancy, there are new and important opportunities to improve outcomes for both the mother and her baby by identifying and managing risks before conception. Most women enter prenatal care several weeks into the pregnancy, even with the most earnest attempts to initiate care after missing one, and sometimes two, menstrual periods. Meanwhile, the conceptus has completed a critical interval that includes uterine implantation, organogenesis, and early system development. For the health care provider, this means that the length of care for such patients is 7 or 8 months at best, with no opportunity to have influenced fetal development during the first 1 or 2 months.

Certain specific diagnostic and clinical interventions become less effective or appropriate in later pregnancy; even more important, the opportunity for prepregnancy planning, including emotional preparation, has disappeared.

To understand the possible impact of preconception knowledge and care on reproductive behavior, and therefore to understand the opportunity lost by unintended pregnancy, it is important to review the content, promise, and limitations of preconception care. A number of authorities and professional groups have published recommendations for the content of preconception care (Cefalo and Moos, 1995; March of Dimes Birth Defects Foundation, 1993; Jack and Culpepper, 1990; Public Health Service Expert Panel on the Content of Prenatal Care, 1989). These recommendations have a high degree of commonality and for the most part focus on optimizing the woman's health and identifying pregnancy risks and negative habits that may influence fetal development. The approach involves active patient participation, individualized management plans, and a commitment to educational needs addressing both medical and psychosocial issues. Topics typically addressed in preconception care include diet and weight, exercise, smoking, use of alcohol and drugs, stopping contraception, identifying and reducing environmental risks (such as exposure to toxoplasmosis), evaluating vaccination history and immunity status, managing pelvic inflammatory disease and various STDs, if present (including chlamydia, gonorrhea, herpes simplex virus, syphilis, HIV infection, and AIDS), and managing such medical conditions as diabetes, hypertension, and cardiovascular disease.

The need for attention to these issues is supported by a study that collected data on the planning status of the births of over 12,000 women and on certain aspects of the women's behavior in the months preceding conception and during the first few weeks of pregnancy—smoking, drinking, being underweight, or delaying initiation of prenatal care (Adams et al., 1993). The investigators found that, even using a relatively narrow definition of need for preconception care, 38 percent of the women had risk profiles that suggested the potential value of such intervention; for women whose pregnancies were unintended, the percentage was higher; for women whose pregnancies were intended, it was lower. To date, however, no large-scale prospective intervention trial has conclusively demonstrated the health benefits to mother or child from a broad program of preconception counseling and care.

For several specific medical problems, however, there is strong evidence that initiating care before conception is critical to both infant and maternal well-being. For example, maternal diabetes is associated with teratogenic and other complications of pregnancy; strict metabolic control both before and during pregnancy has been shown to reduce the risk to the developing fetus. Fuhrman and colleagues (1983) followed 420 pregnant women with insulin-dependent diabetes. Of these women, 292 began strict metabolic control after 8 weeks of pregnancy; among the infants born to this group, 22 had congenital malformations, yielding an incidence rate of 7.5 percent. The other 128 women began strict metabolic control before conception; only one infant was born with a congenital malformation, yielding a 0.8 percent incidence rate. Other studies confirm the importance of pre- and periconceptional metabolic control (Fuhrman et al., 1984; Ylinen et al., 1984; Miller et al., 1981).

Similarly, current data suggest that the risk of neural tube defects (NTDs), such as spina bifida, may be decreased when folic acid is consumed before conception and through the early months of pregnancy. The Medical Research Council Vitamin Study Research Group (1991), which examined the value of folic acid supplementation around the time of conception, showed a 72 percent protective effect among a group of women at risk of a recurrence of fetal NTD—a finding that led, among other things, to the Centers for Disease Control recommendation that women with a history of NTDs who are planning another pregnancy take 4 milligrams of folic acid daily beginning 1 month before conception and continuing through the first 3 months of pregnancy (Centers for Disease Control, 1991). Although some controversy exists regarding the utility of peri-conceptional administration of folic acid to prevent NTDs in women with no history of such problems, the U.S. Public Health Service has recommended the use of folic acid by all women to reduce the chances of NTDs (Centers for Disease Control and Prevention, 1992).

Unintended pregnancies also mean that individuals may not be able to take the fullest advantage of the explosion of research in human genetics. A recent Institute of Medicine (1994) report explores the broader social implications of advances in the ability to detect genetic diseases, advances that are emerging from the Human Genome Project in particular. When completed, the project will make it possible to detect more diseases—some that are uniformly fatal early in life as well as some that emerge later in life and that are not as life-threatening or for which treatments are or will become available. In addition, it will increasingly be possible to identify an individual's carrier status. Such increased genetic knowledge holds promise for reducing the emotional pain, trauma, and expense that genetic defects can cause families; it also carries the possibility of decreasing the need for second-trimester abortion, which remains one of the major options available to couples who learn that their developing fetus carries a serious genetic defect—knowledge that often is available only after many weeks of gestation are completed.[6]

---

[6]Although preconception care offers the opportunity to reduce the prevalence of malformations related to known genetic (or environmental) influences, the causes of most malformations are currently unknown. Early start of prenatal care offers the opportunity to initiate surveillance for malformations through ultrasound and other techniques. Such surveillance may reduce the incidence of births with malformations among those parents who elect induced abortion; for those who continue the pregnancy, early diagnosis offers

Preconception assessment and care, including attention to genetic risk, is not only a woman's issue. Data from laboratory animals in particular suggest that reproductive outcomes are also affected by the male's preconception health status and behavior (Davis et al., 1992). In a comprehensive review of various influences on spermatogenesis and male fertility—spanning nutrition, alcohol and drug use, medical history, exposure to chemicals, and related areas—Cefalo and Moos (1995:240) conclude that involving men in preconception care is important not only for identifying particular risks to male reproductive success but also for encouraging "cooperation and support between the prospective father and mother" in anticipation of pregnancy and then beyond.

For the full potential of preconception intervention to be realized, however, access to such care will need to be more widespread than it is at present, and provider training will need to be increased. Too often, preconception care is an advantage of the privileged few whose private insurance or personal finances make such care affordable and accessible. For many of the women who might benefit the most from preconception care, such as those with a history of poor health maintenance or abuse of alcohol or drugs, it remains only a theoretical benefit that is rarely available and perhaps not even understood.

THE DEMOGRAPHIC IMPLICATIONS OF REDUCING UNINTENDED PREGNANCY

This section suggests how the profile of the childbearing population in the United States would change if unintended pregnancies were eliminated altogether. Such a statistical exercise helps in understanding the consequences of current demographic patterns of unintended pregnancy and subsequent childbearing.

Data presented earlier in this chapter and in Chapter 2 indicate that the incidence of childbearing from unintended pregnancies is higher among unmarried than married women; it has also been shown that, on average, risks of poor outcomes are greater for children of one-parent families than children of two-parent families. Furthermore, the risks of poor child outcomes are particularly high when the child is born to a woman who wanted no children at all or no more children (i.e., a birth from an unwanted pregnancy). It follows from these observations that reducing the proportion of births derived from unintended pregnancies could have a significant impact on the well-being of children in U.S. society by increasing the proportion of children who are the products of intended pregnancies to married mothers.

---

the opportunity to plan perinatal and pediatric management.

How much of a change in children's family contexts could possibly be achieved by reducing the number of births derived from unintended pregnancies? To address this question, information on the relationship between maternal marital status and whether births resulted from unwanted or mistimed pregnancies (using data on births from the 1982 and 1988 NSFG) was applied to the estimated proportion of births to unmarried women in 1994. Births from unwanted and mistimed pregnancies figure differently in this estimation. Births from unwanted pregnancies, by definition, would simply not occur, whereas births that were mistimed at conception would occur, but would occur later—some in marriage and some not. Logit simulation was used to model this redistribution of mistimed pregnancies, as described in more detail in Appendix E.

The results of this simulation show that eliminating unintended pregnancy decreases dramatically the proportion of children who are born to unmarried women. Specifically, the proportion of all births in 1994 that were either to unmarried women or were the result of an unwanted pregnancy would decrease from 38 to 21 percent—a 45 percent reduction overall. The percentage of all births to teenage mothers would also decrease, given the disproportionate representation of teenagers in the pool of unmarried women giving birth, but the precise shape of the age redistribution was not calculated.

The complete elimination of all unintended fertility is an unrealistic goal. However, this statistical exercise adds to the evidence presented earlier in this chapter that an appreciable reduction in the number of unintended pregnancies would improve the well-being of future generations. The fact that other industrialized countries report fewer unintended pregnancies than the United States suggests that progress in the desired direction is a realistic, feasible goal.

CONCLUSION

The data and perspectives presented in this chapter demonstrate that unintended pregnancy has serious consequences. These consequences are not confined only to unintended pregnancies occurring to teenagers or unmarried women and couples; in fact, unintended pregnancy can carry serious consequences at all ages and life stages. First, unintended pregnancy often leads to abortion, a fact that underscores a point made at the outset of this report: reducing unintended pregnancy would dramatically decrease the incidence of abortion. Although it is quite clear that abortion has few if any long-term negative consequences on a woman's medical or psychological well-being, it is nonetheless true that resolving an unintended pregnancy by abortion may be an emotionally difficult experience for a woman and others close to her; in particular, abortion providers, women, and their partners as well may find that abortion poses difficult moral or ethical problems; and there continue to be major political and social tensions, including violence and even murder, associated with abortion in the United States.

Second, a disproportionate share of the women bearing children who were unintended at conception are unmarried and/or at either end of the reproductive age span. These demographic attributes themselves carry increased medical and social burdens for children and their parents. At the same time, it is important to reiterate that although women who are unmarried and/or at either end of the reproductive age span are disproportionately represented among those having births that were unintended at conception, the majority of such births are to women without these attributes (Chapter 2).

Third, a complex and extensive group of studies has attempted to measure the impact of a pregnancy's intention status on a wide variety of child and parental outcomes. These studies show that unintended pregnancies—especially those that are unwanted (as distinct from mistimed)—carry appreciable risks for children, women, men, and families. That is, unintendedness itself poses an added, independent burden beyond whatever might be present because of other factors, including the demographic attributes of the mother in particular. For an unwanted pregnancy, prevention of ill effects on the child is not dependent on whether the unintendedness itself caused the negative outcome. If the unwanted pregnancy can be prevented, any associated ill effects will also be prevented.

With an unwanted pregnancy especially, the mother is more likely to seek prenatal care after the first trimester or not to obtain care. She is more likely to expose the fetus to harmful substances by smoking tobacco and drinking alcohol. The child of an unwanted conception is at greater risk of weighing less than 2,500 grams at birth, of dying in its first year of life, of being abused, and of not receiving sufficient resources for healthy development. The mother may be at greater risk of physical abuse herself, and her relationship with her partner is at greater risk of dissolution. Both mother and father may suffer economic hardship and fail to achieve their educational and career goals. The health and social risks associated with a mistimed conception are similar to those associated with an unwanted conception, although they are not as great.

For some risks, such as low birthweight, an independent effect of planning status cannot be established. That is, the milieu in which the mistimed conception occurs may be the causal link to the adverse outcome. For other risks, such as child abuse and neglect, assisting families in having their children when they are ready for them may attenuate the effects of resource deficits.

Too little is known about the impact of unintended conceptions on family formation, parent–child interactions, and parental well-being. Much more research is needed into the role of family formation on parents' attainments as well as on the development of their children. Research should identify predictors of unintended childbearing within marriage that can be employed to develop programs designed to prevent unwanted pregnancies and assist parents in timing their wanted conceptions. Among married couples who experience unintended conceptions, more research is needed into the long-term consequences to the couples as well as their children.

Fourth, it is also apparent that pregnancy begun without some degree of planning and intent often precludes individual women and couples from participating in preconception risk identification and management and may also mean that they are unable to take full advantage of the rapidly expanding knowledge regarding human genetics. Certain specific diseases and conditions with serious consequences, such as diabetes, are best managed among pregnant women when care is begun before conception. Increased access to such care and increased provider training in this field will help more individuals take advantage of this developing area of clinical practice.

Finally, a recalculation of what the childbearing population in the United States would look like if unintended pregnancy did not occur (unwanted conceptions eliminated and mistimed ones redistributed) shows that a larger proportion of children would be the product of intended conceptions born to married women, thereby improving the life circumstances of children and contributing to the well-being of future generations.

REFERENCES

Adams MM, Bruce C, Shulman HB, et al. Pregnancy planning and preconception counseling. Obstet Gynecol. 1993;82:955–959.

Adler N, David HP, Major BN, Roth SH, Russo NF, Wyatt GE. Psychological responses after abortion. Science. 1990;248:41–44.

Altemeier WA, Vietze PM, Sherrod KA, Sandler HM, Falwey S, O'Connor SM. Prediction of child maltreatment during pregnancy. J Am Acad Child Psychiatry. 1979;18: 201.

American College of Obstetricians and Gynecologists. Special Needs of Pregnant Teens. ACOG Patient Education Pamphlet No. AP103. Washington, DC; 1993.

Astone N, McLanahan S. Family structure, parental practices, and high school completion. Am Sociol Rev. 1991;56:309–320.

Atrash HK, Koonin LM, Lawson HW, et al. Maternal mortality in the United States, 1979–1986. Obstet Gynecol. 1990;76:1055–1060.

Bacon L. Early motherhood, accelerated role transition, and social pathologies. Social Forces. 1974;52:333–341.

Baumrind D. Optimal Caregiving and Child Abuse: Continuities and Discontinuities. National Academy of Sciences Study Panel on Child Abuse and Neglect. Washington, DC: National Academy Press; 1993.

Baydar N, Grady W. Predictors of Birth Planning Status and Its Consequences for Children. Seattle, WA: Battelle Public Health Research and Evaluation Center; 1993.

Blendon RJ, Benson JM, Donelan K. The public and the controversy over abortion. JAMA. 1993;270:2871–2875.

Blomberg S. Influence of maternal distress during pregnancy on postnatal development. Acta Psychiatr Scand. 1980;62:402–417.

Buehler JW, Schulz KF, Grimes DA, Hogue CJR. The risk of serious complications from induced abortion: Do personal characteristics make a difference? Am J Obstet Gynecol. 1985;153:14–20.

Bumpass L, Sweet J. Children's experience in single-parent families: Implications of cohabitation and marital transitions. Fam Plann Perspect. 1989;21:256–260.

Byrd T. Correlates of Prenatal Care Initiation Among Low-Income Hispanic Women. Unpublished doctoral dissertation, Health Sciences Center, The University of Texas School of Public Health, Houston, TX; 1994.

Card JJ, Wise L. Teenage mothers and teenage fathers: The impact of early childbearing on the parents' personal and professional lives. Fam Plann Perspect. 1978;10:199–205.

Cartwright A. Unintended pregnancies that lead to babies. Soc Sci Med. 1988;27:249–254.

Cates W, Grimes DA. Morbidity and mortality of abortion in the United States. In Abortion and Sterilization: Medical and Social Aspects. Hodgson SE, ed. London: Academic Press Inc.; 1981:155–180.

Cates W, Rochat RW, Grimes DA, Tyler CW. Legalized abortion: Effect on national trends of maternal and abortion related mortality. Am J Obstet Gynecol. 1978;132: 211– 214.

Cefalo RC, Moos MK. Preconception Health Care: A Practical Guide. 2nd ed. St. Louis, MO: Mosby; 1995.

Centers for Disease Control and Prevention, Reproductive Epidemiology Unit. The Health Consequences of Induced Abortion. Paper prepared for the Institute of Medicine Committee on Unintended Pregnancy. Washington, DC; 1994.

Centers for Disease Control and Prevention. Recommendations for use of folic acid to reduce the number of cases of spina bifida and other neural tube defects. MMWR. 1992;41:1–7.

Centers for Disease Control. Use of folic acid for the prevention of spina bifida and other neural tube defects. MMWR. 1991;40:513–516.

Cherlin AJ, Furstenberg FF, Chase-Lansdale PL, Kiernan KE, Robins PK, Morrison DR, Teitler JO. Longitudinal studies of effects of divorce on children in Great Britain and the United States. Science. 1991;252:1386–1389.

Child Trends, Inc. Data derived from public use files of the National Longitudinal Survey of Youth, 1979–1988 data, under Contract N01-HD-9-2919 from the National Institutes of Health.

Condon JT, Watson TL. The maternity blues: Exploration of a psychological hypothesis. Acta Psychiatr Scand. 1987;76:164–171.

Cooney TM, Pedersen FA, Indelicato S. Timing of fatherhood: Is on-time optional? J Marriage Fam. 1993;55:205–215.

Council on Scientific Affairs, American Medical Association. Induced termination of pregnancy before and after Roe v Wade: Trends in the mortality and morbidity of women. JAMA. 1992;268:3231–3239.

Cron T. The Surgeon General's Workshop on Violence and Public Health: Review of the recommendations. Public Health Rep. 1986;101:8–14.

Daling JR, Malone KE, Voigt LF, White E, Weiss NS. Risk of breast cancer among young women: Relationship to induced abortion. J Natl Cancer Inst 1994;86:1584–1594.

David HP, Dytrych Z, Matejcek Z, Schuller V. Born Unwanted: Developmental Effects of Denied Abortion. New York/Prague: Springer Publishing Company/Avicenum-Czechoslovak Medical Press; 1988.

Davis DL, Friedler G, Mattison D, Morris R. Male-mediated teratogenesis and other reproductive effects: Biologic and epidemiologic findings and a plea for clinical research. Reprod Toxicol. 1992;6:289–292.

DeMuylder X, Wesel S, Dramix M, Candeir M. A woman's attitude toward pregnancy: Can it predispose her to preterm labor? J Reprod Med. 1992;37:339–342.

DePersio SR, Chen W, Blase D, Lorenz R. Unintended Pregnancy and its Consequences on Live Birth Outcomes and Maternal Behaviors During Pregnancy. Unpublished data analyses; 1994.

Egeland B, Brunnquell D. An at-risk approach to the study of child abuse. J Am Acad Child Psychiatry. 1979;18:219–235.

Erickson JD, Bjerkedal T. Interpregnancy interval: Association with birth weight, still birth and neonatal death. J Epidemiol Community Health. 1978;32:124–130.

Fergusson DM, Horwood LJ, Kershaw KL, Shannon FT. Factors associated with reports of wife assault in New Zealand. J Marriage Fam. 1986;48:407–412.

Forssman H, Thuwe I. Continued follow-up study of 120 persons born after refusal of application for therapeutic abortion. Acta Psychiatr Scand. 1981;64:142–149.

Forssman H, Thuwe I. One hundred and twenty children born after application for therapeutic abortion refused. Acta Psychiatr Scand. 1966;42:71–88.

Franks AL, Kendrick JS, Olson DR, et al. Hospitalization for pregnancy complications, United States, 1986 and 1987. Am J Obstet Gynecol. 1992;166:1339–1344.

Frye AA, Atrash HK, Lawson HW, McKay T. Induced abortion in the United States: A 1994 update. JAMWA. 1994;49:131–136.

Fuhrman K, Reiher HR, Semmler K, et al. The effect of intensified conventional insulin therapy before and during pregnancy on the malformation rate in offspring of diabetic mothers. Exp Clin Endocrinol. 1984;83:173–177.

Fuhrman K, Reiher HR, Semmler K, et al. Prevention of congenital malformations in infants of insulin-dependent diabetic mothers. Diabetes Care 1983;6:219–223.

Furstenberg FF. Premarital pregnancy and marital instability. J Soc Issues. 1976;32:67–86.

Furstenberg FF, Cherlin A. Divided Families. Cambridge, MA: Harvard University Press; 1991.

Furstenberg FF, Morgan SP, Allison PD. Paternal participation and children's well-being. Am Sociol Rev. 1987;52:695–701.

Gazmararian JA, Adams M, Saltzman L, et al. The Relationship Between Intendedness of Pregnancy and Physical Violence. EIS Conference, Centers for Disease Control and Prevention, Atlanta, GA; 1994.

Geronimus AT. Teenage childbearing and social disadvantage—unprotected discourse. Fam Relat. 1992;41:244–248.

Geronimus AT, Korenman S. The socioeconomic consequences of teen childbearing reconsidered. Q J Econ. 1992;107:1187–1214.

Gold RB. Abortion and Women's Health: A Turning Point for America. New York, NY: The Alan Guttmacher Institute; 1990.

Goldenberg RL, Fei S, Cliver SP, Poole VL, Hoffman HJ, Copper RL. Planned/Wanted Status and Pregnancy Outcome. Unpublished manuscript; 1991.

Graham J, Beller AH, Hernandez PM. The effects of child support on educational attainment. In Child Support and Child Well-Being. Garfinkel I, McLanahan S, Robins P, eds. Washington, DC: The Urban Institute; 1994.

Grimes DA, Schulz KF, Cates W Jr, Tyler CW. The Joint Program for the Study of Abortion/CDC: A preliminary analysis. In Abortion in the Seventies. Hern W, Andrikopoulos B, eds. New York, NY: National Abortion Federation; 1977.

Grogger J, Bronars S. The economic consequences of unwed motherhood: Using twin births as a natural experiment. Am Econ Rev. 1994;84:1141–1156.

Grogger J, Bronars S. The socioeconomic consequences of teenage childbearing: Findings from a natural experiment. Fam Plann Perspect. 1993;25:156–161, 174.

Grossman M, Jacobowitz S. Variations in infant mortality rates among counties of the United States: The roles of public policies and programs. Demography. 1981;18: 695–713.

Haaga J. Mechanisms for the association of maternal age, parity, and birth spacing with infant health. In Contraceptive Use and Controlled Fertility: Health Issues for Women and Children. Background papers. Parnell AM, ed. Committee on Population, National Research Council. Washington, DC.: National Academy Press; 1989.

Hakim-Elahi E, Tovell HM, Burnhill MS. Complications of first-trimester abortion: A report of 170,000 cases. Obstet Gynecol. 1990;76:129–135.

Hansen JP. Older maternal age and pregnancy outcome: A review of the literature. Ob Gyn Surv 1986;41:726.

Haveman R, Wolfe B. Succeeding Generations. New York, NY: Russell Sage Foundation; 1994.

Haveman R, Wolfe B, Spaulding J. Childhood events and circumstances influencing high school completion. Demography. 1991;28:133–157.

Hayes C, ed. Risking the Future. Vol. 1. Washington DC: National Academy Press; 1987.

Hoffman SD, Foster EM, Furstenberg FF Jr. Reevaluating the costs of teenage childbearing: Response to Geronimus and Korenman. Demography. 1993;30:291–296.

Hogue CJ, Yip R. Preterm delivery: Can we lower the black infant's first hurdle? JAMA. 1989;262:548–550.

Hook K. The unwanted child: Effects on mothers and children of refused applications for abortion. In Society, Stress, and Disease. Oxford: Oxford Medical Publications; 1975.

Hook K. Refused abortion: A follow-up study of 249 women whose applications were refused by the National Board of Health in Sweden. Acta Psychiatr Scand. 1963;39: suppl. 168.

Hotchner T. Pregnancy and Childbirth. New York, NY: Avon Books; 1990.

Hunter RS, Kilstrom N, Kraybill EN, Loda F, et al. Antecedents of child abuse and neglect in premature infants: A prospective study in a newborn intensive care unit. Pediatrics. 1978;61:629–635.

Institute of Medicine. Assessing Genetic Risks. Washington, DC: National Academy Press; 1994.

Institute of Medicine. Legalized Abortion and the Public Health. Washington, DC: National Academy Press; 1975.

Jack B, Culpepper L. Preconception Care. In New Perspectives on Prenatal Care. Merkatz IR, Thompson JE, eds. New York, NY: Elsevier; 1990.

Jaffe FS, Lindheim BL, Lee PR. Abortion Politics: Private Morality and Public Policy. New York, NY: McGraw-Hill; 1981.

Joyce T. The demand for health inputs and their impact on the black neonatal mortality rate in the US. Soc Sci Med. 1987;24:911–918.

Kendrick JS, Gargiullo PM, Williams LB, Bruce FC. Unintended Pregnancy and the Risk of Low Birth Weight: Data from the 1988 National Survey of Family Growth. Annual Meeting of the American Public Health Association; 1990.

Kiernan K. The impact of family disruption in childhood on transitions made in young adult life. Popul Stud. 1992;46:213–234.

Klebanoff MA. Short interpregnancy interval and the risk of low birthweight. Am J Public Health. 1988;6:667–670.

Klerman LV, Klerman JA. More evidence for the public health value of family planning. Am J Public Health. 1994;84:1377–1378.

Knox V, Bane MJ. Child support and schooling. In Child Support and Child Well-Being. Garfinkel I, McLanahan S, Robins P, eds. Washington, DC: The Urban Institute; 1994.

Kogan MD, Alexander GR, Kotelchuck M, et al. Relation of the content of prenatal care to the risk of low birth weight. JAMA. 1994;271:1340–1345.

Koonin LM, Atrash HK, Lawson HW, Smith JC. Maternal mortality surveillance, United States, 1979–1986. MMWR. 1991;40:1–13.

Koop, CE. Testimony before the Human Resources and Intergovernmental Relations Subcommittee of the Committee on Government Operations, U.S. House of Representatives, 101st Congress; 1989.

Kost K, Forrest J. Intention status of U.S. births in 1988: Differences by mother's socioeconomic and demographic characteristics. 1995;27:11–17.

Kost K, Forrest JD, Singh S. Investigation of the Impact of Pregnancy Intention Status on Women's Behavior During Pregnancy and Birth Outcomes. Paper prepared for the Institute of Medicine Committee on Unintended Pregnancy. Washington, DC; 1994.

Kotelchuck M. Child abuse and neglect: Prediction and misclassification. In Child Abuse Prediction: Policy Predictions. Starr R Jr, ed. Cambridge, MA: Ballenger Publishing Company; 1982.

Kubicka L, Matejcek Z, David HP, Dytrych Z, Miller WB, Roth Z. Prague children from unwanted pregnancies revisited at age thirty. Submitted for publication, October 1994.

Lawson HW, Frye A, Atrash HK, et al. Abortion mortality, United States, 1972–1987. Am J Obstet Gynecol. 1994:1365–1372.

Lee K, Ferguson RM, Corpuz M, Gartner LM. Maternal age and incidence of low birth weight at term: A population study. Am J Obstet Gynecol. 1988;158:84–89.

Lehmann DK, Chism J. Pregnancy outcome in medically complicated and uncomplicated patients aged 40 years or older. Am J Obstet Gynecol. 1987;157:738–742.

Lerman RI. Who Are the Young Absent Fathers? Paper prepared for Assistant Secretary for Policy and Evaluation, Department of Health and Human Services. Boston, MA: Brandeis University; 1985.

Lubarsky SL, Schiff E, Friedman SA, Mercer BM, Sibai BM. Obstetric characteristics among nulliparas under age 15. Obstet Gynecol. 1994;84:365–368.

Luker K. Dubious conceptions: The controversy over teen pregnancy. Am Prospective. 1991;Spring:73–83.

Luker K. Abortion and the Politics of Motherhood. Berkeley, CA: University of California Press; 1984.

Manski C, Sandefur GD, McLanahan S, Powers D. Alternative estimates of the effect of family structure during adolescence on high school graduation. J Am Stat Assoc. 1992;87:23–37.

March of Dimes Birth Defects Foundation. Toward Improving the Outcome of Pregnancy: The 90s and Beyond. New York, NY; 1993.

Marsiglio W. Teenage fatherhood: High school accreditation and educational attainment. In Adolescent Fatherhood. Elster AB, Lamb ME, eds. Hillsdale, NJ: Lawrence Erlbaum Associates; 1986.

Marsiglio W, Mott FL. Does wanting to become pregnant with a first child affect subsequent maternal behaviors and infant birth weight? J Marriage Fam. 1988:1023–1036.

Matejcek Z, Dytrych Z, Schuller V. Children from unwanted pregnancies. Acta Psychiatr Scand. 1978;57:67–90.

McAnarney ER, Hendee WR. Adolescent pregnancy and its consequences. JAMA. 1989; 262:74–77.

McCormick MC, Brooks-Gunn J, Shorter T, Wallace CY, Holmes JH, Heagarty MC. The planning of pregnancy among low-income women in central Harlem. Am J Obstet Gynecol. 1987;156:145–149.

McLanahan S. Family structure and dependency: Early transitions to female household headship. Demography. 1988;25:1–16.

McLanahan S. Family structure and the reproduction of poverty. Am J Sociol. 1985;90: 873–901.

McLanahan S, Bumpass L. Intergenerational consequences of family disruption. Am J Sociol. 1988;93:130–152.

McLanahan S, Sandefur G. Growing Up with a Single Parent. Cambridge, MA: Harvard University Press; 1994.

Medical Research Council Vitamin Study Research Group. Prevention of neural tube defects: Results of the Medical Research Council Vitamin Study. Lancet. 1991;338: 131–137.

Meier KJ, McFarlane DR. State family planning and abortion expenditures: Their effect on public health. Am J Public Health. 1994;84:1468–1472.

Miller E, Hare JW, Cloherty JP, et al. Elevated maternal HbA (1c) in early pregnancy and major congenital anomalies in infants of diabetic mothers. N Engl J Med. 1981; 304:1331–1335.

Moore KA. Bivariate analyses: Age at first birth and well-being at ages 23, 27, and 35. In The Consequences of Early Childbearing in the 1980s, Final Report to National

Institute of Child Health and Human Development, Contract No. N01-HD-9-219. 1992.

Moore KA, Myers DE, Morrison DR, Nord CW, Brown B, Edmonston B. Age at first childbirth and later poverty. J Res Adol. 1993;3:393–422.

Morris L, Warren CW, Aral SO. Measuring adolescent sexual behaviors and related health outcomes. Public Health Rep. 1993;108:31–36 (suppl. 1).

Morris NM, Udry JR, Chase CL. Reduction of low birth weight birth rates by the prevention of unwanted pregnancies. Am J Public Health. 1973;65:935–938.

Mott F, Maxwell NL. School-age mothers: 1968 and 1979. Fam Plann Perspect. 1981;6: 287–292.

Murphy S, Orkow B, Nicola RM. Prenatal prediction of child abuse and neglect: A prospective study. Child Abuse Negl. 1985;9:225–235.

Myhrman A. Family relation and social competence of children unwanted at birth. Acta Psychiatr Scand. 1988;77:187–191.

Najman JM, Morrison J, Williams G, Andersen M, Keeping JD. The mental health of women six months after they give birth to an unwanted baby: A longitudinal study. Soc Sci Med. 1991;32:241–247.

National Abortion and Reproductive Rights Action League. 1994 Update to Who Decides? A State by State Review of Abortion Rights. Washington, DC; 1994.

National Center for Health Statistics. Advance report of final natality statistics, 1992. Monthly Vital Statistics Report. 1994;43(5) (suppl.).

National Research Council, Committee on Population. Contraception and Reproduction: Health Consequences for the Developing World. Washington, DC: National Academy Press; 1989a.

National Research Council, Committee on Population. Contraceptive Use and Controlled Fertility: Health Issues for Women and Children. Background papers. Washington, DC: National Academy Press; 1989b.

Oates K, Davis A, Ryan M. Predictive factors for child abuse. Aust Paediatr J. 1980;16: 239.

O'Reilly-Green C, Cohen WR. Pregnancy in women aged 40 and older. Obstet Gynecol Clin North Am. 1993;20:313–331.

Orr S, Miller CA. Psychosocial and behavioral factors and intendedness of pregnancy. Unpublished manuscript. Johns Hopkins University School of Hygiene and Public Health. 1995.

Pamuk ER, Mosher WD. Health Aspects of Pregnancy and Childbirth, United States, 1982. (PHS)89-1992. Hyattsville, MD: U.S. Department of Health and Human Services; 1988.

Parke RD, Beitel A. Hospital-based interventions for fathers. In Fatherhood: Applied Perspectives. Lamb M, ed. New York, NY: John Wiley & Sons; 1986.

Parke RD, Neville B. Teenage fatherhood. In Risking the Future: Adolescent Sexuality, Pregnancy, and Childbearing. Vol. II. Working Papers and Statistical Appendixes. Hofferth SL, Hays CD, eds. Washington, DC: National Academy Press; 1987.

Parke RD, Tinsley BJ. Fatherhood: Historical and contemporary perspectives. In Life Span Developmental Psychology: Historical and Generational Effects. McCluskey KA, Reese HW, eds. New York, NY: Academic Press; 1984.

Powers D. Transitions into idleness among white, black, and Hispanic youth: Some determinants and policy implications. Sociol Perspectives. 1994;37:183–210.

Prysak M, Lorenz RP, Kisly A. Pregnancy outcome in nulliparous women 35 years and older. Obstet Gynecol. 1995;85:65–70.

Public Health Service Expert Panel on the Content of Prenatal Care. Caring for Our Future: The Content of Prenatal Care. Washington, DC: U.S. Public Health Service; 1989.

Rawlings JS, Rawlings VB, Read JA. Prevalence of low birthweight and preterm delivery in relation to the interval between pregnancies among white and black women. N Engl J Med. 1995;332:69–74.

Resnick MD, Chambliss SA, Blum RW. Health and risk behaviors of urban adolescent males involved with pregnancy. Fam Soc. 1993:366–374.

Rosenfield A. The difficult issue of second trimester abortion. NEJM. 1994;331:324–325.

Ryder NB. The predictability of fertility planning status. Stud Fam Plann. 1976;7:294–307.

Ryder NB. Consistency of reporting fertility planning status. Stud Fam Plann. 1979;10: 115–128.

Sable MR. Pregnancy timing and wantedness and adverse pregnancy outcomes: Results of a population-based retrospective study in Missouri. Paper presented at the American Public Health Association meeting, Washington, DC; 1992.

Salmon P, Drew NC. Multidimensional Assessment of Women's Experience of Childbirth: Relationship to Obstetric Procedure, Antenatal Preparation and Obstetric History. J Psychosom Res. 1992;36:317–327.

Sandefur G, McLanahan S, Wojtkiewicz R. The effects of parental marital status during adolescence on high school graduation. Soc Forces. 1992;71:103–122.

Scott JR, et al. Danforth's Obstetrics and Gynecology. 6th ed. Philadelphia, PA: Lippincott; 1989.

Seltzer J. Consequences of marital disruption for children. Ann Rev Sociol. 1994;20: 235–266.

Smith S, Hanson R, Noble S. Social aspects of the battered baby syndrome. Br J Psychiatry. 1974;125:568.

Stevens-Simon C, White MM. Adolescent pregnancy. Pediatr Ann. 1991;20:322–331.

St. John C, Winston TJ. The effect of social support on prenatal care. J Appl Behav Sci. 1989;25:79–98.

Teachman JD. Early marriage, premarital fertility, and marital dissolution. J Fam Issues. 1983;4:105–126.

Thomson E, Hanson T, McLanahan S. Family structure and child well-being: Economic resources vs. parental behaviors. Soc Forces. 1994;73:221–242.

Thornton A. Influence of the marital history of parents on the marital and cohabitational experiences of children. Am J Sociol. 1991:96:868–894.

Tietze C, Lewit S. Joint program for the study of abortion (JPSA): Early medical complications of legal abortion. Stud Fam Plann. 1972;3:97–122.

Vercellini P, Guglielmo Z, Rognoni MT, et al. Pregnancy at forty and over: A case-control study. Eur J Obstet Gynecol. 1993;48:191–195.

Waite LJ, Moore KA. The impact of an early first birth on young women's educational attainment. Soc Forces. 1978;56:845–865.

Watkins E. Low income negro mothers—their decision to seek prenatal care. Am J Public Health. 1968;58:655–667.

Wells RH, Everstein IW, Bailey M. Pregnancy wantedness and maternal behavior during pregnancy. Demography. 1987;24:407–412.

Westoff CF, Ryder NB. The predictive validity of reproductive intentions. Demography. 1977;14:431–453.

Wineberg H. Childbearing and dissolution of the second marriage. J Marriage Fam. 1992;54:879–887.

Wineberg H. Intermarital fertility and dissolution of the second marriage. Soc Sci Res. 1991;75:62–65.

Wojtkiewicz R. Simplicity and complexity in the effects of parental structure on high school graduation. Demography. 1993;30:701–717.

World Health Organization Collaborating Center in Perinatal Care & Health Service Research in Maternal and Child Care. Unintended pregnancy and infant mortality/morbidity. In Closing the Gap: The Burden of Unnecessary Illness. Ambler RW, Dull HB, eds. New York, Oxford: Oxford University Press; 1987.

Wright NH. Family planning and infant mortality rate decline in the United States. Am J Epidemiol. 1975;101:182–187.

Wu L, Martinson B. Family structure and the risk of a premarital birth. Am Sociol Rev. 1993;58:210–232.

Ylinen K, Aula P, Stenman UH, et al. Risk of minor and major fetal malformations in diabetes with high haemoglobin A (1c) values in early pregnancy. Br Med J 1984; 289:345–346.

Zill N, Morrison D, Coiro MJ. Long-term effects of parental divorce on parent-child relationships, adjustment, and achievement in young adulthood. J Fam Psychology. 1993;7:91–103.

Zimicki S. The relationship between fertility and maternal mortality. In Contraceptive Use and Controlled Fertility: Health Issues for Women and Children. Background papers. Parnell AM, ed. Committee on Population, National Research Council. Washington, DC.: National Academy Press; 1989.

Zuravin SJ. Unplanned childbearing and family size: Their relationship to child neglect and abuse. Fam Plann Perspect. 1991;23:155–161.

4

Patterns of Contraceptive Use

Chapters 2 and 3 summarized the demography of unintended pregnancy and its consequences. The composite picture that emerges is that unintended pregnancy is common in the United States and that much would be gained if a higher proportion of pregnancies were intended at conception. This surely is not a new thought, nor is it particularly controversial.

The complexities begin to mount, however, when the next issue is approached—namely, understanding why there are such high rates of unintended pregnancy in the United States. What is it about our culture, our education and values, our methods of contraception, or our health care system that produces the patterns described in Chapter 2? This is more than a rhetorical question. It is, in fact, the essence of the challenge for policy leaders and others who are searching for ways to decrease the proportion of pregnancies that are unintended.

The direct cause of unintended pregnancy, of course, is sexual activity accompanied by contraceptive misuse, failure, or nonuse altogether. Accordingly, this chapter explores patterns of contraceptive use as they bear on unintended pregnancy. Trends in the use of different contraceptive methods are discussed, including both sterilization and reversible contraception. A discussion of contraceptive use among men is also included, covering use at first intercourse as well as at different stages of the reproductive life span; this discussion is followed by commentary on so-called dual-method contraception—that is, the use of two methods of contraception simultaneously. The chapter also includes with a brief discussion of the intersection of unintended pregnancy with sexually transmitted diseases (STDs). The next three chapters, Chapters 5–7, consider the many factors that influence contraceptive use and therefore the occurrence of unintended pregnancy.

PATTERNS OF CONTRACEPTIVE USE AND UNINTENDED PREGNANCY

In 1988, there were more than 3 million unintended pregnancies in the United States. Slightly fewer than half of these unintended pregnancies occurred among women who reported using reversible contraception, and slightly more than half among women who reported not using contraception despite no apparent intent to become pregnant (Harlap et al., 1991). In absolute numbers, this means that, in 1988, approximately 21 million women who reported using reversible methods of contraception experienced 1.5 million unintended pregnancies. And approximately 4 million women who reported that they were not actively seeking pregnancy and not using contraception at the time that they became pregnant experienced an additional 1.7 million unintended pregnancies (Mosher, 1990).

Figure 4-1 was developed to help provide a better understanding of this complicated connection between contraceptive use and unintended pregnancy. Using data from the National Survey of Family Growth (NSFG), this figure shows that in 1988[1] there were approximately 58 million women of reproductive ages 15–44[2] in the United States (Tier 1). Six out of 10 of these women reported using contraception; 4 out of 10 reported that they were not currently using contraception (Tier 2). The women who reported using contraception are divided into two groups: those who relied on contraceptive sterilization, either their own or their partner's (Group A), and those who used reversible contraception (Group B). Of these two groups, only the women in Group B have an appreciable risk of becoming pregnant unintentionally, inasmuch as sterilization is so effective.

Similarly, women who reported that they were not currently using contraception are divided into two groups. The first—Group C—is comprised of women who were currently sexually active (i.e., they reported having had

---

[1]As this volume was being completed, data on contraceptive use from the 1990 National Survey of Family Growth (NSFG) telephone reinterview survey were published (Peterson, 1995). These data are used sparingly through this chapter because of concerns about the response rates among some subpopulations.

[2]This number is slightly different from the comparable number in Table 2-1 which is for 1990, not 1988, and includes 13- and 14-year-old girls. Data from 1988 (which exclude 13- and 14-year-olds) are used here because this chapter relates contraception to unintended pregnancy, and 1988 data on unintended pregnancy are more complete than 1990 data.

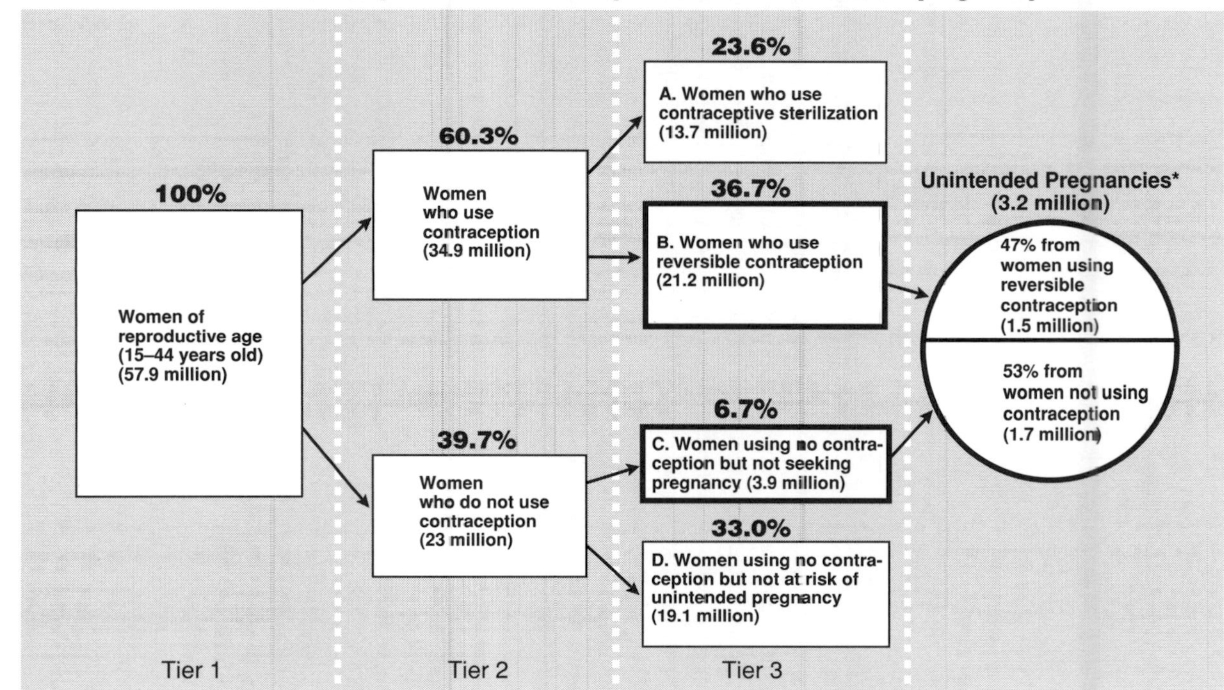

FIGURE 4-1 Contraceptive status of women experiencing unintended pregnancies, 1988. As noted in Chapter 2, the best available estimate of the pregnancies that are unintended is 57 percent. This estimate is based on the 1988 NSFG and supplemented by abortion data from 1987 compiled by The Alan Guttmacher Institute and the Centers for Disease Control. Sources: Harlap S, Kost K, Forrest JD. Preventing Pregnancy, Protecting Health: A New Look at Birth Control Choices in the United States. New York, NY: The Alan Guttmacher Institute; 1991; Mosher WD. Contraceptive practice in the US, 1982–1988. Fam Plann Perspect. 1990;22:198–205.

intercourse in the 3 months before the survey interview),[3] were fertile (neither they nor their partner had been contraceptively sterilized and they did not believe they were infertile for other reasons), and were not pregnant, postpartum, or trying to conceive. That is, they were clearly at risk of experiencing an unintended pregnancy because they used no contraception, but at the same time, they report that they were not actively planning for, or desiring, a pregnancy at that time. The other group, Group D, includes women who were not using contraception, but who were highly unlikely to experience an unintended pregnancy. These women were sterile for noncontraceptive reasons, sterile for reasons other than surgery, already pregnant or in the immediate postpartum period, trying to conceive, had never had intercourse, or were not currently sexually active (Mosher, 1990).

Thus, unintended pregnancy derives almost entirely from two groups. It occurs among women using reversible contraception (Group B), because contraceptive methods may fail or be used improperly, as discussed later in this chapter. It also occurs frequently among the relatively small group of women using no contraception who nonetheless are not actively seeking pregnancy (Group C), simply because sexual intercourse without the protection of contraception often leads to pregnancy.

Table 4-1 shows how women who do not intend to become pregnant are distributed between Groups B and C, according to several demographic variables. The table shows, for example, that among all sexually active women ages 40–44 who do not intend to become pregnant and who are not contraceptively sterilized, almost one-fourth (23.8 percent) use no contraceptive method, a finding that helps to explain the high rates of unintended pregnancy observed among older women.

It is important to stress, however, that women typically move back and forth between these two groups, making the distinction between them one that only applies at a given point in time. In particular, the category of contraceptive nonuse (Group C) includes a wide variety of women. It clearly includes women who consistently use no contraception over months or even years, many of whom have experimented with nonuse, have not become pregnant, and have gradually come to believe that they are subfecund—and in fact sometimes are. But it also includes women exhibiting only occasional periods of nonuse. Indeed, the majority of women in this nonuse category have used contraception at some previous time (Forrest, 1994b). For example, a woman may use a reversible method for a year and then, for a variety of reasons, stop using it for several months, perhaps intending to try a different method shortly. This is illustrated

[3]This definition of sexual activity is slightly more constrained than the definition in Chapter 2, in that it includes only those women who are currently sexually active, not those who have *ever* had sexual intercourse.

TABLE 4-1 Sexually Active Women Who Reported No Intent to Become Pregnant, and Were Either Using Reversible Contraception (Group B), or Not Using Contraception (Group C), by Age, Marital Status, and Poverty Level, 1988[a]

	Percentage of Women		
Characteristics	Reversible Contraception (Group B)	No Contraception (Group C)	Total
Total	84.7	15.3	100.0
Age			
15–19	78.5	21.5	100.0
20–24	87.0	13.0	100.0
25–29	86.8	13.2	100.0
30–34	87.2	12.8	100.0
35–39	84.3	15.7	100.0
40–44	76.2	23.8	100.0
Marital Status			
Never married	80.2	19.8	100.0
Married	89.4	10.6	100.0
Formerly married	84.5	15.5	100.0
Poverty level			
<100%	71.1	28.9	100.0
100–199%	82.1	17.9	100.0
≥200%	88.2	11.8	100.0

[a]The denominator for these percentages is women who reported that they did not intend to become pregnant minus women who reported that they used contraceptive sterilization (i.e., all of the women in Groups B and C, but not those in Group A).

SOURCE: Forrest JD. Contraceptive use in the United States: Past, present and future. Adv Popul. 1994a;2:29–48.

by the finding that 28 percent of contraceptive-using married women discontinue their contraceptive method during any given year without the intention of becoming pregnant. Approximately 50 percent of these women immediately switch to another method of birth control, and the other half go through a period of contraceptive nonuse (Grady et al., 1988; Henshaw and Silverman, 1988). Of course, even temporary nonuse may result in an unintended pregnancy, especially if the nonuse interval is extensive.

From a practical point of view, however, it is important to recognize that unintended pregnancy results both from spells of contraceptive nonuse and from contraceptive failure or misuse, and that the strategies needed to reduce the incidence of unintended pregnancy in each of these two groups may well be different. For example, encouraging women who are currently using contraception (Group B) to be even more careful with their methods of contraception or to use more effective methods (e.g., to switch from foam to oral contraceptives) will be quite a different task from helping a woman to confront the risks of being sexually active, not desiring pregnancy, and using no contraception at all (Group C).

Unintended Pregnancy Among Women Using No Contraception (Group C)

As shown in Figure 4-1, only 6.7 percent of women of reproductive age can be described as not intending pregnancy, yet not using contraception. This small group (Group C) contributed a full 53 percent of all unintended pregnancies in 1988, demonstrating how risky it is to engage in sexual intercourse without contraception when pregnancy is not being actively sought. Table 4-2 highlights the demographic attributes of the women in Group C. It reveals, among other things, that contraceptive nonuse is seen among women of all ages.

Nonuse among teenagers merits an additional comment. Some portion of this phenomenon reflects the common experience of having used no contraception at first intercourse, which is related to the age at first intercourse. The age of first intercourse has declined in recent years: higher proportions of adolescent men and women reported being sexually experienced at each age between the ages of 15 and 20 in 1988 than in the early 1970s. The percentage of women who had had intercourse before their 18th birthday rose from 35 to 56 percent during this time period; for men the percentage increased from 55 to 73 (The Alan Guttmacher Institute, 1994; see also Laumann et al., 1994). This is significant for unintended pregnancy because the younger the age of first intercourse, the less likely that contraception will be used at that first intercourse or in the months directly following the event. Again, though, as shown in Table 4-2, the majority of nonusers are not adolescents.

TABLE 4-2 Sexually Active Women Who Reported No Intent to Become Pregnant and Were Not Using Contraception (Group C), by Age, Marital Status, Poverty Level, and Race and Ethnicity, 1988[a]

Characteristics	Percentage
Age	
15–19	20.6
20–24	20.1
25–29	21.1
30–34	15.2
35–39	11.5
40–44	11.5
Total	100.0
Marital Status	
Never married	52.1
Married	33.7
Formerly Married	14.2
Total	100.0
Poverty Level	
$<150\%$	38.2
150–299%	23.5
$\geq 300\%$	38.3
Total	100.0
Race/ethnicity	
White	61.1
Black	19.7
Hispanic	13.8
Other	5.4
Total	100.0

[a]The denominator for these percentages is sexually active women who reported not intending to become pregnant and not using contraception.

SOURCE: National Center for Health Statistics. Unpublished tables from the 1988 National Survey of Family Growth. Tables 1-1, 1-2, 1-4, and 1-6 for 1988.

Unintended Pregnancy Among Women Using Contraception (Groups A and B)

Women who report using contraception—a much larger group than those who do not—also experience unintended pregnancy and, as noted in Figure 4-1, contribute nearly half of all unintended pregnancies. Unintended pregnancies occur almost exclusively among women reporting use of *reversible* contraception (Group B). Women who have been sterilized for purposes of contraception or who are relying for protection against pregnancy on their partner's sterilization (Group A) contribute virtually not at all to the pool of unintended pregnancy. Nonetheless, it is important to note several aspects of this group because so many women and couples rely on sterilization to prevent pregnancy, particularly in the later phases of the reproductive life span.

Contraceptive Sterilization

Nearly 40 percent of all women who report using contraception relied on contraceptive sterilization (either their own or their partner's) to avoid unintended pregnancy in 1988. Female sterilization is used much more frequently than male sterilization. Although male and female sterilization rates were nearly equivalent in the 1970s, by 1988, 28 percent of women using contraception relied on female sterilization and only 12 percent relied on their partner's use of vasectomy (Mosher and Pratt, 1990). The 1990 NSFG telephone reinterview survey and the 1992 and 1994 Ortho Birth Control Studies indicate that heavy reliance on sterilization has continued into the early 1990s, and female sterilization has continued as the predominate form (Forrest and Fordyce, 1993; Ortho Pharmaceutical Company, 1994; Peterson, 1995).[4]

Several factors probably account for the growing preference for female rather than male sterilization, despite the fact that the male sterilization procedure is safer and less expensive. The growing availability of quick and safe procedures such as laparoscopy during the 1970s and 1980s made it easier for women to choose sterilization, and the legacy of medical reticence, exemplified

---

[4]Because data from the 1988 and 1990 NSFG predate the introduction of both injectable and implantable hormonal contraceptives, they are supplemented in this chapter by data from the 1992 and 1994 Ortho Birth Control Studies. The Ortho Birth Control Studies are an annual survey by the Ortho Pharmaceutical Corporation of contraceptive attitudes and the contraceptive methods used. The value of this survey is somewhat limited, however. Random sampling is not used, and the surveys tend to underrepresent black women and households with annual incomes greater than $50,000. Nevertheless, they do provide some insight into contraceptive use in the 1990s.

by the "120 rule,"[5] eased as well. The sterilization decision has come to be based more on client request and preference rather than provider opinion, and female sterilization has increasingly come to be seen as the most foolproof method of contraception by women who become tired or distrustful of other methods and who appreciate the control that sterilization provides. Women also may choose sterilization because the burden of contraception most often falls on them. In addition, obstetricians and gynecologists may be more likely to discuss female sterilization with women than internists (or other clinicians) are to discuss male sterilization with men.

Reversible Contraception

Women currently using reversible contraception—approximately 21 million in 1988—contribute slightly less than half of all unintended pregnancies (Group B). Their demographic attributes are shown in Table 4-3.

The dynamics of pregnancy occurring despite the use of contraception are unclear, and both method failure (i.e., the condom broke because of manufacturing problems) and user failure (i.e., the condom broke because it was used incorrectly) must be taken into account. It is often difficult, as a practical matter, to distinguish clearly between a genuine contraceptive failure and the failure of an individual or couple to use a method properly and consistently. Only with methods that require no specific action once they are established, such as a contraceptive implant, can these distinctions be made with certainty.

One of the most important and difficult problems faced in understanding how pregnancy can occur in the presence of contraception is that the primary data source for computed rates is interviews (and questionnaires) with women and men in which the respondents are asked about their patterns of contraceptive use at the time that an unintended pregnancy occurred. Most people being interviewed understand intuitively that to admit that no contraception at all was being used or that it was being used improperly, despite no desire to become pregnant at the time, is in some sense an embarrassing admission, however honest it might be. The socially desirable answer, of course, is to say that contraception was being used carefully and consistently, but that an unintended pregnancy occurred anyway. Because of this problem, estimates of genuine contraceptive failure (the method was used perfectly, but pregnancy occurred nonetheless) are probably inflated by some unknown, but real factor. This is not

---

[5]Clinicians used to refuse to sterilize women until the patient's age multiplied by the number of live births she had had equaled 120; for example, a physician might refuse to sterilize a 30-year-old woman who had had three live births (30 x 3 = 90), but might agree to do so if she had had four live births (30 x 4 = 120)—hence the "120 rule."

TABLE 4-3 Women Who Reported No Intent to Become Pregnant and Were Using Reversible Methods of Contraception (Group B), by Age, Marital Status, Poverty Level, and Race and Ethnicity, 1988[a]

Characteristics	Percentage
Age	
15–19	13.6
20–24	24.5
25–29	25.3
30–34	18.8
35–39	11.2
40–44	6.6
Total	100.0
Marital Status	
Never married	38.2
Married	52.3
Formerly Married	9.5
Total	100.0
Poverty Level	
<150%	20.1
150–299%	23.2
≥300%	56.6
Total	100.0
Race/ethnicity	
White	75.8
Black	12.2
Hispanic	8.4
Other	3.6
Total	100.0

[a]The denominator for these percentages is women who reported using reversible contraception.

SOURCE: National Center for Health Statistics. Unpublished tables from the 1988 National Survey of Family Growth. Tables 1-1, 1-2, 1-4, and 1-6 for 1988.

to say that method failures never occur because they do. Rather it is to suggest that some unintended pregnancies ascribed to method failure may in fact be due to user failure and even to nonuse.

There is also no doubt that using many of the reversible contraceptive methods correctly and consistently can be very challenging. For example, Oakley (1994) has sketched the chain of events that using an oral contraceptive requires a woman to master: obtaining pills, taking them in the correct order, taking each pill within the appropriate time window, abstaining from sex or using a backup method when necessary, obtaining refills on time, stopping one cycle and starting the next at the right time, interpreting problems correctly (neither over-reacting nor under-reacting), and taking effective action to resolve problems (see Chapter 5 for more discussion of the skills required for contraceptive use). The point is that many reversible methods are difficult to use perfectly all of the time, and therefore user failure should be seen as reflecting both the skills of the user as well as the inherent complexity of many available reversible methods themselves.

Recognizing these realities, researchers studying contraceptive failure rates often distinguish between typical use and perfect use, thus providing some context for separating mechanical failure from user foible. Perfect use reflects contraceptive use that is consistently performed according to the specified instructions; all pregnancies occurring in the presence of perfect use are classified as method failures. Typical use, on the other hand, reflects a combination of actual method failure and user failure—a more real-world, everyday measure. Rates of failure are substantially higher with typical use than with perfect use.

Not surprisingly, in typical use, coitus-dependent methods are significantly less effective than coitus-independent methods, especially those that are longer-acting. For example, the first-year contraceptive failure rate for condoms and diaphragms ranges from 12 to 20 percent (Hatcher et al., 1994), and the 6-month failure rate of the female condom is estimated to be 12 percent (Trussell et al., 1994). By contrast, contraceptive implants and injections have less than a 1 percent failure rate (Ross, 1989; Hatcher et al., 1994). Overall, those reversible methods that are nearly impervious to user shortcomings are most effective in day-to-day life.

Jones and Forrest (1992) computed failure rates of several commonly used methods based on the 1982 and 1988 NSFG. These rates, shown in Table 4-4, were calculated on the basis of the first 12 months of use, and therefore may not reflect failure rates over longer periods of time. The investigators suggest that rates of contraceptive failure may have increased during the 1980s, especially for some methods. Failure rates for oral contraceptives, for example, increased from 6 to 8 percent between 1982 and 1988—a trend that is particularly worrisome given the fact that under conditions of perfect use, oral contraceptives yield only about one pregnancy in 1,000 women in the first year of use. This increase can also be seen in less reliable methods; for example, the failure rate for periodic abstinence increased from 16 to 25 percent during the 1980s.

It is important to emphasize that, given the imperfect array of contraceptives available to both men and women and the years of exposure to the risk of unintended pregnancy, some appreciable number of unintended pregnancies will inevitably occur over the life course. One simple computation suggests that this accumulates to a large risk over time. Ross (1989) offers the example of a young

TABLE 4-4 Percentages of Women Experiencing Contraceptive Failure During the First 12 Months of Use, Corrected for Underreporting of Abortion, by Method, 1982 and 1988 NSFG[a]

	Percentage	
Method	1982	1988
Oral contraceptive	6.2	8.3
Condom	14.2	14.8
Diaphragm	15.6	15.9
Periodic abstinence	16.2	25.6
Spermicides	26.3	25.2
Other	22.2	27.8

[a]Correction for underreporting of abortion is based on 1987 data from The Alan Guttmacher Institute and the Centers for Disease Control.

SOURCE: Jones EF, Forrest JD. Contraceptive failure rates based on the 1988 NSFG. Fam Plann Perspect. 1992;24:12–19:Table 1.

couple of undiminished fertility who use a contraceptive that is 95 percent effective. In this example, the couple experiences a monthly risk of pregnancy of about 1 percent. Over 10 years, that risk accumulates to a 70 percent probability that an unintended pregnancy will occur at some point during the decade. Similarly, Trussell and Vaughn (1989) have estimated that the average woman will experience one contraceptive failure for every 2.25 live births, a number that increases substantially if women who are in relationships in which at least one partner has been sterilized are excluded from the analysis (see also Harlap et al., 1991). These data underscore the fact that an appreciable part of both a woman's and a man's reproductive life span is spent at risk of unintended pregnancy, using a variety of reversible contraceptive methods that are rarely, if ever, 100 percent effective. In fact, Forrest (1993) has estimated that about 75 percent of a woman's reproductive years are spent trying to avoid pregnancy.

Contraceptive misuse and failure are not evenly distributed across all ages and stages of the reproductive life span. They are higher among unmarried women (and formerly married women in particular) and those whose incomes are 200 percent or less of the poverty level (Forrest, 1994a). The concentration of these contraceptive failures in certain groups of women is undoubtedly part of the underlying explanation for the concentration of unintended pregnancy in these same groups, as noted in Chapter 2.

Current Choices Among Reversible Methods

Women and their partners have a broad array of reversible contraceptive methods from which to choose, and the popularity of various methods has changed over time. Table 4-5 presents information about the results of these choices in 1988, showing the use of both contraceptive sterilization and reversible contraception (i.e., the women in Groups A and B in Figure 4-1). Table 4-6 supplements Table 4-5 by displaying contraceptive choices within the group of reversible methods only over the 1982–1990 interval.

Three issues stand out in reviewing Table 4-5. First, coitus-independent methods are the most popular among the women surveyed. Oral contraceptives were the most frequently used method in 1988; this was followed closely by female sterilization. Other methods, ranked in order of popularity, were condoms, male sterilization, the diaphragm, periodic abstinence, withdrawal, the IUD, and foam. Second, the rank order changes somewhat with the age of the user. For example, oral contraceptives were the most frequently used method among those 15–29 years old, but female sterilization was the most frequently used method among those 30–44 years old. Third, condom use was dramatically higher among adolescents than among older women. Data from the 1990 NSFG suggest a change in the rank order: female sterilization was the most frequently used method; this was followed by oral contraceptives. Data from the 1988 and 1990 NSFG do not reflect the current increase in the use of hormonal implants and injections; however, data from the 1994 Ortho Birth Control Study indicate the growing popularity of these methods (Peterson, 1995; Ortho Pharmaceutical Company, 1994).

It is probable that condom use is higher than is indicated by these data. The 1988 NSFG reported the more effective method when condoms were stated as being used with sterilization, oral contraceptives, IUDs, or diaphragms, thereby partially obscuring the importance of condoms. Concomitant use of condoms and any method other than these four was coded as condom use. When the data are retabulated to include all methods used, the number of women using condoms rises to 5.8 million, or approximately 17 percent of all users in 1988 (Mosher and Pratt, 1990). In addition, occasional use of condoms is not reported in the NSFG. Women are asked to report all methods they have used for 1 month or more, and thus may fail to report episodic condom use. A separate question about condom use suggests that 14 percent of women who reported condom use in response to this question did not report condoms as their current method (either alone or with another method), and this was especially true among younger women (Hatcher et al., 1994).

Because women at either end of the reproductive age span have relatively high rates of unintended pregnancy, it is useful to discuss their contraceptive use in more detail. Roughly, these two groups are women under age 20 and women age 40 and over.

TABLE 4-5 Choice of Contraceptive Methods Among Women Who Use Either Contraceptive Sterilization or Reversible Contraception by Age, Marital Status, Poverty Level, Race and Ethnicity, Education, and Religion, 1988[a] (in percent)

Characteristics	All Methods	Sterilization: Female	Sterilization: Male	Oral Contraceptive	Condom	Diaphragm	IUD	Other[b]
Total	100	28	12	31	15	6	2	6
Age								
15–19	100	2	0	59	33	1	0	5
20–24	100	5	2	68	15	4	0	6
25–29	100	17	6	45	16	6	1	9
30–34	100	33	14	22	12	9	3	7
35–39	100	45	20	5	12	8	3	7
40–44	100	51	22	3	11	4	4	5
Marital Status								
Never married	100	6	2	59	20	5	1	7
Married	100	31	17	21	14	6	2	9
Formerly married	100	51	4	25	6	5	4	5
Poverty Level								
<150%	100	37	4	36	13	2	3	5
150–299%	100	32	12	29	14	5	2	6

≥300%	100	22	14	30	16	8	2	8
Race/ethnicity								
White	100	26	14	30	15	7	2	6
Black	100	38	1	38	10	2	3	8
Hispanic	100	32	4	33	14	2	5	10
Education								
≤11 years	100	52	7	23	6	1	4	7
12 years	100	34	15	29	11	3	2	6
≥13 years	100	21	13	29	16	10	2	9
Religion								
Protestant	100	32	12	29	13	4	NA	10
Catholic	100	22	12	33	16	6	NA	11
Jewish	100	12	13	15	22	27	NA	10
None	100	18	11	37	18	10	NA	6

[a]The denominator for these percentages is all women who use contraceptives in each category; for example, among women ages 15–19 who reported using some type of contraception, 59 percent used oral contraceptives.
[b]"Other" contraceptive methods include periodic abstinence, foam, withdrawal, douche, sponge, jelly or cream alone, and other methods.

SOURCES: Goldsheider C, Mosher WD. Patterns of contraceptive use in the United States: The importance of religious factors. Stud Fam Plann. 1991;22:102–115;Table 3; Mosher WD. Contraceptive practice in the US, 1982–1988. Fam Plann Perspect. 1990;22:198–205:Table 4.

TABLE 4-6 Trends in Choice of Reversible Contraceptive Methods Among Women, by Age, Marital Status, Poverty Level, and Race and Ethnicity, 1982 through 1990[a]

	1982					1988					1990				
Characteristics	Oral Contraceptive	Condom	Diaphragm	IUD	Other[b]	Oral Contraceptive	Condom	Diaphragm	IUD	Other	Oral Contraceptive	Condom	Diaphragm	IUD	Other
Total	42.5	18.2	12.3	10.8	16.2	50.6	24.1	9.4	3.3	12.6	49.2	30.6	4.8	2.4	13.0
Age															
15–19	64.2	20.9	6.0	1.3	7.6	59.8	33.4	1.0	0.0	5.8	52.0	44.0	0.0	0.0	4.0
20–24	60.0	11.6	11.1	4.6	12.8	72.9	15.5	4.0	0.3	7.3	61.4	28.0	0.7	1.1	8.8
25–29	43.2	13.4	14.5	12.9	15.0	57.8	20.3	7.1	1.7	13.1	61.0	24.5	3.0	0.5	11.0
30–34	29.6	22.3	14.7	16.5	16.9	40.2	22.4	16.6	5.4	15.4	44.0	29.3	8.6	1.7	16.4
35–39	14.2	28.9	9.7	18.7	28.6	14.7	33.3	21.8	7.6	22.6	29.4	28.6	9.2	2.8	30.0
40–44	3.7	34.1	12.7	18.9	30.7	12.0	39.3	14.6	13.9	20.2	10.2	42.8	17.7	8.4	20.9
Marital status															
Never Married	56.1	12.3	14.2	5.7	11.7	64.3	21.4	5.3	1.4	7.6	56.6	33.7	0.9	0.7	8.1
Married	33.5	24.5	11.3	1.7	18.8	39.8	27.9	12.1	3.9	16.3	43.6	29.6	8.7	3.0	15.1
Formerly married	49.6	16.1	11.7	20.1	16.1	55.4	12.9	11.6	7.9	12.2	49.7	21.5	2.0	5.5	21.3

Poverty level															
<150%	52.4	13.0	8.8	11.9	13.9	60.2	19.6	4.4	6.4	9.4	53.2	32.0	1.3	2.4	11.1
150–299%	39.5	18.1	11.1	10.3	21.0	50.8	21.8	9.5	4.6	13.3	53.5	30.0	2.0	5.0	9.5
≥300%	39.3	20.9	15.0	10.6	14.1	45.3	23.6	13.0	2.8	15.3	46.7	28.7	7.2	1.7	15.7
Race/ethnicity															
White	40.6	20.1	14.1	8.9	16.3	49.1	25.3	11.0	2.5	12.1	49.8	29.7	5.2	2.3	13.0
Black	55.2	9.2	4.7	13.6	17.2	62.2	16.5	3.3	5.2	12.8	49.4	33.6	2.8	2.4	11.8
Hispanic	41.7	9.5	6.5	26.5	15.7	52.2	21.3	3.8	7.8	14.9	51.9	28.3	2.5	3.1	14.2

[a]In each category, the denominator is women using reversible contraceptives. For example, 64.2 percent of 15–19-year-old women who reported using reversible contraception in 1982 used oral contraceptives, 59.8 percent used oral contraceptives in 1988, and 52.0 percent used oral contraceptives in 1990.

[b]"Other" contraceptives include periodic abstinence, foam, withdrawal, douche, sponge, jelly or cream alone, and other methods.

SOURCES: National Center for Health Statistics. Unpublished tables from the 1982 and 1988 National Survey of Family Growth. Tables 1-7, 1-8, 1-10, 1-12, for 1982. Peterson L. Contraceptive use in the United States: 1982–1990. Advance Data. National Center for Health Statistics. 1995(260):1–15. Tables 4 and 5.

Adolescents Nearly 80 percent of sexually active teenage women (i.e., those who have had intercourse within the last 3 months) reported using some type of contraception in 1988, and as noted above, they most frequently used oral contraceptives and condoms (Forrest, 1994a). To get a more refined picture of this group, it is helpful to separate the broad category of adolescents into early (12–14), middle (15–17), and late (18–19) adolescence, because contraceptive use varies dramatically across these age groups. Very little is known about the contraceptive use of early adolescents because girls under age 15 are often excluded from surveys on sexual activity, and moreover, a substantial portion of sexual activity among this group is unanticipated or non-voluntary, which makes the use of any method unlikely (see Chapter 7) (Moore et al., 1989).

More information is available about contraceptive use by older teens. In 1988, most sexually active 15–17-year-olds who used contraception reported using oral contraceptives (53 percent); this was followed by the use of condoms (40 percent). The rank order of popularity of these contraceptives apparently switched by 1990, when condoms became the most popular contraceptive among 15–17-year-olds (52 percent); this was followed by oral contraceptives (41 percent). Oral contraceptives have consistently been the most popular choice among 18–19-year-olds, with condoms a distant second (Peterson, 1995).

Women 40 and Over With regard to women at the other end of the reproductive life span, 92 percent of sexually active women aged 40–44 reported using some method of contraception in 1988, with a heavy reliance on contraceptive sterilization (primarily female sterilization) (Forrest, 1994a). Nonetheless, unintended pregnancy is quite common among those women who use reversible methods, primarily because the nonsurgical methods that they choose are the least effective: for example, only 12 percent of women who use reversible methods choose oral contraceptives. The most popular method after sterilization is the condom (39 percent), which has an appreciable failure rate, as noted earlier (Table 4-4).

Although in the past women in this age group were considered to be at greater risk than younger women of adverse side effects from oral contraceptives, that is no longer the case for most women (Kaeser, 1989). Data from the 1994 Ortho Birth Control Study suggest that use of oral contraceptives among women is this age category may have risen very slightly in the early 1990s (Ortho Pharmaceutical Company, 1994).

Reversible Contraceptive Methods: Types and Trends

In general, methods that are both long-acting[6] and coitus-independent (such as contraceptive implants) have the highest effectiveness rates but are used by relatively few women; less than 10 percent of all women who report using reversible methods of contraception use methods that are both long-acting and coitus-independent. Methods that are coitus-independent but require complicated compliance regimens (that is, oral contraceptives) are often less effective in typical use than those that are long-acting; nonetheless, oral contraceptives in particular remain the most popular method of reversible contraception. Although methods that are coitus-dependent are generally the least effective in preventing pregnancy, they are important to highlight because they are so popular among women at especially high risk of unintended pregnancy (such as younger women, unmarried women, and older women who are not relying on their own or their partner's sterilization to avoid pregnancy) and because they are often one part of a dual method system, as discussed later in this chapter. Table 4-6 presents data on contraceptive choices over the 1982–1990 interval within the group of reversible methods only.

Long-Acting Coitus-Independent Methods There are three broad classes of contraceptive methods that are both long-acting and coitus-independent: implantable hormones, injectable hormones, and IUDs. Given their high rates of effectiveness, they are very important in preventing unintended pregnancy. Few survey data are available to describe the patterns of use of contraceptive implants and injectables because they are such recent arrivals in the United States. Norplant, a contraceptive implant that releases the synthetic progestin levonorgestrel through capsules that are placed in the upper arm, provides highly effective contraceptive protection for up to 5 years; it was approved for use in the United States in 1990. Four percent of reproductive-age women who report using reversible contraception currently use this method (Ortho Pharmaceutical Company, 1994), and about half of the Norplant users are unmarried (The Alan Guttmacher Institute, 1993). The issue of implant removal has gained added visibility recently, as exemplified by a class action liability lawsuit based on alleged removal problems. (Additional material on Norplant is in Chapters 5 and 7.)

Depo-Provera is an injectable progestin, recently approved for use in the United States, that provides contraceptive protection for at least three months (Hatcher et al., 1994). In 1994, approximately 3 percent of reproductive-age

---

[6]Long-acting means that the method itself is effective for an extended period of time, as is the case, for example, with contraceptive implants (5 years of effectiveness) or the CuT 380A (Paraguard) IUD (8 years of effectiveness). These methods have the added advantage that the individual user need take only minimal action to maintain the method once it is in place.

women who reported the use of a reversible method relied on Depo-Provera (Ortho Pharmaceutical Company, 1994). Although the injectable contraceptive was licensed for sale in the United States later than contraceptive implants, it is rapidly increasing its market share, and informal reports from clinic directors confirm that current demand for Depo-Provera is high (R. Wisman, pers. com., 1994).

Even though the IUD is long-acting and coitus-independent, use of this method decreased in all age groups during the 1980s. This decrease has been attributed to the withdrawal of the IUD from the U.S. market by two major manufacturers in 1985 and 1986 because of various concerns about liability exposure (Forrest, 1986). By 1988, only 700,000 women were using this method (3.3 percent of those women using reversible contraception), and by 1990, this level had dropped to 2.4 percent (Table 4-6) (Mosher, 1990; Peterson, 1995). Although IUDs are currently available in the United States, the association with a litigious past and the paucity of clinicians with experience in inserting IUDs continues to hamper a renewal of their widespread use.

Other Coitus-Independent Methods Although their popularity has waned slightly since the 1960s, oral contraceptives were the leading method of reversible contraception during the 1980s, especially among never-married women and women under 30 years old. Oral contraceptive use decreased in the 1970s, but rose again in the 1980s (Mosher and Pratt, 1990). The increase in oral contraceptive use during the 1980s was primarily due to uptake among women in their 20s; use among adolescent women reporting contraceptive use declined during this period (from 64.2 to 59.9 percent). Between 1988 and 1990, oral contraceptive use appeared to decrease among women in their early 20s, but increase among women in their late 20s. Oral contraceptive use among women aged 35–39 who reported using reversible contraceptives also rose in 1990, from 14.7 to 29.4 percent. Oral contraceptive use was higher among low-income women than more affluent women early in the 1980s, but by 1990, economic status did not appear to affect the likelihood of oral contraceptive use among women using reversible contraception.

Coitus-Dependent Methods During the 1980s, reliance on condoms increased both overall and among certain subpopulations, but most notably among adolescent women, never-married women, and minority women. Condom use increased significantly among 15–19-year-olds who reported using reversible contraception, from 20.9 to 33.4 percent between 1982 and 1988 and to 44.0 percent in 1990. Among 20–24-year-olds who reported using reversible contraception, condom use rose from 11.6 to 15.5 to 28.0 percent, respectively. Condom use did not change among married couples using reversible contraception, but it did increase significantly among never-married and formerly married women. For example, condoms were the second leading method of choice among never-married women who reported using reversible contraception in 1988 and 1990, increasing from 12.3 percent in 1982 to 21.4 percent in 1988 and to 33.7 percent in 1990.

The popularity of other coitus-dependent methods, such as the diaphragm, cervical cap, contraceptive sponge, spermicides, periodic abstinence, and withdrawal, declined in the 1980s (Mosher, 1990). The decline was not uniform, however. For example, the decline in diaphragm use among women who reported use of reversible contraception was most apparent among younger women. In 1982, 6.0 percent of 15–19-year-olds, 11.1 percent of 20–24-year-olds, and 14.5 percent of 25–29-year-olds reported using diaphragms; by 1990, those proportions had decreased to 0.0, 0.7, and 3.0, respectively.

Risks and Benefits of Reversible Contraceptive Methods Reversible methods vary in their abilities to prevent unintended pregnancy, as noted in Table 4-4, and each is also associated with different risks and side effects. In addition, each has significant noncontraceptive benefits that are discussed much less frequently in the popular literature. This material is presented in Table 4-7.

CONTRACEPTIVE USE AMONG MEN

Much of the information about contraception, as noted earlier, is based on reports from women. Although women are often asked what methods their male partners use, it is important to review data derived from men themselves, because men have consistently contributed to their partners' protection against unintended pregnancy through their own use of contraceptive methods. This section discusses men's use of contraception at various stages of their reproductive lives, reflecting in particular the increase in men's use of condoms in the 1980s.

Use of Male Methods of Contraception at First Intercourse

Data from the National Survey of Adolescent Men suggest that condom use accounts for more than half of the contraception that occurs at first intercourse (Pleck et al., 1993). Among teenage men in 1988, for example, 55 percent used condoms and 38 percent used less effective methods such as withdrawal or no method; only 7 percent used an effective female method such as oral contraceptives. Condom use at first intercourse rose dramatically in this age group during the 1980s, and at the same time, use of ineffective methods or no contraception at first intercourse fell from 71 to 38 percent between 1979 and 1988 (Pleck et

TABLE 4-7 Noncontraceptive Benefits, Risks, and Side Effects of Various Reversible Contraceptive Methods

Method	Noncontraceptive Benefits	Risks	Side Effects
Implantable contraceptives	Decreased risk of PID,[a] ovarian cancer, and endometrial cancers; lactation not disturbed; decreased menstrual blood loss and risk of anemia; decreased menstrual pain; suppression of pain associated with ovulation	Infection at implant site	Tenderness at implant site, menstrual cycle disturbance (amenorrhea becomes less common over time), weight gain, breast tenderness, headaches, ovarian enlargement, dizziness, nausea, acne, dermatitis, hair loss
Injectable contraceptives	Decreased risk of PID, ovarian cancer, and endometrial cancers; decreased menstrual blood loss and risk of anemia; decreased menstrual pain; suppression of pain associated with ovulation; decreased frequency of seizures	Decreased bone density	Menstrual cycle disturbance (amenorrhea becomes more common over time), weight gain, breast tenderness, depression, delay in return of fertility, decreased HDL cholesterol levels, headaches
IUDs	None known; however progestin-releasing IUDs may decrease menstrual blood loss and pain	PID, perforation of the uterus, anemia	Menstrual cramping, spotting, increased bleeding

Oral contraceptives	Protects against acute infection of the fallopian tubes, PID, ovarian cancer, endometrial cancer, choriocarcinoma, benign breast masses, fibroids, ovarian cysts; decreased menstrual blood loss and risk of anemia; decreased menstrual pain; suppression of pain associated with ovulation	Estrogen-associated: blood clot complications, stroke, liver tumors, hypertension, heart attacks, cervical erosion or ectopia Progestin-associated: diabetes-related changes, hypertension, heart attacks Possible risks: breast cancer, cervical cancer, liver cancer	Estrogen-associated: nausea, headaches, fluid retention, weight gain, increased breast size, breast tenderness, stimulation of breast tumors, watery vaginal discharge, rise in cholesterol concentration in gallbladder bile, uterine fibroids Progestin-associated: weight gain, depression, fatigue, headaches, decreased libido, acne, increased breast size, breast tenderness, increased LDL cholesterol level, decreased HDL cholesterol level, chronic itch
Male condoms	Protects against STDs,[b] including HIV-AIDS; delays premature ejaculation; erection enhancement; prevention of sperm allergy	None known	Decreased sensation during intercourse, allergy to latex, possible interference with erection
Female condoms	Protects against STDs, including HIV-AIDS	None known	Decreased sensation during intercourse, allergy to polyurethane

Continued

TABLE 4-7 Continued

Method	Noncontraceptive Benefits	Risks	Side Effects
Barrier methods (diaphragm and cervical cap)	Protects against STDs, prevention against HIV-AIDS not proven; diaphragm protects against PID and cervical neoplasia	Vaginal trauma, toxic shock syndrome	Vaginal and urinary tract infection; vaginal discharges if not removed appropriately; allergy to spermicide, rubber, or latex; bladder or rectal pain, penile pain
Spermicides	Protects against STDs, prevention against HIV-AIDS not proven	None proven	Vaginal irritation, yeast vaginitis, allergy to spermicidal agents

[a]Pelvic inflammatory disease.
[b]Sexually transmitted diseases.

SOURCE: Hatcher RA, Trussell J, Stewart F, et al. Contraceptive Technology, 16th revised ed. New York, NY: Irvington Publishers, Inc.; 1994.

al., 1993). This increase may reflect deepening concern over HIV-AIDS transmission. Since 1988, there appears to have been no further growth overall in the use of condoms at first intercourse among men (Ku et al., 1993c; Pleck et al., 1993).

Withdrawal is also a method frequently used early in a man's reproductive life span, although it is being reported less often in recent years. It is useful to note that withdrawal, although not very effective, is still much more effective than failing to withdraw altogether, because the 1-year pregnancy rate of withdrawal is 19 percent and the 1-year pregnancy rate of no contraception at all is 85 percent (Hatcher et al., 1994).

Use of Male Methods by Married Men

Although the role of men in providing contraceptive protection at first intercourse is somewhat well known, less attention has been paid to the use of male contraceptive methods by married men. Since nationally representative data about the contraceptive practices of married women were first collected in 1973, male partners have been found to provide at least one-fourth of the contraception that is reported. As measured at three points in time (1973, 1988, and 1990), condom use among married men has remained stable at 14 percent. Sterilization, however, rose from 11 to 19 percent between 1973 and 1990 (Mosher, 1990; Peterson, 1995).

Although vasectomy is an important contraceptive method, few data are available in the literature to help provide an understanding of the dynamics of its use. Miller and colleagues (1991) report that married couples who are less traditional and more egalitarian are more likely to choose male over female sterilization; in addition, when the wife feels that communication between the spouses is effective, vasectomy is again more likely to be chosen over female sterilization. As shown in Table 4-5, there are also racial and ethnic differences in the reliance of women on male versus female sterilization. For example, very few minority women report that they rely on their partner's sterilization to protect them against unintended pregnancy. As noted earlier, vasectomy is a highly effective contraceptive method, but unfortunately, nearly 40 percent of men fail to return for a post-vasectomy semen analysis. If sperm are still present in the *vas deferens* of these men who lack follow-up care, they remain at risk of causing an unintended pregnancy for some time (J.M. Haws, pers. com., July 1994).

Age and Condom Use

Condom use has increased in the past decade, reaching especially high levels among adolescents. However, data from the 1991 Follow-up of the National

Survey of Adolescent Males and the 1991 National Survey of Men suggest that condom use decreases as men grow older (see Figure 4-2) (Pleck et al., 1993). Although the measures are not completely comparable across the two data sets, there is clearly a negative association between condom use and age. Although older men are part of an earlier cohort who initiated sexual activity before the age of AIDS and safe sex, there are also indications that the decline in condom use reflects the maturation of relationships and the transition to female methods of contraception (including sterilization) that are often more effective in preventing pregnancy (Landry and Camelo, 1994).

Even among adolescents aged 15 to 19, there appears to be a decrease in condom use by age, reflecting movement to female methods after initial sexual experiences during which condoms are often used. One study reports that 16-year-old men who are sexually active use condoms more than 19-year-olds (Sonenstein et al., 1989). Figure 4-3 provides an example of this by showing the contraceptive method used at last intercourse for sexually active adolescent men in 1988 and for the same young men nearly 3 years later, in 1991.

Race, Ethnicity, and Condom Use

Condom use varies by racial and ethnic affiliation. Black men are the most likely to report using condoms at all ages. Among adolescents, black men use condoms at higher rates than either Hispanic men or non-Hispanic white men (Pleck et al., 1991). The average percentage of times condoms were used increased among adolescent men of all ages between 1988 and 1991, but particularly among Hispanics (nearly 6 percent increase) and whites (nearly 5 percent increase) (Centers for Disease Control and Prevention, 1993). Nationally representative data about condom use among adult Hispanic men are not available.

Although condom use among black adolescent men is higher at last intercourse than among white men of comparable age, condom use at first intercourse is lower. Since black men, on average, initiate sex about 1 year earlier than white men, and since earlier ages of first intercourse are associated with less use of contraception, some of the racial difference in condom use at first intercourse is attributable to differentials in age at initiation (Sonenstein et al., 1989). However, after age at initiation is controlled along with other confounding variables, being a young black man continues to be associated with lower condom use at first intercourse (Ku et al., 1993a).

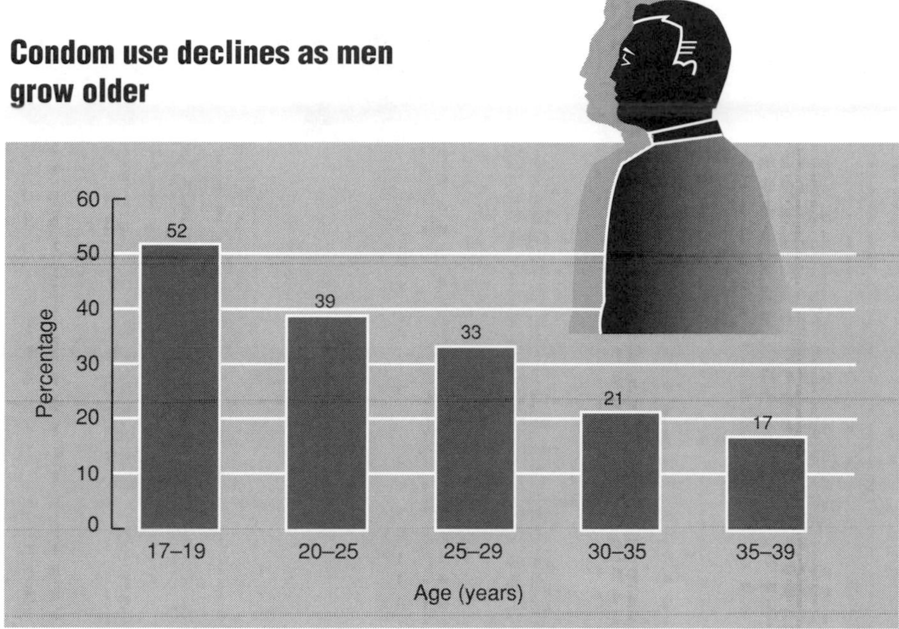

FIGURE 4-2 Condom use among men, by age, 1991. Source: Pleck JH, Sonenstein FL, Ku L. Changes in adolescent males' use of and attitudes toward condoms, 1988–1991. Fam Plann Perspect. 1993:25:106–110, 117.

Socioeconomic Status and Condom Use

Among adolescents, significant associations have been found in one study between socioeconomic measures and the use of effective contraception. However, the direction of the association was unanticipated by the researchers. Adolescent men with lower socioeconomic status were expected to report lower rates of effective contraceptive use, yet it was found that, net of other variables, use of effective contraception was higher among sexually experienced men living in neighborhoods with high poverty rates and lower among more affluent men (Ku et al., 1993b; Sonenstein et al., 1992). Multivariate analyses have not uncovered any systematic associations between the socioeconomic status of adolescent men and their use of condoms. Measures of family income, parental education, and welfare receipt are not significantly related to recent condom use among sexually experienced men (Pleck et al., 1991; Ku et al., 1992). By contrast, adult men with more education report greater condom use than those with less education (Tanfer et al., 1993).

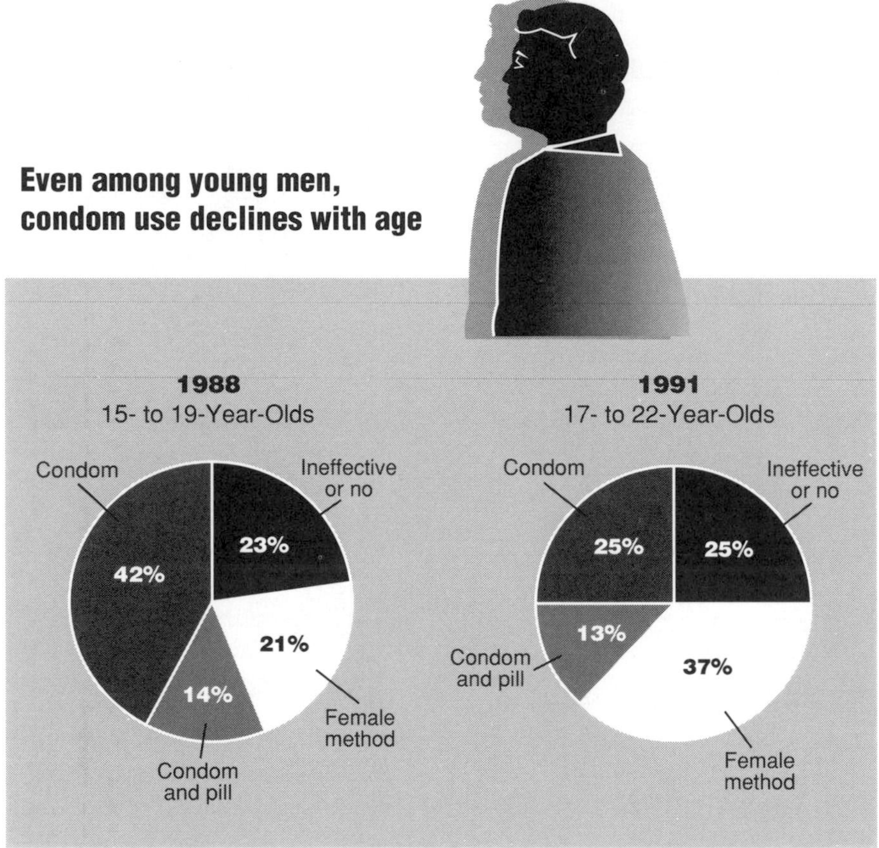

FIGURE 4-3 Form of contraception used at last intercourse as teen males grow older. Source: Pleck JH, Sonenstein FL, Ku L. Changes in adolescent males' use of and attitudes toward condoms, 1988–1991. Fam Plann Perspect. 1993:25:106–110, 117.

USE OF DUAL CONTRACEPTIVE METHODS

Given the appreciable failure rates of single reversible methods, it is important to consider the use of two methods simultaneously to prevent unintended pregnancy. Dual methods often involve the active participation of both male and female partners (particularly if one of the two methods chosen is a condom), and use of dual methods can expand the role of men in preventing unintended pregnancy.

Depending on the combination of methods selected, the use of two methods simultaneously can also reduce the risk of STDs. For example, the use of two female methods, such as oral contraceptives and foam, provides more complete protection against unintended pregnancy than the use of either method alone. The use of both a female method and a condom, however, not only provides added protection against unintended pregnancy but is also a more effective way for women and men to protect themselves from the risk of contracting an STD.

There is some evidence that the use of dual methods is increasing. For example, in 1979 a mere 3 percent of sexually active urban men aged 17–19 reported using both a condom and a female method of contraception simultaneously; this rate rose to 16 percent by 1988 (Zelnick and Kantner, 1980; Pleck et al., 1993). More recently, 25 percent of all women in the 1992 Ortho Birth Control Study reported using condoms concurrently with another method, and more than half of the women using less effective methods such as periodic abstinence reported using condoms as well (Forrest and Fordyce, 1993). Dual usage appears to have increased between 1992 and 1994; 46 percent of the women surveyed in the 1994 Ortho Birth Control Study reported using condoms in addition to their primary contraceptive. Among this group of dual-method users, nearly half claim that they are doing so solely for the prevention of unintended pregnancy (Ortho Pharmaceutical Company, 1994).

SEXUALLY TRANSMITTED DISEASES

As just noted, sexual activity can result not only in unintended pregnancies but also in the transmission of STDs. However, there are other links between unintended pregnancy and STDs as well: many risk factors for STDs and unintended pregnancy are the same; unintended pregnancy precludes the opportunity to resolve an STD before conception; and the desire to achieve protection against both STDs and unintended pregnancy may influence the choice of contraceptive methods, including dual methods.

STDs are spread by the transfer of infectious organisms from one person to another during sexual contact. Although it is difficult to calculate the prevalence of STDs, there are currently an estimated 56 million cases of viral STDs in the United States, and approximately 12 million new cases of both viral and nonviral STDs occur annually (Centers for Disease Control and Prevention, 1993). Two-thirds of new cases occur to people under 25 years of age, a cohort that also contributes heavily to unintended pregnancy, and approximately 3 million adolescents acquire an STD every year (Donovan, 1993). More than 20 organisms and syndromes are now recognized as STDs, including curable nonviral infections (e.g., chlamydia, gonorrhea, syphilis, or chancroid) and viral infections that are not curable, but are treatable (e.g., human papillomavirus or genital herpes) or preventable (e.g., hepatitis B virus through the hepatitis B vaccine) (Centers for Disease Control and Prevention, 1993; Alan Guttmacher Institute, 1994). Many of these STDs, if left untreated, can result in serious health repercussions not only for the man or woman who is infected, but also for a developing fetus.

Of great concern at present is HIV, a relatively new viral STD. HIV infection results in AIDS. AIDS is currently both incurable and fatal, although antiretroviral therapies are available for treatment. Nearly 1 million people in the United States were estimated to be infected with HIV in 1993—approximately 1 in 100 men and 1 in 800 women (Centers for Disease Control and Prevention, 1993). Perinatal transmission of HIV occurs in approximately 20 to 30 percent of births to infected mothers (Hatcher et al., 1994). Nearly 80 percent of AIDS cases are to people between the ages of 20 and 44, the prime childbearing years (Centers for Disease Control and Prevention, 1993).

The risk factors for STD infection overlap those for unintended pregnancy. For example, the risk of both unintended pregnancy and STD infection is greater for women and men who initiate sexual intercourse at lower ages, for those who have a greater number of both current and lifetime sexual partners, and for those who have a higher frequency of intercourse (Centers for Disease Control and Prevention, 1993; see also Kost and Forrest, 1992).

One particularly unfortunate consequence of unintended pregnancy is that it often precludes the chance to resolve an STD before conception or to consider avoiding pregnancy altogether because of the presence of an incurable STD that poses serious risks to a fetus, such as HIV-AIDS (Chapter 3 includes additional discussion of other opportunities for health promotion that are missed because a pregnancy is unintended). STDs left untreated in pregnant women can result in premature delivery, infection in the newborn, or infant death (Centers for Disease Control and Prevention, 1993).

Finally, because sexual activity often carries a risk of both unintended pregnancy and STD transmission, the choice of contraceptive methods has become more complicated. As suggested in the previous section on dual-method use, it is often necessary to use more than one method to prevent both STDs and unintended pregnancy. But individuals and couples may attach differing priorities to these two goals, and their priorities may change over time and across relationships. Moreover, couples may find it difficult to use two methods simultaneously. In this era of AIDS and the increasing incidence of other STDs, research on the determinants of contraceptive behavior has yet to take into consideration this complicated calculus. Two notable exceptions are the research by Kost and Forrest (1992), in which contraceptive decision-making was examined from the perspective of preventing both pregnancy and STDs, and the research by Landry and Camelo (1994), who reported on discussions with young, unmarried people about their use of contraception in both preventing pregnancy and avoiding STDs.

In this context, it is important to note that although condoms are the most effective contraceptive method for reducing STD transmission, other methods can also provide some protection against selected pathogens (Table 4-8). Unfortunately, no single method at present provides maximum protection against both unintended pregnancy and all STDs.

TABLE 4-8 Effects of Contraceptives on Bacterial and Viral STDs

Contraceptive Methods	Bacterial STD	Viral STD
Condoms	Protective	Protective
Spermicides with nonoxynol-9	Protective against gonorrhea and chlamydia	Undetermined in vivo
Diaphragms	Protective against cervical infection; associated with vaginal anaerobic overgrowth	Protective against cervical infection
Oral contraceptives	Associated with increased cervical chlamydia; protective against symptomatic pelvic inflammatory disease	Not protective
IUDs	Associated with pelvic inflammatory disease in first month after insertion	Not protective
Rhythm method	Not protective	Not protective

SOURCES: Ehrhardt AA, Wasserheit JN. Age, gender, and sexual risk behaviors for sexually transmitted diseases in the United States. In Research Issues in Human Behavior and Sexually Transmitted Diseases in the AIDS Era. Wasserheit JN, Aral SO, Holmes KK, Hitchcock PJ, eds. Washington, DC: American Society for Microbiology; 1991. Hatcher RA, Trussell J, Stewart F, et al. Contraceptive Technology, 16th revised ed. New York, NY: Irvington Publishers, Inc.; 1994: Table 4-2.

CONCLUSION

Several interesting conclusions emerge from an exploration of the patterns of contraceptive use as they relate to unintended pregnancy. First, women who report using reversible means of contraception (a large group) and women who report using no contraception at all despite having no clear intent to become pregnant (a small group) contribute roughly equally to the pool of unintended pregnancies. That is, about half of all unintended pregnancies derive from women who are not actively seeking pregnancy and who are using reversible contraception; the other half derive from women who are also not actively seeking pregnancy but who nonetheless are not using contraception. Many women and couples who are not intending to become pregnant move between these two groups, sometimes practicing contraception and sometimes not.

Contraceptive use has increased in recent years, primarily because of a rise in contraceptive female sterilization; moreover, the participation of men in providing reversible contraceptive protection is increasingly important, particularly at first intercourse. Nonetheless, unintended pregnancy continues to occur among couples who use reversible methods of contraception because many reversible methods are of only limited effectiveness even under conditions of perfect use, and because of the misuse of these same methods, some of which can be explained by the difficult compliance regimens that many require. Overall, coitus-dependent methods are much more susceptible to user failure than are long-acting coitus-independent methods, and thus couples relying on coitus-dependent methods are at greater risk of unintended pregnancy.

To reduce the risk of unintended pregnancy to the bare minimum, short of sterilization, couples are increasingly using two methods at once. Depending on which two methods are selected, dual-method use can help to reduce the risk of both STD transmission and unintended pregnancy. Indeed, the whole process of method selection has been complicated by the increasing presence of STDs and the importance of sexually active couples protecting themselves against both threats.

REFERENCES

The Alan Guttmacher Institute. Sex and America's Teenagers. New York, NY; 1994.

The Alan Guttmacher Institute. Norplant: Opportunities and Perils for Low-Income Women. Special Report No. 2. New York, NY; 1993.

Centers for Disease Control and Prevention. Division of STD/HIV Prevention Annual Report. Atlanta, GA; 1993.

Donovan P. Testing Positive: Sexually Transmitted Disease and the Public Health Response. New York, NY: The Alan Guttmacher Institute; 1993.

Ehrhardt AA, Wasserheit JN. Age, gender, and sexual risk behaviors for sexually transmitted diseases in the United States. In Research Issues in Human Behavior and Sexually Transmitted Diseases in the AIDS Era. Wasserheit JN, Aral SO, Holmes KK, Hitchcock PJ, eds. Washington, DC: American Society for Microbiology; 1991.

Forrest JD. Contraceptive use in the United States: Past, present and future. Adv Popul. 1994a;2:29–48.

Forrest JD. Epidemiology of unintended pregnancy and contraceptive use. Am J Obstet Gynecol. 1994b;170(5):1485–1489.

Forrest JD. Timing of reproductive stages. Am J Obstet Gynecol. 1993;82:110.

Forrest JD. The end of IUD marketing in the United States: What does it mean for American women? Fam Plann Perspect. 1986;18:52–56.

Forrest JD, Fordyce RR. Women's contraceptive attitudes and use in 1992. Fam Plann Perspect. 1993;23:175–179.

Forrest JD, Singh S. The sexual and reproductive behavior of American women, 1982–1988. Fam Plann Perspect. 1990;22:206–214.

Goldsheider C, Mosher WD. Patterns of contraceptive use in the United States: The importance of religious factors. Stud Fam Plann. 1991;22:102–115.

Grady WR, Haywood MD, Florcy FA. Contraceptive discontinuation among married women in the United States. Stud Fam Plann. 1988;19:227–235.

Harlap S, Kost K, Forrest JD. Preventing Pregnancy, Protecting Health: A New Look at Birth Control Choices in the United States. New York, NY: The Alan Guttmacher Institute; 1991.

Hatcher RA, Trussell J, Stewart F, Stewart GK, Kowal D, Guest F, Cates W, Policar MS. Contraceptive Technology, 16th revised ed. New York, NY: Irvington Publishers, Inc.; 1994.

Henshaw SK, Silverman J. The characteristics and prior contraceptive use of US abortion patients. Fam Plann Perspect. 1988;20:158–168.

Jones EF, et al. Unintended pregnancy, contraceptive practice and family planning services in developed countries. Fam Plann Perspect. 1988;20:53–67.

Jones EF, Forrest JD. Contraceptive failure rates based on the 1988 NSFG. Fam Plann Perspect. 1992;24:12–19.

Kaeser L. Reconsidering the age limits of pill use. Fam Plann Perspect. 1989;21:273–274.

Kost K, Forrest JF. American women's sexual behavior and exposure to risk of sexually transmitted diseases. Fam Plann Perspect. 1992;24:244–254.

Ku L, Sonenstein FL, Pleck JH. The dynamics of condom use among young men during and between sexual relationships. In press.

Ku L, Sonenstein F, Pleck J. Factors influencing first intercourse for teenage men. Public Health Rep. 1993a;108:680–694.

Ku L, Sonenstein FL, Pleck JH. Neighborhood, family and work: Influence on the premarital behaviors of adolescent males. Soc Forces. 1993b;72:479–503.

Ku L, Sonenstein FL, Pleck JH. Young men's risk behaviors for HIV infection and sexually transmitted diseases, 1988 through 1991. Am J Public Health. 1993c;83:1609–1615.

Ku L, Sonenstein F, Pleck JH. The association of AIDS education and sex education with sexual behavior and condom use among teenage men. Fam Plann Perspect. 1992;24: 100–106.

Landry DJ, Camelo TM. Young unmarried men and women discuss men's role in contraceptive practice. Fam Plann Perspect. 1994;26:222–227.

Laumann EO, Gagnon JH, Michael RT, Michaels S. The Social Organization of Sexuality: Sexual Practices in the United States. Chicago, IL: University of Chicago Press; 1994.

Miller WB, Shain RN, Pasta DJ. Tubal sterilization of vasectomy: How do married couples make the choice? Fertil Steril. 1991;56:278–284.

Moore KA, Nord CW, Peterson JL. Nonvoluntary sexual activity among adolescents. Fam Plann Perspect. 1989;21:110–114.

Mosher WD. Contraceptive practice in the US, 1982–1988. Fam Plann Perspect. 1990; 22:198–205.

Mosher WD, Bachrach CA. Contraceptive use, United States, 1980. Vital and Health Statistics, Series 23, No. 12. DHHS Pub. No. (PHS) 86-1988. Washington, DC: U.S. Government Printing Office; September 1986.

Mosher WD, McNally JW. Contraceptive use at first premarital intercourse: United States, 1965–1988. Fam Plann Perspect. 1991;23:108–116.

Mosher WD, Pratt WF. Contraceptive use in the United States, 1973–88. Advance Data from Vital and Health Statistics; No. 182. Hyattsville, MD: National Center for Health Statistics; 1990.

National Center for Health Statistics. Unpublished tables from the 1982 and 1988 National Survey of Family Growth.

Oakley D. Rethinking patient counselling techniques for changing contraceptive behavior. Am J Obstet Gynecol. 1994;170:1585–1590.

Ortho Pharmaceutical Company. Unpublished data from the 1994 Ortho Birth Control Study; 1994.

Peterson L. Contraceptive use in the United States: 1982–1990. Advance Data from Vital and Health Statistics; No. 260. Hyattsville, MD: National Center for Health Statistics; 1995.

Pleck JH, Sonenstein FL, Ku L. Changes in adolescent males' use of and attitudes toward condoms, 1988–1991. Fam Plann Perspect. 1993:25:106–110, 117.

Pleck JH, Sonenstein FL, Ku LC. Adolescent males' condom use: Relationships between perceived cost-benefits and consistency. J Marriage Fam. 1991;53:733–746.

Ross JA. Contraception: Short-term vs. long-term failure rates. Fam Plann Perspect. 1989;21:275–277.

Sonenstein FL, Pleck JH. The male role in family planning: What do we know? Paper prepared for the Committee on Unintended Pregnancy, Institute of Medicine. Washington, DC; 1994.

Sonenstein FL, Pleck JH, Ku LC. Sexual activity, condom use and AIDS awareness among adolescent males. Fam Plann Perspect. 1989;21:152–158.

Sonenstein FL, Pleck JH, Ku LC. Cost and Opportunity Factors Associated with Pregnancy Risk Among Adolescent Males. Paper presented at the Annual Meeting of the Population Association of America. Denver, CO; April 30, 1992.

Statistical Abstract of the United States, 1993. Table No. 109. Washington, DC: U.S. Department of Commerce; 1993.

Tanfer K, Grady WR, Klepinger DH, Billy JOG. Condom use among US men, 1991. Fam Plann Perspect. 1993;25:61–66.

Trussell J, Sturgen K, Strickler J, Dominik R. Comparative contraceptive efficacy of the female condom and other barrier methods. Fam Plann Perspect. 1994;26:66–72.

Trussell J, Vaughn B. Aggregate and lifetime contraceptive failure in the United States. Fam Plann Perspect. 1989;21:226.

Zelnik M, Kantner JF. Sexual and contraceptive experience of young unmarried women in the United States, 1976 and 1971. Fam Plann Perspect. 1977;9:55–61.

Zelnik M, Kantner JF. Sexual activity, contraceptive use and pregnancy among metropolitan-area teenagers: 1971–1979. Fam Plann Perspect. 1980;12:230–1, 233–237.

5

Basic Requirements: Contraceptive Knowledge and Access

The patterns of contraceptive use, misuse, and nonuse described in the previous chapter are troubling because a common result is unintended pregnancy. These patterns are also quite puzzling; with so many different contraceptive devices in existence, some widely available, even in drugstores, what is the explanation for inadequate contraceptive vigilance?

This chapter reviews two factors that might help to explain these observed patterns. The first is that inadequate use of contraception may be traceable in part to insufficient knowledge about methods of birth control and related issues of human reproduction, as well as to difficulty in mastering the skills that many reversible methods of contraception require. This section also considers the adequacy of school-based education and information about contraception.

The second issue considered is that access to contraceptive services and supplies—particularly for the more effective methods—may be limited. Later chapters discuss various personal and interpersonal factors that affect contraceptive use and therefore unintended pregnancy (Chapter 6), as well as the broader sociocultural and economic environments in which decisions about contraception and pregnancy are made (Chapter 7).

This focus on knowledge, skills, and access is not meant to obscure another possible explanation for unintended pregnancy, which is the relatively limited and often unsatisfactory array of contraceptive methods available to men and women in the United States. Experts in contraception and family planning, as well as men and women themselves, have long noted that the existing array of methods is often ill suited to the varying needs of couples and individuals over time, and that some methods are too difficult or unpleasant to use consistently, while others are too expensive or unsatisfactory in some other way. This underlying discontent with current contraceptive technology is at the heart of repeated calls for expanded research to develop new forms of contraception (Chapter 9).

It is also important to emphasize here that the committee considers knowledge about methods of birth control, as well as access to them, to be basic requirements for effective contraceptive use. This view is consistent with observations about such other preventive interventions as prenatal care and immunizations, where the point has been made that both knowledge and access are necessary preconditions to use (Institute of Medicine, 1994, 1988). However, as subsequent material suggests, these basic elements, on their own, may not be enough to produce careful and consistent use of contraception; they are necessary but may not always be sufficient to prevent unintended pregnancy. Put another way, it is unreasonable to expect widespread, careful use of contraception in the absence of basic knowledge and access to services, but this does not mean that when such pieces are in place good contraceptive use is guaranteed. This perspective is developed in more detail in Chapter 6.

KNOWLEDGE, SKILLS, AND SCHOOL-BASED EDUCATION

One of the explanations most often given for unintended pregnancy is that men and women, especially those who are teenagers, are poorly informed about contraception and related topics in reproductive health. Accordingly, this section considers that explanation and also addresses the skills needed to use many reversible methods. The section concludes with a discussion of school-based education and information about contraception.

Contraceptive Knowledge

Individuals learn about contraceptive methods, including their risks and benefits, as well as how to use them, from a wide variety of sources: friends and family, the electronic and print media, health professionals and the educational materials that they distribute, such institutions as schools and colleges, and numerous community resources. Unfortunately, few data are available to assess carefully the content and quality of the information provided in each of these settings. There are data about school-based sex education programs, summarized later in this chapter, but little on the content and quality of information available through the adolescent grapevine, for example. Few studies have addressed the education that parents offer their children about contraception, although some studies suggest that parents often do not discuss contraception with their children and that, in any event, such communication may not exert much of an effect on the child's subsequent use of contraception (Tanfer, 1994). Moreover, the information about media content—especially television—pertains more to its overall sexual content than to its information about contraception (Chapter 7).

There is, however, clear evidence that many Americans are misinformed about the risks and benefits of particular contraceptive methods—exaggerating the former and underestimating the latter, especially in the case of oral contraceptives. For example, a 1993 Gallup poll found that more than half of American women believe there are "substantial risks" (mainly cancer) involved in using the birth control pill, and 4 in 10 erroneously believe that the health risks of taking oral contraceptives are greater than those of childbearing (Gallup Organization, 1994). The widespread lack of knowledge among both providers and potential users regarding emergency contraception[1] is another indication that many Americans lack basic information about all available means of contraception (Grossman and Grossman, 1994; Trussell and Stewart, 1992).

Numerous smaller studies confirm this general picture. Balassone (1989), for example, conducted a prospective study of 76 sexually active teenaged women securing oral contraceptives at several private family planning clinics, and found that, in general, the young women underestimated the chances of pregnancy in the absence of contraception, and had inaccurate knowledge regarding the effectiveness of various contraceptive methods. In 1991, 247 women (mean age of 30.2 years) receiving care at a university health center were queried about their views of the benefits and risks of the pill. Almost half believed that oral contraceptives carry substantial risks, cancer in particular. Large percentages—between 80 and 95 percent—were unaware of the health benefits of oral contraceptives other than pregnancy prevention (e.g., the protective effect against benign breast disease, the reduced risk of both ovarian and endometrial cancer, and the lowered risk of pelvic inflammatory disease) (Peipert and Gutmann, 1993). Similarly, Lowe and Radius (1987) reported that "dangerous misconceptions" prevailed among unmarried college students with regard to knowledge of anatomy, physiology, and the appropriate use of effective contraception. And in their study sample of low-income black adolescents, Poland and Beane (1980) reported that teenagers articulated the common mythology that IUDs, for example, can "get lost in the body," and that

---

[1]Emergency contraception refers to using oral contraceptives or other hormones up to 72 hours after unprotected intercourse or inserting an intrauterine device (IUD) up to 7 days after unprotected intercourse. Emergency contraception via oral contraceptives reduces the risk of pregnancy by about 75 percent; emergency contraception accomplished via the post-coital insertion from an IUD is even more effective, approaching 100 percent. Though not recommended as a routine method of pregnancy prevention, emergency contraception can serve as an entry point for regular contraceptive care and use (Hatcher et al., 1995; Trussell and Stewart, 1992).

if pregnancy occurs with an IUD in place, the baby will be born with the device in it somewhere.

One reason that Americans are misinformed about contraception generally may be that the electronic media tend to report more of the bad news than the good news about various methods. Some data support this widely held view—especially the notion that the protective health benefits offered by various contraceptives are often underpublicized compared with the modest risks (Peipert and Gutmann, 1993; Adams Hillard, 1992). Clinic personnel report, for example, that adverse media coverage of Norplant has led to requests for removal of the implant, even among women who were experiencing no problems (Herman, 1994). Additional material is presented in Chapter 7 suggesting that although the electronic media present copious amounts of sexually enticing material, they rarely air complementary information on how to prevent such consequences of sexual activity as unintended pregnancy or sexually transmitted diseases (STDs).

Numerous studies of adolescents have clearly shown that many also have very limited and often faulty information about when fertility begins, the timing of fertility within the menstrual cycle, and the probability of conception (see, for example, Clark et al., 1984; Cvetkovich and Grote, 1983; Oskamp and Mindick, 1983; Foreit and Foreit, 1981). A common reason given by adolescents for nonuse of contraception is that on a given occasion, the risk of pregnancy was judged to be low because of the "time of month." Yet research has confirmed that a substantial proportion of those who cite time of month as the reason for foregoing contraception could not correctly identify the period of greatest risk (Tanfer, 1994).

It is not just adolescents who have incorrect information about human sexuality and contraception, however; adults may as well. When the Annie E. Casey Foundation began working in the early 1990s with groups of parents to improve their communication with young people about sex, contraception, and related topics to reduce teenage pregnancy (as part of the foundation's Plain Talk initiative), program leaders quickly learned that the parents themselves had major gaps in their knowledge about the topics at hand and that they needed help not only in communicating about sexual issues, but also in mastering basic information (S.L. Edwards, pers. com., 1994).

Polling data on STDs also suggest a widespread lack of accurate information regarding sexual health. In 1993, the Campaign for Women's Health and the American Medical Women's Association sponsored a poll (via telephone interviews with 1,000 randomly selected women aged 18–60) to learn more about American women's knowledge about STDs generally. Key findings included the following: 84 percent said they are not worried about contracting an STD (including 78 percent of those with multiple partners); 66 percent knew virtually nothing about STDs other than HIV and AIDS; only 1 in 10 reported being "very knowledgeable" about STDs; only 11 percent knew that many STDs can be more harmful to women's health than to men's; and 53 percent viewed STDs as a "dirty" disease that represents either shame or punishment (Campaign for Women's Health and American Medical Women's Association, 1994).

Such misinformation can lead to poor contraceptive use and therefore unintended pregnancy. A study in the mid-1980s, for example, probed reasons that sexually active teenage women delay making a first visit to a family planning clinic. Information was collected from more than 400 sexually active young women under age 19 attending family planning clinics and from about 400 sexually active female students at two junior and two senior high schools. Across all groups, one of the most commonly cited reasons for delay in attending a family planning clinic was that contraception is "dangerous." For example, among those who had never gone to a clinic at all, 19 percent cited this reason as the most important factor explaining their delay, and an additional 45 percent listed it as a "contributing" factor (Zabin et al., 1991). Similarly, in the Balassone (1989) study mentioned earlier, the subjects least likely to continue using oral contraceptives at 3 months' follow-up were those who believed that there were appreciable health-related problems associated with using oral contraceptives, felt that their risk of pregnancy was less than that of their peers, and had poor problem-solving skills. Chapter 6 presents more detailed information on the fears, attitudes, and feelings that can influence contraceptive use.

In sum, there is significant misinformation among both adults and adolescents about the risks and benefits of contraception. This lack of knowledge can limit efforts to obtain contraception and continue using it, thereby increasing the risk of unintended pregnancy.

Contraceptive Skills

Knowledge about contraception is particularly important because many reversible methods of contraception require considerable skill for proper use. Patient package inserts, education and counseling sessions at many birth control clinics, and various popular books attempt to educate users about the nitty-gritty of how to use specific methods and how to manage problems that are commonly encountered. But practitioners in the field, such as workers in family planning clinics, report that there is great variation in the abilities of clients to use methods properly and that there may not be adequate appreciation of the difficulty faced in mastering the mechanics of contraception (Quint et al., 1994). To use a diaphragm correctly, for example, one must know at a minimum where to go to get the method, how to insert the device properly and to check its position, how much spermicide to apply, how many hours after intercourse to remove it, how to insert additional spermicide into the vagina if repeated intercourse will occur while the diaphragm is still in place, and how to check for holes or tears in the device. Moreover, this information must be used properly each time that the diaphragm is employed, and the user must be willing to forego intercourse or use alternative methods of contraception if the diaphragm is unavailable for some reason. An equally long list of complexities is attached to oral contraceptive use (Oakley, 1994), as noted in Chapter 4. Rarely do contraceptive counselors have the time to cover all of these issues or to reinforce key messages through follow-up, which is one of the reasons that the longer-acting methods (such as hormonal implants and injections) continue to attract interest. Reflecting these difficulties, Adams Hillard (1992) reports that adolescents miss taking an average of three pills monthly and between 20 and 30 percent of all users of oral contraceptives miss a pill every month.

The complexity of the contraceptive task may also be one of the reasons that some studies have shown a link between education, cognitive functioning, and unintended pregnancy—specifically, that contraceptive use increases with education. With more years of schooling, a woman may be better equipped to understand the risks and benefits of becoming pregnant, to make plans to reduce that risk, and then to execute those plans. Consistent with this view, in a national sample of never-married women in their 20s at risk of pregnancy, when the effects of other social and demographic variables were controlled, education was found to be associated not only with better contraceptive use but also with the choice of more effective methods (Tanfer et al., 1992). Among urban female adolescents attending family planning clinics, the stage of cognitive development was found to be the best predictor of contraceptive decision-making (Sachs, 1985). Several studies have also shown that better educated or high-income women who use less effective methods use them more effectively than less educated or low-income women who use the same methods (Jones and Forrest, 1992, 1989; Grady et al., 1986, 1983; Schirm et al., 1982).

School-Based Education and Information

One source of contraceptive information and education that has been studied more thoroughly than others is schools. Most school-based sex education programs can be categorized into one of four types: (1) those that try to increase knowledge about reproductive health and especially about all methods of pregnancy prevention including abstinence, and emphasize the risk and consequences of pregnancy; (2) those that do the same and add material on "values clarification" and skills in communicating and decision-making; (3) those that advocate abstinence but do not discuss contraception; and (4) those that accompany comprehensive education in reproductive health with clinical services including family planning care. In both this section of the report and elsewhere (Chapter 8 especially), various aspects of these approaches are discussed.

Public opinion and public policy both support a strong role for schools in educating young people about human sexuality, whatever the controversies in some communities. The American College of Obstetricians and Gynecologists, for example, commissioned the Gallup Organization to conduct a study of public knowledge of and attitudes toward contraception. This 1985 study of 1,036 women and 520 men aged 18 and over showed that approximately 90 percent of the adult population wanted sex education to be taught in schools. Fifty-four percent of women and 47 percent of men wanted it to start in elementary school; 81 percent of women and 74 percent of men wanted sex education to start before high school (American College of Obstetricians and Gynecologists, 1985). Similarly, the Sexuality Information and Education Council of the United States reports that there is strong public support for sexuality education, including explicit instruction about contraception and STD prevention. More than 8 in 10 adults support teaching about sexuality in the public schools; more than 9 in 10 want AIDS education for their children. Seventy-seven percent think that courses for 12-year-olds should include information about birth control. Almost two-thirds say that courses should include information about abortion, sexual intercourse, and premarital sex (Debra and DeMauro, 1990). Parents of students show their support for sexuality education in other ways. When given the option of excusing their children from sexuality education classes, less than 5 percent do so (Haffner, 1994).

Mirroring public opinion, 47 states either recommend or mandate sexuality education; every state recommends or mandates AIDS education; and 38 states plus the District of Columbia and Puerto Rico have developed either state curricula or guidelines to shape the implementation of programs at the local level. Almost all state curriculum guides include abstinence messages as well as positive and affirming statements about human sexuality; topics most commonly covered are body image, reproductive anatomy, puberty, decision-making skills, families, abstinence, STDs, HIV and AIDS, sexual abuse, and gender roles (Haffner, 1994).

Despite the public support and state policies, available school-based information and education about human sexuality in general and contraception in particular are insufficient in a number of ways. First, while it is true that many states require schools to provide sexuality education and HIV/AIDS education to students at different grade levels, it is also the case that in many states, the content of those educational programs is limited by statute or by state policy or both (The Alan Guttmacher Institute, 1989). The precise nature of these restrictions can serve to limit the effectiveness of the educational programs by, for example, prohibiting explicit discussion of topics directly related to pregnancy prevention, such as contraception.

Second, a recent survey of state sexuality education curricula and guidelines revealed important gaps. The survey found that although contraception is included in a majority of the state guides, the coverage is often incomplete. Only

10 states have unambiguous messages about contraception at the junior high school level, and Iowa alone clearly includes introductory material at the elementary grade level. Only three states include coverage of contraception at both the junior and senior high levels, and condoms are mentioned in just five state curriculum guides. States vary as to which details they discuss concerning contraception, from simply identifying the concept to explaining the range of contraceptive techniques and relative effectiveness. Discussing contraceptive use with a partner is rarely covered. A 1992 study of HIV and AIDS education programs nationwide found a similar lack of prevention information; only five states adequately discussed condom use (Haffner, 1994). Moreover, it is apparent that many of the available instructional materials, particularly those provided by state agencies, are inadequate, as is the training provided to teachers of sexuality education (The Alan Guttmacher Institute, 1989). For example, a 1987 survey of secondary school sex education teachers found clear evidence of misinformation about various methods of contraception; 77 percent held the erroneous belief that women taking oral contraceptives should stop from time to time to "give the body a rest" (Forrest and Silverman, 1989).

A different, slightly dated analysis, the National Longitudinal Survey of Youth (NLSY)—a survey of a nationally representative sample of more than 12,000 young people aged 14–22 in 1979, who were reinterviewed in 1984 at ages 19–27—paints an equally checkered picture. Marsiglio and Mott (1986) found that by age 19, a bare majority (60 percent of the men and 52 percent of the women) reported that they had taken a sex education course in school, although the probability of having taken a sex education course in early adolescence was seen to increase over time. Even those who had taken a course, however, revealed important gaps in knowledge about such basic issues as when in a woman's menstrual cycle she is relatively more and less fertile.

One of the most important and sobering findings of the NLSY is that many teenagers become sexually active before having taken a sex education class. The investigators concluded: "Among young people who waited until age 18 to start having sex, 61 percent of women and 52 percent of men had already been exposed to a sex education course . . . ; but among those who started at 16 or younger, fewer than half—in the case of males, considerably fewer—had taken a course. Furthermore, only 35 percent of young people who became sexually active at age 18 had previously received course instruction about where to obtain contraceptives, and only about 57 percent of the more limited group of course takers had received such instruction" (Marsiglio and Mott, 1986:160).

The issue of the *effects* of such instruction on the sexual and reproductive behavior of young people has been passionately debated, with opponents claiming that it actually increases the level of sexual activity which in turn leads to nonmarital pregnancy and other problems, and proponents denying any such effect and claiming that it probably reduces the rate of pregnancy by promoting more effective contraceptive practice. It is difficult for research to resolve this debate definitively because of the wide variation in the content and depth of the sex education offered, differences in the research definitions of "sex education," the reluctance of schools and agencies to allow evaluation of the effects of such courses, and deficiencies in some study designs (Furstenberg et al., 1985; Kirby, 1984; Scales, 1981; Spanier, 1976).

There are, however, several bodies of information that shed light on this topic. National survey data present mixed results, but indicate that adolescents who receive sex education are more likely to use contraception than those who do not receive such instruction (Ku et al., 1993, 1992; Dawson, 1986; Marsiglio and Mott, 1986; Furstenberg et al., 1985; Zelnik and Kim, 1982). Retrospective surveys, however, cannot provide causal associations; such associations can only be made through evaluations with experimental or quasi-experimental designs. Unfortunately, few evaluations are so methodologically rigorous, and most fail to measure behavior change and long-term program effects (Chapter 8).

In an attempt to address the lack of rigorous assessment, Kirby (1984) used quasi-experimental designs to evaluate 15 well-regarded sex education curricula from the 1970s and early 1980s. He concluded that the programs did increase knowledge about various topics in reproductive health, but did not change sexual behavior or contraceptive use.

This discouraging picture appears to be changing. In a 1994 review, Kirby and colleagues suggest that both programs and evaluation methods have improved. Evidence from more than 20 surveys and studies of school-based sex and HIV and AIDS education programs indicates that specific programs delayed the initiation of intercourse, reduced the frequency of intercourse, reduced the number of sexual partners, or increased the use of contraceptives. In addition, available data indicate clearly that participation in these sexuality education programs has not been found to encourage adolescents to initiate sexual intercourse, or to increase the frequency of intercourse among adolescents who were sexually active before the program.

The sex education programs reviewed by Kirby and colleagues (1994) clustered into three types: (1) abstinence-only programs that do not discuss contraception, (2) sexuality or AIDS education programs that discuss both abstinence and contraception, and (3) programs that provide comprehensive reproductive health education covering many topics including contraception and abstinence, as well as clinical services. Abstinence-only programs appear to affect attitudes regarding premarital intercourse, but the few evaluations that measure behavior change are limited by methodological problems, and there is insufficient evidence to determine whether abstinence programs delay the age of first intercourse or affect other sexual and contraceptive behaviors. Effects of programs of the second type are mixed, but those that most successfully delay sexual intercourse or increase contraceptive use appear to focus on the "particular facts, values, norms, and skills necessary to avoid sex or unprotected sex" (Kirby et al., 1994:355). The impact of school-based or school-linked reproductive health services is inconclusive, but the largest behavioral effects are observed in sites with strong educational components. Although these programs may not represent the average school-based sex education curriculum in current use (see, for example, Firestone, 1994), many communities are attempting to replicate the more effective models in new sites. In Chapter 8, several of these carefully evaluated programs are discussed in more detail.

A final point needs to be made. Whatever the merits of the various school-based programs being developed around the country, there are virtually no parallel programs for older men and women. Perhaps there is an unstated national belief that adults already know enough about reproduction, contraception, and related topics, or that what they do not know they can find out. Perhaps the absence of an institutional base, like the school system, for offering education about reproductive health to adults explains the gap. Whatever the reason, inadequate contraceptive use is seen in all age groups, not just adolescents, and therefore adults too may benefit from better information and education in this area.

ACCESS TO CONTRACEPTION

To what extent is inconsistent or nonuse of contraception, and therefore unintended pregnancy, due to a lack of access to birth control services and supplies? In particular, to what extent is there limited access to the more effective methods of birth control, leading couples to rely on less effective methods which, by definition, have higher failure rates?

Unfortunately, answering these questions is difficult because access varies by the method being considered (condoms versus hormonal implants, for example), and because contraception can be secured through a variety of sources and systems—from pharmacies and condom boutiques to clinics, hospital centers, and private physician offices. Nonetheless, this topic attracts strong opinions on both sides. On the one hand, some have argued that, with condoms and spermicides available in virtually every drugstore, allegations of limited access to contraception are clearly fatuous. On the other hand, public health analysts point with alarm to the decline in constant dollar support for the Title X program (the family planning grant program authorized under the Public Health Service Act that targets reproductive health services to low-income women and adolescents) (Ku, 1993; Gold and Daley, 1991), and to the major financial barriers to care that women may experience, both those with private health insurance and those without, when they try to obtain the more effective methods of contraception (Kaeser and Richards, 1994).

There is widespread agreement, however, that whatever access problems exist, they pertain more to methods requiring a medical visit, such as oral contraceptives, than to nonprescription methods such as condoms or spermicides, which can be secured from many different types of facilities. Condoms in particular are increasingly available through a particularly wide variety of sources, including vending machines, largely in response to concern over the spread of various STDs including AIDS. Unfortunately, these nonprescription methods have significant failure rates and therefore appreciable rates of unintended pregnancy are associated with them. Nonetheless, they do provide more protection against unintended pregnancy than no method at all, and as such are an important part of pregnancy prevention. In this context, it is important to note that the number of nonprescription contraceptive devices—never very large—has recently been depleted by the removal of the contraceptive sponge from the market, leaving condoms and spermicides as the only nonprescription methods now available.

The importance of inquiring carefully into contraceptive access is suggested by international comparisons of contraceptive use and various markers of unintended pregnancy and abortion. For example, a cross-national study completed by The Alan Guttmacher Institute considered the factors that might help to explain the higher rates of adolescent pregnancy, abortion, and childbearing in the United States as compared with those in various other industrialized countries (Chapter 2). One of the main conclusions of that analysis was that in those countries reporting more favorable rates, contraceptive services were apparently widely available, confidential, and very inexpensive, if not free (Jones et al., 1986). An additional analysis that examined adults as well as adolescents elaborated on this observation. The investigators concluded that contraceptive use—and, in particular, use of the more effective methods—was favorably affected by such factors as the presence of a national health plan or health care system that includes family planning services and that covers all citizens; the full integration of family planning services into general health care services, rather than such services being separate or specialist-based; the fact that family planning clinics are seen as serving all women, not just those who are poor or adolescent; the availability of free or subsidized supplies (oral contraceptives in particular); and supportive attitudes among providers (especially relevant to the prevalence of sterilization) (Jones et al., 1989). The importance of ease of access to contraceptive care also emerged from a comparison of U.S. and Danish family planning policies and practices. David and colleagues (1990) report that all people born or living in Denmark are entitled to free contraceptive counseling from a variety of sources, including the network of general practitioners who encourage the use of the more effective methods of contraception and make them readily available.

Other cross-national comparisons are consistent with these perspectives (Klaus, 1993). Miller (1993, 1988), for example, suggests that the more favorable rates reported by numerous Western European and other industrialized countries on such maternal and child health measures as infant mortality reflect, in part, the more generous policies and benefits that these countries offer pregnant women and young families. It may be that these supportive policies also make women less inclined to recall pregnancies as unwanted or mistimed. They may also help to encourage better contraceptive use, as evidenced by their lower rates of unintended pregnancy (Chapter 2), both by enhancing access to family planning services and by strengthening the consensus that pregnancy and childbearing are too important to be undertaken casually, accidentally, or unintentionally.

Data on Overall Access

A variety of data sets are available to consider recent trends in access to contraceptive services. In the aggregate they give a mixed picture. Using the National Survey of Family Growth (NSFG), Mosher (1990) concluded that the proportion of all women aged 15–44 who have had one or more "family planning visits" in the preceding year did not change significantly between 1982 (37 percent) and 1988 (35 percent), and that this evidence of little or no change held across all age and income groups.

However, investigators at the Center for Health Economics Research, using the same data set, recalculated the proportions who had had a family planning visit on the basis of the number of women in each category who were estimated to be sexually active (or were planning to be), and concluded that, among this subset, there was an important decline in family planning visits among teenagers and among both poor (below 200 percent of the poverty level) and nonpoor women between 1982 and 1988. For example, they calculated that of sexually active women under age 20 in 1982, 65 percent had had a family planning visit in the preceding year, versus 57 percent in 1988; for poor women, the figure was 46 percent in 1982 and 42 percent in 1988 (Robert Wood Johnson Foundation and the Center for Health Economics Research, 1993). The investigators believe that these data reflect increased problems with access to contraceptive services (although they may also reflect decreased interest in securing contraception).

Bits of information from various parts of the country suggest that access to the more effective methods of contraception—that is, those requiring some sort of contact with the health care system—may be constrained, particularly in the public sector. For example, in December 1992 and January 1993, a team from the New York City Mayor's Advisory Council on Child Health called 115 service sites that offer family planning care in the city to request an appointment for contraceptive services; one-third of the callers were not able to make an appointment at all, and the rest confronted significant difficulties and delays. The authors concluded that because the family planning system was so underfunded and poorly organized, access was very limited and that, in addition, succeeding in the task of making a family planning appointment in the New York City system requires "motivation, persistence, and fortitude" (Mayor's Advisory Council on Child Health, 1993). Additional material on this study appears later in this chapter.

A somewhat similar 1994 report of Colorado family planning clinics noted an average wait of three weeks for a contraceptive appointment; reducing this wait by, for example, opening weekend or evening clinics, was not possible given available resources (J. Henneberry to J. DeSarno, pers. com., 1994). And in the District of Columbia, some family planning clinics report waiting times of over 25 working days between the first call and an appointment (R.S. Guy, pers. com., 1994).

Adolescents may face particular barriers in obtaining the more effective methods of contraception owing to variations among providers regarding the circumstances under which they will provide family planning services to adolescents, especially if there is no parental involvement. Some providers, for example, decline to offer contraceptive care to adolescents because of insufficient knowledge about legal requirements in this area; others may object to offering contraceptive care to minors without parental consent. Although the Title X program was designed in part to increase access to contraception among adolescents, the limited financing and reach of that program means that access barriers continue to exist for this age group in some communities.

Nonetheless, it is important to mention again that most women not actively seeking pregnancy use contraception, and as a general matter, contraceptive use has increased in recent years, including among men (Chapter 4). Among those few women who are not seeking pregnancy but are not using any method of contraception, the vast majority have used a method at some point. Based on a 1993 follow-up telephone interview of women aged 20–41 from the 1993 National Survey of Women (NSW), Sonenstein and colleagues (1994) recently reported that 80 percent had had a "reproductive health visit" (defined to include contraceptive care, if desired) in the past year—a figure that rose to 90 percent for a visit in the past two years. Data such as these suggest that, in one way or another, most women and men have found ways to secure and use one or more methods of birth control.

The problem with this more favorable picture is that even if most people use contraception most of the time, and even if access to the best methods of contraception is more or less adequate in most places, the net result will be an appreciable level of unintended pregnancy, given the relative ease with which pregnancy occurs. Preventing pregnancy requires scrupulous use of the best methods—not some of the time but all of the time. Therefore, even modest problems in access to contraception, as available data certainly suggest, are enough to facilitate unintended pregnancy.

In the next several subsections, some specific factors that may limit access to contraception are explored: various financial issues including contraceptive pricing and public investment in family planning services, problems in the provider base for contraception, and general bureaucratic complexities. The next main section explores the proposition that many opportunities to provide contraceptive information and services are being missed.

Financial Barriers

As is the case for a wide variety of health care interventions (see, for example, Stoddard et al., 1994), insurance coverage affects access to contraception (Kirkman-Liff and Korenfeld, 1994). For example, in the 1993 NSW survey of more than 1,000 women aged 21–40 mentioned earlier, Sonenstein and colleagues (1994) found that whether or not a reproductive health visit had occurred was heavily influenced by the presence of health insurance and a regular source of care. Overall, 20 percent of the sample had not had a reproductive health visit in the past year; however, for those without a regular source of care, the figure was 39 percent; for those without health insurance altogether, the figure was 42 percent.

Private Insurance

With regard to private insurance, the 1988 NSFG revealed that, overall, private insurance does not lie behind most family planning visits. In that year, about 41 percent of all women who received family planning services reported paying for their most recent visit out of their own pockets. Another 17 percent said they used insurance with a copayment or deductible. Insurance completely covered only 25 percent of recent visits, and 7 percent of visits were covered by Medicaid. The remaining services were provided at no charge to the client (Kaeser and Richards, 1994).

This modest presence of private insurance as a financing source for contraceptive services is consistent with the historic traditions of private-sector health insurance coverage—providing coverage of surgical services but not covering preventive care. A 1994 study by The Alan Guttmacher Institute of the coverage of reproductive health services in various insurance and financing plans concluded that although 85 percent or more of typical private health insurance policies cover sterilization services and 66 percent cover abortion, coverage of reversible contraception was appreciably thinner. None of the five reversible methods included in the study—intrauterine devices (IUDs), diaphragms, hormonal implants and injectables (e.g., Norplant and Depo-Provera), and oral contraceptives—is routinely covered by more than 40 percent of typical plans. Furthermore, half of the large-group plans cover no methods at all, and only 15 percent cover all five. Notably, even though oral contraceptives, the most commonly used reversible method, are routinely covered by only one-third of large-group plans, this did not result from a failure to cover prescription drugs. Although virtually all of the plans typically cover prescription drugs, two-thirds of these do not routinely cover oral contraceptives. Similarly, although more than 90 percent of the plans typically cover medical devices in general, less than 20 percent of these plans cover IUDs or diaphragms and 25 percent cover hormonal implants. In addition, the study found that less than a fourth of the plans routinely cover contraceptive counseling (The Alan Guttmacher Institute, 1994). Thus, many privately insured women who need contraceptive care must go out of plan and pay for it themselves, use over-the-counter methods that may be less effective, or not use any method at all.

Health Maintenance Organizations

Demonstrating their emphasis on preventive care, many health maintenance organizations (HMOs)—although not all—provide more comprehensive coverage for contraception than do typical fee-for-service plans. Only 7 percent of HMOs provide no coverage at all, and 40 percent cover all five methods noted above. Still, coverage of the various methods is far from uniform or complete, from 59 percent for Norplant insertion, to 84 percent for oral contraceptives, to 86 percent for IUD insertion. However, coverage of contraceptive counseling is routinely covered by at least 90 percent of HMOs. Even though HMOs cover a wider range of contraceptive services than do private plans, they nonetheless frequently require copayments for those services, which may serve as a deterrent for some women (The Alan Guttmacher Institute, 1994). In addition, adolescents especially may be reluctant to obtain contraceptive care as a dependent in a managed care setting, fearing that confidentiality will not always be maintained.

It is important to stress that these data on HMOs do not necessarily reflect the practices of all managed care arrangements, including both Medicaid managed care systems and for-profit networks. There are an increasing number and variety of such arrangements, but no data are available to assess how they address contraceptive services and supplies. Particularly in systems that are highly cost-competitive, coverage of both preventive services and prescription drugs (within which many of the more effective reversible methods of contraception fall) may be limited.

Public Sector Programs

In contrast to private insurance coverage and HMOs, the Medicaid programs of all 50 states and the District of Columbia provide reimbursement for contraceptive services, as required by law. Moreover, since the late 1980s,

Medicaid has become the principal source of public funding for contraceptive services, accounting for 58 percent of all federal family planning expenditures (and 43 percent of all public family planning expenditures), or approximately $270 million in 1990. Between 1984 and 1991, Medicaid spending for family planning services increased 41 percent and the number of clients served increased 31 percent (Ku, 1993). Nevertheless, as noted earlier, only 7 percent of all family planning visits are covered by Medicaid (Kaeser and Richards, 1994).

Women who use Medicaid to obtain family planning services do so in a wide variety of settings, from private physician offices to public clinics. Unfortunately, no systematic data are available to determine whether Medicaid-enrolled women who try to obtain prescription-based methods of contraception have appreciable difficulty in finding a provider who will accept them and their payment source. However, this problem has clearly affected access to prenatal care and to many other services as well. Although federal law requires states to set reimbursement rates in the Medicaid program that are adequate to ensure the participation of sufficient numbers of providers, particularly those providing pediatric services and services to pregnant women, this requirement has not been enforced effectively (Institute of Medicine, 1988). The increasing tendency to place the Medicaid population in managed care networks has undoubtedly affected their overall ability to obtain health services, but the direction of the change, and how access to contraception in particular has been affected, is not yet well understood (National Academy of Social Insurance, 1994).

Not all low-income women qualify for Medicaid. In most states, Medicaid coverage is tied to eligibility for Aid to Families with Dependent Children (AFDC), which usually means that a woman must be single and have at least one child. Furthermore, Medicaid eligibility levels in many states are extremely low—nationwide, the average income eligibility level is an income that is 50 percent of the poverty level, or $5,945 a year for a family of three. In recent years, Congress has passed a series of measures that were intended to help break the link between AFDC and Medicaid by allowing pregnant, low-income women and their young children with incomes up to 133 percent of the poverty level (and, at the state's option, up to 185 percent) to qualify for Medicaid, even if they were not receiving AFDC. The recent increases in Medicaid as a financing source for contraceptive services may reflect, in part, these eligibility expansions. Pregnant women who would not otherwise qualify for Medicaid (i.e., non-AFDC recipients) remain eligible for 60 days postpartum; thus, during that period, women are covered by Medicaid for family planning services. After 60 days, however, their coverage ends, unless states cover these services themselves, meaning that Medicaid cannot be relied on as a steady source of contraceptive financing for the most effective methods, except for the poorest women (Kaeser and Richards, 1994).

Adolescents may find it especially difficult to rely on Medicaid as a financing source for contraception. Even after the eligibility expansions of the 1980s, noted just above, states are only required to cover individuals (who are not pregnant, postpartum, under age six, or linked through a categorical program such as AFDC or Supplemental Security Income [SSI]) up to 100 percent of the federal poverty level if they are born after September 30, 1983. This means that all adolescents up to age 19 do not have to be covered until the year 2002. Even in those states that have chosen to provide Medicaid coverage to the poor and low-income adolescent population at an earlier date, adolescents may experience particular difficulty establishing Medicaid eligibility or utilizing Medicaid coverage independently of their parents and thus may be unable or unwilling to rely on Medicaid as a source of funding for the family planning services they need. The limited enrollment of adolescents in the Early and Periodic Screening, Diagnosis and Treatment program within Medicaid also suggests that the full potential of this part of the Medicaid program for providing teenagers with contraceptive services, including on-going assessment and counseling, has not yet been realized.

Many women with Medicaid coverage, as well as women with neither private health insurance nor Medicaid coverage, secure family planning care through a network of almost 5,500 clinics that obtain an appreciable portion of their funds from public sources, including the Title X program, and the Maternal and Child Health Services Block Grant, as well as the Title XX Social Services Block Grant, and federal, state, and local funds. Of these clinics, more than 4,000 receive some Title X funds (Henshaw and Torres, 1994). Anyone may seek services at a Title X-funded clinic; lower-income women may receive free services depending on their ability to pay. By law, women, including adolescents, whose incomes fall below 100 percent of the poverty level must receive fully subsidized services; women whose incomes are between 100 and 250 percent of the poverty level may receive services on a sliding-scale basis. Women whose incomes are above that level must pay the clinic's full fee, which is usually less than would be charged by a private practitioner.

A recent study of this network of clinics assessed trends in their sources and amounts of public support. Major conclusions included the following: for these clinics, Title X funding fell by roughly half between 1981 and 1991, after adjusting for inflation, and their overall level of federal revenue (including Medicaid and several other federal sources as well) fell 38 percent over this same interval; Title XX (Social Services Block Grant) funding for these clinics took a particularly sharp decline. This loss of federal funds was cushioned by growth in various other revenue sources; for example, funding from state and local sources grew by 112 percent and private revenue climbed 82 percent (again, in constant dollars). The net effect of these many changes was that the total revenue available to this clinic system from all sources, both public and private, fell 6 percent, from $518 million in 1981 to $485 million in 1991 (using

1991 constant dollars) (Ku, 1993). These findings are generally consistent with an earlier analysis, using a somewhat different set of data and definitions, which found that public expenditures for family planning declined by a third between 1980 and 1990 (Gold and Daley, 1991). Unfortunately, data are not available on trends in the total dollar amount spent in the United States for family planning services in general.

Curiously, this net decline in public investment was not reflected in declining numbers of clients receiving care in this clinic system. Ku (1993) reports that the number of women receiving care rose 17 percent between 1981 and 1991, from 3.8 million to 4.5 million. Although there is much speculation about the meaning of serving more clients through family planning clinics with less money (was the quality of care compromised? did clinics become more efficient? were important ancillary services reduced?), the precise impact is still under investigation.

The decline in public support, variously measured, is troubling given the evidence that, as Donovan (1991) has noted, clinics are "facing higher costs and sicker patients." For example, the Family Planning Council of Southeastern Pennsylvania reported in 1991 that it now spends more on medicines to treat STDs than on contraceptive methods—just the opposite of the case 5 to 8 years ago; and in the state of New York, visits to family planning clinics for treatment of STDs since 1984 have risen almost 80 percent. These reports are mirrored around the nation as the number and spread of STDs escalate.

Moreover, the costs incurred by family planning clinics have risen sharply in recent years. In 1992, new rules were issued to implement the Clinical Laboratories Improvement Act, a sweeping reform of the nation's clinical laboratory system. Depending on the complexity of the tests performed at a clinic, compliance with the new regulations on hiring of new personnel, retraining, new administrative costs, and annual registration and inspection fees that in many cases had not been budgeted, costs rose by up to $3,000 per site. Pap smears in particular reflect these rising costs. For example, 25 agencies in Colorado funded by the state health department to do family planning paid $200,000 to $300,000 more in 1991 for Pap tests than they did in 1990. Another set of regulations implementing the new Occupational Safety and Health Act standards on blood-borne diseases may also have added new costs to family planning clinics. One Title X grantee, Planned Parenthood of Wisconsin, estimated the total costs of complying with the regulations for its clinic network at $64,425, or approximately $1,611 per clinic for each of its 40 clinics (Kaeser and Richards, 1994).

Contraceptive Pricing

One particular aspect of financial barriers that merits mention is the possibility that the cost to consumers of various methods of contraception may affect method choice and, in particular, limit access. Common sense suggests that pricing affects choice of method, but few data are available from the United States to understand the dimensions of this influence on contraceptive use generally or on the choice of method in particular (see Appendix G for a discussion of selected cost issues).

Policymakers and family planning program administrators believe that consumer cost affects access and use, as demonstrated by the policy of "public sector pricing" of contraceptive devices. Some U.S. pharmaceutical companies offer oral contraceptives (OCs) at a significantly reduced price to various nonprofit and public family planning programs (e.g., Planned Parenthood, Title X programs, and other public sector clinics), thereby allowing them to provide OCs to clinic clients at well below market price or provide them for free. Program leaders believe that offering such prescription methods at low or no cost increases their use, particularly given the heavy representation in these clinics of low-income women and adolescents.[2]

Recently, the pricing of contraceptives has been questioned in relationship to both the cost of manufacturing some methods and the relative public–private investment in their development. With regard to the first issue, for example, the production cost for each monthly cycle of OCs is typically in the range of $0.15, based on the cost of bulk purchasing by the U.S. Agency for International

---

[2]This special pricing arrangement is one of the reasons that concern has been raised about approving OCs for over-the-counter sale, as has recently been proposed by a number of groups (Samuels et al., 1994). Under such a new arrangement, the special pricing system would undoubtedly end because clinics would presumably be much less involved in purchasing and providing OCs. This would translate into a loss of income to public sector clinics inasmuch as the special arrangement does provide these clinics with limited funds to help cover the expenses incurred in providing OCs to their patients. There is also concern that without the requirement of a medical visit, women would seek out and receive less counselling about contraception and perhaps less medical care as well, such as screening for STDs. Moreover, OCs are currently covered by Medicaid and some private insurance companies (although not by most); were OCs to be provided over-the-counter, this coverage would no longer apply, thereby increasing the out-of-pocket cost of obtaining OCs for women who had previously relied on these payment sources to help cover the costs of their OCs (A. Rosenfield, pers. com., 1994). Despite these many concerns, over-the-counter sale would undoubtedly increase access to this highly effective method.

Development, yet the current market price to consumers in New York and elsewhere is around $20 per cycle (A. Rosenfield, pers. com., 1994).

With regard to the second issue, a number of critics have argued that the pricing of Norplant (about $365) may not adequately reflect the substantial investment of the U.S. government in developing the method, and that the original price per Norplant kit was in excess of costs and seemed to be based only on what a consumer would pay for five years of OCs (which are roughly similar in effectiveness to Norplant) (A. Rosenfield, pers. com., 1994). Although a public sector pricing structure for Norplant is now being developed, its details are not yet clear, and field experience continues to suggest that the high cost of the device remains a barrier to its use (Frost, 1994), particularly because the base charge of $365 is often supplemented by additional insertion fees and other charges, which may bring the total to well over $500 or more. Although all 50 states and the District of Columbia offer Medicaid financing for Norplant insertion, many low-income women are not eligible for Medicaid and have no private health insurance coverage. For them, Norplant is accessible only if sliding fee scales are available, typically in publicly subsidized clinics, or the out-of-pocket costs are manageable (Kaeser, 1994). Moreover, as noted above, private insurance coverage as well as the coverage offered by HMOs and other systems can be spotty.

The issue of Norplant removal has recently become more visible as exemplified by a recent class action liability lawsuit based on alleged removal problems. For a variety of reasons, including recent television programming that has stressed the undesirable side effects of Norplant, many facilities are reporting an increase in requests for removal. Some state Medicaid programs will not pay for the removal of a device inserted while a woman was on Medicaid if, at the time she requests removal, she is no longer enrolled in Medicaid; other restrictions may apply as well. In response, some clinics serving predominantly low-income women (such as the Los Angeles Regional Family Planning Council) have created special funds to help finance the removal of the implants.

The Provider Base for Contraception

This section considers the possibility that access to contraception may be constrained by the limited training offered to physicians and other health professionals regarding contraception. The importance of provider training is confirmed by data on access to Norplant. Frost (1994) reported that of those organized family planning providers (i.e., clinics, not private physicians) who were not able to offer the implant to their clients, 60 percent suggested that the absence of a person trained in insertion and removal was a major contributing factor.

Even though obstetrician-gynecologists, internists, and general and family practitioners are the most common physician providers of contraceptive information and services to women and men, the guidelines for these specialties include very little *required* training in the general area of pregnancy prevention. Moreover, there is limited attention in training programs to the special needs or preferences of various groups at especially high risk of unintended pregnancy. Adolescents, for example, often require carefully designed, age-appropriate services and counseling that may be appreciably different from the services offered to adult men and women. Although specialists in adolescent medicine receive training about just these sensitivities, most physicians do not. Accreditation requirements for postgraduate training, established by the Accreditation Council for Graduate Medical Education (ACGME), are often vague regarding knowledge necessary to offer comprehensive contraceptive services, including adequate counseling and education for various groups who may have special needs. For example, the current requirements for residency training in obstetrics and gynecology state only that education must include "clinical skills in family planning," leaving the content of the curriculum open to variation (American Medical Association, 1994). ACGME has recently revised these requirements to be more comprehensive, stating that programs "must provide a structured didactic and clinical training experience in all methods of family planning" (Accreditation Council for Graduate Medical Education, 1995). These new provisions will become effective in January 1996.

Because the ACGME requirements are presently so nonspecific, residency programs have inconsistent standards for their contraceptive training. The repercussions of these varied standards are evident in a 1993 survey of obstetrics and gynecology residency program directors and chief residents across the country. In that survey, less than two-thirds (63 percent) of program directors indicated the presence of a faculty member associated with their program having a special interest in family planning, and only 13 percent of surveyed programs included an official family planning rotation. Although some programs allowed students to seek training in contraception and abortion in affiliated or nearby clinics, time constraints and other reasons prevented many students from doing so. Consequently, 38 percent of the students queried had never inserted an intrauterine device, 11 percent had never fitted a diaphragm, and an additional 43 percent had fitted a diaphragm less than 10 times. Clinical experience with oral contraceptives and sterilization is apparently rich, but obstetrician–gynecologists trained solely in these methods are unlikely to prescribe other methods that their patients may find preferable for any number of reasons (Westoff et al., 1993). And training—even basic information—about the uses of emergency contraception is exceedingly thin (F.H. Stewart, pers. com., 1994). A recent study of internal medicine and family practice residents indicates that they may also be inadequately trained to care for women of reproductive age.

Of those surveyed, over 40 percent failed to indicate that they would provide female patients with information about family planning options, STDs, and safer sex (Conway et al., 1995). The closely related issue of training in abortion is discussed in Chapter 7.

Despite low minimum competency requirements in the area of family planning, some graduate programs recognize the need for providers to be well trained in contraception and therefore offer thorough preparation as part of their curricula. For example, the University of California at San Francisco, the University of Pittsburgh, and the University of Maryland have each established fellowship programs that provide intensive training in family planning to obstetrician-gynecologists who have completed their residencies (M. Creinin, pers. com., 1994).

The fact that some programs provide adequate training, of course, does not guarantee that a graduated resident will go on to provide contraception. Some general and family practitioners choose to offer no contraceptive services, and about one in five general and family practitioners does not provide reversible contraceptive services because of such factors as the relatively low pay for such services, religious or moral objections, or simply a discomfort with sexuality and related issues (Orr and Forrest, 1985). A recent Centers for Disease Control and Prevention (1994) survey on HIV prevention practices revealed that 25 percent of all physicians felt their patients would be offended by questions regarding their sexual behavior. Physicians who are reluctant to discuss sexual behavior in the context of something as perilous as the HIV epidemic may be even less likely to raise the issue in regard to pregnancy prevention. Additional data confirm this general finding. A recent Harris survey commissioned by the Commonwealth Foundation found that although the vast majority of Americans had seen a health care provider in the last year, only a small portion reported that either contraception or prevention of STDs was mentioned by the provider (Commonwealth Foundation, 1994).

It is important to pinpoint an additional reason that some providers may approach contraception gingerly—fear of liability exposure and litigation. Liability concerns within both the pharmaceutical and provider communities not only decreased the variety of intrauterine devices available in the U.S. market in the 1980s but currently also limit the number of physicians, including obstetrician-gynecologists, willing to insert the few now on the market (Forrest, 1986). Emergency contraception shares some of the same burden. Oral contraceptive manufacturers have not applied for U.S. Food and Drug Administration approval to market oral contraceptives for use as emergency contraceptives, citing, among other reasons, that they are concerned about the liability issues that such use might raise (F.H. Stewart, pers. com., 1994). Whatever the merits of this concern, the main barrier to wider use appears to be the lack of knowledge about the method among both providers and the women they care for, as noted above (Trussell et al., 1992).

Although there seems to be an emerging consensus that the nation needs more primary care and general practitioners, specialization remains a more profitable and intellectually challenging option for many medical students, and it may well be many years before the supply of primary care and general practitioners catches up with the need. Nurse practitioners and advanced-practice nurses are being relied on in increasing numbers to provide primary care to patients, and many studies have indicated that the basic health care provided by nurses is of high quality (Mundinger, 1994). Nurses' effectiveness in promoting health, communicating with patients, adapting medical regimens according to patient preferences and environments, and using community resources make them prime candidates for encouraging contraceptive use as well. A recent survey confirmed their commitment to contraceptive access: a self-administered questionnaire surveying graduates of five reproductive health nurse practitioner programs in the United States revealed that 56 percent of the respondents were currently employed by a Title X agency (National Association of Nurse Practitioners in Reproductive Health, 1994). Even though many nurses are presently providing selected contraceptive services, the role that nurses play in providing access could undoubtedly be increased.

Bureaucratic Hurdles

In day-to-day life, the specific barriers to access outlined thus far, such as limited insurance coverage and insufficient provider training, can interact with each other and with additional obstacles to produce a bureaucratic tangle that undoubtedly limits access to contraception. After all, the medical services required to secure the more effective forms of contraception in the United States are embedded in the nation's general health care system, with its well-described problems of geographic maldistribution of providers, problems in locating transportation to service sites, bureaucratic delays in arranging for care, difficulty even in finding the telephone number to call for services, seeing different providers at each visit, absence of translators, long waits for appointments and in the waiting rooms once an appointment is in hand, and so forth. These general barriers are not detailed here because they have been well covered in previous reports from the Institute of Medicine (1994, 1988) and from many other sources.

Several case studies specific to contraceptive access illustrate the point, particularly the New York City study noted earlier. As described above, in December 1992 and January 1993, a team from the New York City Mayor's Advisory Council on Child Health called 115 service sites that ostensibly offer family planning care in the city to request an appointment for contraceptive services. In over one-third of the cases, even the English-speaking callers were not able to make an appointment at all, although this figure varied by type of clinic. The two most common reasons for the inability to make an appointment were no one answering the phone at all (five or more attempts were made) and being told that a doctor's referral was necessary before an appointment could be booked. Other reasons included requirements that a woman register at a clinic in person before an appointment for family planning could be made, and the absence of a doctor to offer care. Even those who were successful in making appointments frequently were put on hold repeatedly, sometimes for over 30 minutes. For those able to make an appointment, the mean number of days between the call and the appointment for all types of facilities was 20 working days, with the range in means across facilities being 10–51 working days. When the callers mentioned that they "had no insurance," 4 in 10 were asked to bring cash to cover the full anticipated charges, which averaged $79.00. The authors concluded that because the family planning system was so underfunded and poorly organized, access was very limited and that therefore, as noted earlier, succeeding in the task of making a family planning appointment in the New York City system requires "motivation, persistence, and fortitude" (Mayor's Advisory Council on Child Health, 1993).

Female sterilization offers another example of multiple entanglements. Despite the heavy reliance by American women on sterilization (Chapter 4), data suggest that bureaucratic and institutional barriers may limit access to this procedure. For example, federal regulations for subsidized sterilization mandate a strict set of policies with which a provider must comply, including sterilization counseling, a signed consent form, a required 30-day delay between signing the consent form and performing the sterilization, and performing the procedure not less than 30 but no more than 180 days of the consent being signed. The intent of these policies is to protect women by ensuring informed and timely consent, and with good reason, given the past history of abuses (Chapter 7). But it is also true that the protective policies can sometimes create administrative burdens for hospitals and clinics that may limit the number of facilities offering this procedure—an outcome that may have the effect of placing additional burdens on low-income and minority women, the very women the policies were intended to protect. Physicians themselves may place additional requirements on women, thus hindering access to sterilization. Klerman and colleagues (1993) note that to minimize legal liability, operative risks, or risk of patient regret, physicians may require patients to lose weight prior to surgery, stop smoking, obtain a more extensive laboratory workup, be happily married, have a certain number of children, or be a certain age. Many low-income men also may find it difficult to obtain a sterilization. For example, less then 20 percent of publicly supported family planning clinics report providing male sterilization services (Burt et al., 1994).

Hospitals that accept federal reimbursement for sterilization procedures often have long waiting lists for female sterilization because of the unavailability of physicians or operating rooms, the loss of patient records and consent forms, delayed laboratory tests, payment issues related to Medicaid eligibility, and the requirement in some states that the federal consent form be placed in the record preoperatively (Klerman et al., 1993). These problems can delay the procedure beyond the 60-day postpartum period so that a woman is no longer eligible for postpartum Medicaid coverage, or in some extreme cases, the procedure may be delayed past 180 days, resulting in a woman needing to start the administrative and consent procedure all over again. The 30-day waiting period can also be particularly burdensome. For example, if a woman signs a consent form while she is pregnant, asking to be sterilized at the time of delivery, a full 30 days must pass before the request can be honored. If by chance she delivers before the 30 days are up, the sterilization cannot be performed at the time of delivery, thereby requiring that she return to the hospital at some later time to be sterilized. Not surprisingly, one of the effects of all of these complexities is an increased risk of unintended pregnancy among women whose requests for sterilization cannot be accommodated immediately postpartum (Davidson et al., 1990).

MISSED OPPORTUNITIES

Thus far, this chapter has considered two broad explanations for inadequate contraceptive use: limited knowledge about and insufficient access to contraceptive services and supplies. This section considers another factor that may give some clues about how to increase both contraceptive knowledge and access. The tendency in the United States to offer health and human services in categorical, problem-specific ways may result in missing many opportunities to offer information, education, and services that help couples avoid unintended pregnancies. In a recent editorial advocating increased attention to immunizing children, U.S. Department of Health and Human Services Secretary Donna Shalala stated, "Every encounter of any sort that a physician or provider has with a patient—whether in an office or an emergency department or a hospital room—offers an opportunity to screen children for needed vaccines and administer appropriate vaccines immediately." Such screening "should become as routine as measuring blood pressure in adults" (The Blue Sheet, 1993:9). This perspective has not yet been articulated for contraceptive services, even though, just as for immunizations, many opportunities are present to improve the contraceptive vigilance of adults as well as adolescents.

One example is the disinclination of many clinics that screen for and treat STDs to provide contraceptive services. Two recent investigations reveal clearly that the clients typically seen in STD clinics are often poor users of contraception, frequently have multiple sexual partners, lack much basic information about pregnancy and reproduction, and would be receptive to more information and to additional services to address their contraceptive needs. Upchurch and colleagues (1987) surveyed 516 women attending an STD clinic in an urban, inner-city area to learn about various contraceptive and sexual practices and knowledge. They documented high rates of STDs and STD recurrences and poor use of contraception. They concluded that making contraceptive services available in STD clinics could be of great help to the women typically seen in these clinics who are at high risk of unintended pregnancy and who are known to be poor users of contraception. Similar conclusions were reached in a more recent survey at another STD clinic (Horn et al., 1990).

The categorical, single-problem focus also means that few drug treatment programs for men or women—even for women who are new mothers—emphasize contraception or preventing unintended pregnancies (Gehshan, 1994). For example, since 1988, the federal Center for Substance Abuse and Prevention (CSAP), in conjunction with the Maternal and Child Health Bureau, has funded more than 100 programs targeted to women of childbearing age, especially those who are pregnant or have a child less than 1 year old at the time of enrollment. Although the goals of the program grants could include an emphasis on preventing unintended pregnancy, a recent review of 112 projects receiving CSAP support in 1991 revealed that none had program objectives that included pregnancy prevention, nor did any of the program evaluations focus on this issue (Cartoof, 1994). Although there are many reasons for this state of affairs—not the least being that many drug treatment personnel are not trained in this area and have few extra resources to devote to this topic—several pilot projects have demonstrated that integration of drug treatment and family planning services is not only possible but also leads to better use of contraception (Armstrong et al., 1991).

The practice patterns of pediatricians raise a similar point. Pediatricians' emphasis on preventive care makes them likely candidates to encourage the use of contraception. They are in a unique position to provide information both for their adolescent patients, many of whom have or will soon become sexually active, and for new parents as well in the form of interconceptional care. The subspecialty of adolescent medicine draws attention to the need for training in the health needs of teenagers, including those related to sexuality, but general pediatricians are only beginning to consider whether their work in protecting the health of infants and young children includes counseling mothers and couples about the need for reasonable intervals between births and the importance of being in good health before conception. The American Academy of Pediatrics reports that only 34 percent of surveyed physicians routinely ask their patients, when appropriate, about family planning (Clark, 1993). Klerman and Reynolds (1994) assert that all pediatricians should be educated to ask mothers about their plans for future pregnancies, and should be prepared to give advice about spacing of pregnancies and about contraceptive methods. They speculate that although some physicians may feel they are prying or overstepping their boundaries in discussing these matters, the issue seems very appropriate when it is raised in the context of the physical and emotional health of the infant being examined. For example, extending the interval between pregnancies can help to increase the amount of attention devoted to the present child or children and to improve the health of future children by allowing sufficient time for maternal recovery between pregnancies. The importance of an adequate interpregnancy interval for reducing the risk of low birthweight in subsequent pregnancies has recently been well documented, lending added importance to pregnancy spacing and interconceptional care (Rawlings et al., 1995). This is not to suggest that pediatricians be equipped and prepared to carry out a full examination in preparation for providing prescription-based methods of contraception, but rather that the physician raise the subject, and when appropriate, provide counseling, encouragement, and, at a minimum, a nonprescription contraceptive method or a referral. At the same time, it is important to acknowledge that because relatively few poor or minority children see a pediatrician regularly, only part of the childbearing population would be reached by this strategy.

This notion of missed opportunities is not limited to the health sector. Many others in the helping professions are in a position to raise issues of pregnancy planning and contraception but fail to do so (Tyrer, 1994). The limited commitment of many school systems to education regarding contraception, human reproduction, and related issues has already been mentioned, and in Chapter 7, the potential role of the media in this area is also explored. Other sectors that could become involved include social service agencies, church-affiliated centers, homeless shelters, job training and employment services, and various community and neighborhood centers that provide integrated services to families. Intervention programs working with troubled families offer unique and important opportunities to engage parents in topics of pregnancy spacing and planning; for a wide variety of reasons, however, such opportunities are often passed over. Some case workers feel the subject of family planning is taboo or too controversial; sometimes the case workers sense that the underlying problems of families are so compelling that attempts to discuss family planning will be essentially futile; some perhaps fail to appreciate that improving the life prospects of the child currently in treatment will be compromised if another baby arrives too soon. Whatever the reluctance, there is a newly articulated view in the field of family-centered care, especially that provided to families with infants and toddlers, that contraception and pregnancy planning are important topics to address (Lieberman, 1993).

A somewhat philosophical explanation for these missed opportunities to offer contraceptive information and services is that in the United States and many other countries as well, there may be a tendency to "overmedicalize" family planning—that is, to make contraception (especially the more effective methods) so definitively a medical service that access is, in fact, constrained, inasmuch as access to medical care generally can be difficult (Shelton et al., 1992). This view lies behind the current interest in providing oral contraceptives as over-the-counter rather than prescription drugs; the notion is that easing access to oral contraceptives would increase their use (Samuels et al., 1994). Similarly, some agencies are experimenting with providing the first several cycles of oral contraceptives to adolescents without requiring a pelvic examination at the outset, given that one of the reasons some adolescents are reluctant to begin using highly effective means of contraception is fear of pelvic examinations and medical procedures in general (Zabin and Clark, 1981; see also Beckman et al., 1992, and Chapter 6).

CONCLUSION

The data and perspectives presented in this chapter suggest that one of the reasons contraceptive use is inadequate—and that unintended pregnancy therefore continues to occur—is that Americans have important gaps in their knowledge about contraception in general, and about the risks and benefits of various methods of birth control in particular. The resulting fears and misconceptions can impede the use (including the continuation) of contraception, which in turn contributes to the risk of unintended pregnancy. The complexity of using some contraceptive methods properly may help to explain the observation that education and cognitive ability are positively associated with greater success in contraceptive use. Data suggest that high quality instruction in schools (only one of many information sources) about various aspects of human sexuality, including contraception, is not uniformly available nationwide; moreover, what is available may sometimes be too little and too late, inasmuch as a significant portion of young people begin sexual activity before having had the benefit of any formal education about contraception and related topics. Knowledge is increasing about how to structure school-based curricula to reduce both precocious sexual activity as well as to improve contraceptive use once sexual activity has begun. Nonetheless, all such information centers on adolescents, and little is known about how to improve the knowledge and skills of *adults* regarding contraception.

It is also apparent that, through a combination of financial and structural factors, the U.S. health care system makes access to contraception a complicated, sometimes expensive proposition. Condoms, the most accessible form of contraception, provide valuable protection against STDs but must be accompanied by prescription-based methods to afford maximum protection against unintended pregnancy. Unfortunately, other accessible nonprescription methods (such as foam) neither prevent the transmission of STDs nor offer the best protection against unintended pregnancy. In particular, private health insurance participates poorly in the financing of contraception; eligibility and other restrictions on Medicaid support for contraception make it a source of steady financing only for the poorest women; and the net decline in public investment in family planning services, in the face of higher costs and sicker patients, may have led to a net decline in access to care for women who rely on publicly subsidized contraceptive services.

Finally, too few providers of health care and social services use all available opportunities to discuss contraception and the importance of intended pregnancy to the health and well-being of women and men, children, and families. Within the health care community, this may be due to limited training in contraception as well as to such other factors as personal feelings about birth control and concerns about liability. Outside of the health care community, the lack of attention may be due to a sense that contraception is a medical issue, perhaps a touchy subject, or "not part of my job." The net effect of these missed opportunities is that only a limited range of providers and institutions are involved in helping Americans to know about—and acquire the means to prevent—unintended pregnancy.

REFERENCES

Accreditation Council for Graduate Medical Education. Press Release. February 15, 1995.

Adams Hillard PJ. Oral contraception compliance: The extent of the problem. Adv Contracept. 1992;8:13–19.

The Alan Guttmacher Institute. Uneven and Unequal: Insurance Coverage and Reproductive Health Services. New York, NY; 1994.

The Alan Guttmacher Institute. Risk and Responsibility: Teaching Sex Education in America's Schools Today. New York, NY: The Alan Guttmacher Institute; 1989.

American College of Obstetricians and Gynecologists. News Release. Gallup Poll Shows What Public Knows and Thinks About Birth Control. Washington, DC; March 6, 1985.

American Medical Association. Graduate Medical Education Directory, 1994–1995. Chicago, IL: American Health Information Management Association; 1994:91.

Armstrong KA, Kenen R, Samost L. Barriers to family planning services among patients in drug treatment programs. Fam Plann Perspect. 1991;23:264–271.

Balassone ML. Risk of contraceptive discontinuation among adolescents. J Adol Health Care. 1989;10:527–533.

Beckman L, Harvey S, Murray J. Perceived contraceptive attributes of current and former users of the vaginal sponge. J Sex Res. 1992;29:31–42.

The Blue Sheet. Childhood immunization hearing will be convened jointly by Senate and House committees April 21. F-D-C Reports; April 21, 1993;8–9.

Burt MB, Aaron LY, Schack LR. Family planning clinics: Current status and recent changes in services, clients, staffing, and income sources. In Publicly Supported Family Planning in the United States. Washington, DC: The Urban Institute and Child Trends, Inc.; 1994.

Campaign for Women's Health and the American Medical Women's Association. Women and Sexually Transmitted Diseases: The Dangers of Denial. Washington, DC; 1994.

Cartoof V. Unpublished data. July 1994.

Centers for Disease Control and Prevention. HIV prevention practices of primary care physicians—United States, 1992. MMWR. 1994;42:988-992.

Christopher S, Roosa M. Evaluation of an abstinence only adolescent pregnancy prevention program: Is "Just say no" enough? Fam Relat. 1990;39:68–72.

Clark G. Survey links physicians' age, sex to practice style. Am Acad Pediatrics News. 1993;January:6–7.

Clark SD Jr, Zabin LS, Hardy JB. Sex, contraception, and parenthood: Experience and attitudes among urban black young men. Fam Plann Perspect. 1984;16:77–82.

Commonwealth Foundation. Unpublished data, December 1994.

Conway T, Tzyy-Chyn H, Mason E, Mueller C. Are primary care residents adequately prepared to care for women of reproductive age? Fam Plann Perspect. 1995;27: 66–70.

Cvetkovich G, Grote B. Adolescent development and teenage fertility. In Adolescents, Sex, and Contraception. Byrne D, Fisher WA, eds. Hillsdale, NJ: Lawrence Earlbaum Associates; 1983.

David HP, Morgall JM, Osler M, et al. United States and Denmark: Different approaches to health care and family planning. Stud Fam Plann. 1990;21:1–19.

Davidson AR, Philliber SG, Graves WL, Rulin MC, Cushman LF. Sterilization Decision Making and Regret: The Determinants and Consequences of Unfulfilled Sterilization Plans. Paper presented at the annual meeting of the Population Association of America. Toronto, Canada; 1990.

Dawson D. The effects of sex education on adolescent behavior. Fam Plann Perspect. 1986;18:162–170.

Debra D, DeMauro D. Winning the Battle for Comprehensive Sexuality and HIV/AIDS Education. New York, NY: Sexuality Information and Education Council of the United States; 1990.

Donovan P. Family planning clinics: Facing higher costs and sicker patients. Fam Plann Perspect. 1991;23:198–203.

Family Planning Council of Southeastern Pennsylvania and the Coordinating Office for Drug and Alcohol Abuse Programs, Philadelphia. What We Have Learned. Atlanta, GA: Centers for Disease Control and Prevention, Behavioral and Prevention Research Branch, Division of STD/HIV Prevention; 1991.

Firestone WA. The content and context of sexuality education: An exploratory study in one state. Fam Plann Perspect. 1994;26:125–131.

Foreit JR, Foreit KG. Risk-taking and contraceptive behavior among unmarried college students. Popul Environ. 1981;4:174–188.

Forrest JD. The end of IUD marketing in the United States: What does it mean for American women? Fam Plann Perspect. 1986;18:52–57.

Forrest JD, Silverman J. What public school teachers teach about preventing pregnancy, AIDS and sexually transmitted diseases. Fam Plann Perspect. 1989;21:65–72.

Forrest JD, Singh S. The sexual and reproductive behavior of American women. Fam Plann Perspect. 1990;22:206–214.

Frost JJ. The availability and accessibility of the contraceptive implant from family planning agencies in the United States, 1991–1992. Fam Plann Perspect. 1994; 26:4–10.

Furstenberg FF, Moore KA, Peterson J. Sex education and sexual experience among adolescents. Am J Public Health. 1985;5:1331–1332.

Gallup Organization. Women's Attitudes Towards Contraceptives and Other Forms of Birth Control. Princeton, NJ; January 1994.

Gehshan S. The Provision of Family Planning Services in Substance Abuse Treatment Programs. Paper prepared for the Committee on Unintended Pregnancy, Institute of Medicine. Washington, DC; 1994.

Gold RB, Daley D. Public funding of contraceptive, sterilization and abortion services, fiscal year 1990. Fam Plann Perspect. 1991;23:204–211.

Grady WR, Hayward MD, Yagi J. Contraceptive failure in the United States: Estimates from the 1982 National Survey of Family Growth. Fam Plann Perspect. 1986; 18:200–209.

Grady WR, Hirsch MB, Keen N, Vaughan B. Contraceptive failure and continuation among married women in the United States. Stud Fam Plann. 1983;14:9–19.

Grossman RA, Grossman BD. How frequently is emergency contraception prescribed? Fam Plann Perspect. 1994;26:270–271.

Haffner D. Sexuality Education and Contraceptive Instruction in U.S. Schools. Paper prepared for the Committee on Unintended Pregnancy, Institute of Medicine. Washington, DC; 1994.

Hatcher RA, Trussell J, Stewart F, et al. Emergency Contraception: The Nation's Best Kept Secret. Atlanta, GA: Bridging the Gap Communications; 1995.

Henshaw SK, Torres A. Family planning agencies: Services, policies and funding. Fam Plann Perspect. 1994;26:52–59.

Herman R. Whatever happened to the contraceptive revolution? Washington Post, Health Section; December 13, 1994.

Horn JE, McQuillan GM, Ray PA, Hook EW. Reproductive health practices in women attending an inner-city STD clinic. Sex Transm Dis. 1990;July–September:133–137.

Institute of Medicine. Overcoming Barriers to Immunization. Washington, DC: National Academy Press; 1994.

Institute of Medicine. Prenatal Care: Reaching Mothers, Reaching Infants. Washington, DC: National Academy Press; 1988.

Jones, EF, Forrest JD. Contraceptive failure rates based on the 1988 NSFG. Fam Plann Perspect. 1992;24:12–19.

Jones EF, Forrest JD. Contraceptive failure in the United States: Revised estimates from the 1982 National Survey of Family Growth. Fam Plann Perspect. 1989;21:103–109.

Jones EF, Forrest JD, Goldman N, et al. Teenage Pregnancy in Industrialized Countries. New Haven, CT: Yale University Press; 1986.

Jones EF, Forrest JD, Henshaw SK, Silverman J, Torres A. Pregnancy, Contraception and Family Planning Services in Industrialized Countries. New Haven, CT: Yale University Press; 1989.

Kaeser L. Public funding and policies for provision of the contraceptive implant, fiscal year 1992. Fam Plann Perspect. 1994;26:11–16.

Kaeser L, Richards CL. Barriers to Access to Reproductive Health Services. Paper prepared for the Committee on Unintended Pregnancy, Institute of Medicine. Washington, DC; 1994.

Kirby D. Sexuality Education: An Evaluation of Programs and Their Effects. Santa Cruz, CA: Network Publications; 1984.

Kirby D, Short L, Collins J, et al. School-based programs to reduce sexual risk behaviors: A review of effectiveness. Public Health Rep. 1994;109:339–360.

Kirkman-Liff B, Korenfeld JJ. Access to family planning services and health insurance among low-income women in Arizona. Am J Public Health. 1994;84:1010–1012.

Klaus A. Every Child a Lion: The Origins of Maternal and Infant Health Policy in the United States and France, 1890–1920. Ithaca, NY: Cornell University Press; 1993.

Klerman LV, Phelan ST, Poole VL. Family planning: Can it favorably influence the rate of low birthweight? Unpublished. University of Alabama at Birmingham; 1993.

Klerman LV, Reynolds DW. Interconceptional care: A new role for the pediatrician. Pediatrics. 1994;93:327–329.

Ku L. Financing of family planning services. In Publicly Supported Family Planning in the United States. Washington, DC: The Urban Institute and Child Trends, Inc.; 1993.

Ku LC, Sonenstein FL, Pleck JH. Factors affecting first intercourse among young men. Public Health Report. 1993;108:680–694.

Ku LC, Sonenstein FL, Pleck JH. The association of AIDS education and sex education with sexual behavior and condom use among teenage men. Fam Plann Perspect. 1992;24:100–106.

Lieberman AF. Family planning as a clinical Issue. Zero to Three. 1993;13:1–5.

Lowe CS, Radius SM. Young adults' contraceptive practices: An investigation of influences. Adolescence. 1987;22:291–304.

Marsiglio W, Mott FL. The impact of sex education on sexual activity, contraceptive use and premarital pregnancy. Fam Plann Perspect. 1986; 18:151–162.

Mayor's Advisory Council on Child Health. Family Planning Appointment Study. Department of Health, New York City. August 1993.

Miller CA. Maternal and infant care: Comparisons between Western Europe and the United States. Int J Health Serv 1993;23:655–664.

Miller CA. A review of maternity care programs in Western Europe. Perspect on Prev 1988;2:31–38.

Mosher W. Use of family planning services in the United States: 1982 and 1988. Advance Data. No. 184. National Center for Health Statistics. April 11, 1990.

Mundinger M. Advanced-practice nursing—good medicine for physicians? N Engl J Med. 1994;330:211–214.

National Academy of Social Insurance. Current Research in Managed Care: What Can We Say About Perinatal Services? Washington, DC; 1994.

National Association of Nurse Practitioners in Reproductive Health. Five Nurse Practitioner Programs Graduate Survey Summary; 1994.

Oakley, D. Rethinking patient counseling techniques for changing contraceptive behavior. Am J Obstet Gynecol. 1994;170:1585–1590.

Orr M, Forrest J. The availability of reproductive health services from US private physicians. Fam Plann Perspect. 1985;17:63–69.

Oskamp S, Mindick B. Personality and attitudinal barriers to contraception. In Adolescents, Sex, and Contraception. Byrne D, Fisher WA, eds. Hillsdale, NJ: Lawrence Earlbaum Associates; 1983.

Peipert JF, Gutmann J. Oral contraceptive risk assessment: A survey of 247 educated women. Obstet Gynecol. 1993;82:112–117.

Poland ML, Beane GE. A study of the effects of folklore about the body on IUD use by black adolescent Americans. Contracep Deliv Syst. 1980;1:333–340.

Quint JC, Musick JS, Ladner JA. Lives of Promise, Lives of Pain: Young Mothers After New Chance. New York, NY: Manpower Demonstration Research Corporation; 1994.

Rawlings JS, Rawlings VB, Read JA. Prevalence of low birthweight and preterm delivery in relation to the interval between pregnancies among white and black women. N Engl J Med. 1995;332:69–74.

Robert Wood Johnson Foundation and Center for Health Economics Research. Access to Health Care: Key Indicators for Policy. Princeton, NJ; 1993.

Sachs B. Contraceptive decision making in urban, black female adolescents in relation to cognitive development. Int J Nurs. 1985;22:117–126.

Samuels SE, Stryker J, Smith M. Over-the-counter birth control pills: An overview. In The Pill: From Prescription to Over the Counter. Samuels SE, Smith MD, eds. Menlo Park, CA: The Henry J. Kaiser Foundation; 1994.

Scales P. Sex education in the '70s and '80s: Accomplishments, obstacles, and emerging issues. Fam Relat. 1981;30:557–561.

Schirm AL, Trussell J, Menken J, Grady WR. Contraceptive failure in the United States: The impact of social, economic, and demographic factors. Fam Plann Perspect. 1982;14:68–75.

Shelton JD, Angle MA, Jacobstein RA. Medical barriers to access to family planning. Lancet. 1992;340:1334–1335.

Sonenstein FL, Schulte MM, Levine G. Women's perspectives on reproductive health services. In Publicly Supported Family Planning in the United States. Washington, DC: The Urban Institute and Child Trends, Inc.; 1994.

Spanier GB. Formal and informal sex education as determinants of premarital sexual behavior. Arch Sex Behav. 1976;5:39–47.

Stoddard JJ, St. Peter RF, Newacheck PW. Health insurance status and ambulatory care for children. N Engl J Med. 1994;330:1421–1430.

Tanfer K. Determinants of Contraceptive Use: A Review. Paper prepared for the Committee on Unintended Pregnancy, Institute of Medicine. Washington, DC; 1994.

Tanfer K, Cubbins L, Brewster K. Determinants of contraceptive choice among single women in the United States. Fam Plann Perspect. 1992;24:155–173.

Trussell J, Stewart F. The effectiveness of postcoital hormonal contraception. Fam Plann Perspect. 1992;24:262–264.

Trussell J, Stewart F, Guest F, Hatcher RA. Emergency contraceptive pills: A simple proposal to reduce unintended pregnancies. Fam Plann Perspect. 1992;24:269–273.

Tyrer LB. Obstacles to the use of hormonal contraception. Am J Obstet Gynecol. 1994;170:1495–1498.

Upchurch DM, Farmer MY, Glasser D, Hook EW. Contraceptive needs and practices among women attending an inner-city STD clinic. Am J Public Health. 1987;77: 1429.

Westoff C, Marks F, Rosenfield A. Residency training in contraception sterilization and abortion. Obstet Gynecol. 1993;81:311–314.

Zabin LS, Clark SD. Institutional factors affecting teenagers' choice and reasons for delay in attending a family planning clinic. Fam Plann Perspect. 1981; 15:25–29.

Zabin LS, Stark HA, Emerson MR. Reasons for delay in contraceptive clinic utilization: Adolescent clinic and nonclinic populations compared. J Adolesc Health. 1991; 12:225–232.

Zelnik M, Kim YJ. Sex education and its association with teenage sexual activity, pregnancy and contraceptive use. Fam Plann Perspect. 1982; 14:117–126.

6

Personal and Interpersonal Determinants of Contraceptive Use

The previous chapter concluded that one of the reasons that the United States has high levels of unintended pregnancy is that both knowledge about and access to contraception may be insufficient. The point was also made, however, that the determinants of contraceptive use and of unintended pregnancy are not limited to knowledge and access alone.

In fact, there is persuasive evidence that personal and emotional factors are closely connected to inadequate contraceptive vigilance and therefore unintended pregnancy. For example, in a series of telephone interviews with 760 women aged 18–35 at risk of unintended pregnancy, researchers learned that 23 percent of the women interviewed were sexually active but using no contraception, despite no apparent desire to become pregnant. Most of the reasons given for not using contraception involved feelings about and experiences with specific methods of contraception, issues involving relationships with their partner, and a general discomfort with contraception—all of which have more to do with emotion, attitude, and belief than with the availability of contraception or specific knowledge about individual methods (Silverman et al., 1987). As every current or former dieter or smoker knows, the gap between knowledge and behavior change in particular can be very great. Accordingly, this chapter addresses personal and interpersonal attitudes, feelings, and beliefs that can affect contraceptive use and therefore the risk of unintended pregnancy. It begins with a brief note on some theoretical and methodological problems that burden research in this field and then discusses several cross-cutting themes. Later sections summarize research on how contraceptive use is influenced by several specific attitudes and personality dimensions, and by selected situational factors.

A COMMENT ON AVAILABLE DATA

It is sometimes difficult to draw broad conclusions from research on the relative importance and interaction of the personal and interpersonal factors that affect contraceptive use and unintended pregnancy because the data available are of such variable quality and limited generalizability. For example, the literature often fails to distinguish between those who experience unintended pregnancies despite some attempt to use contraception versus those who use no contraception at all, and rarely is consistent nonuse of contraception distinguished from briefer episodes of nonuse. Few studies have been replicated, and sample sizes tend to be small. Moreover, most of the individual studies in this area do not share the same theoretical orientation or use the same test instruments to probe various personal dimensions related to unintended pregnancy and contraceptive use, thereby impeding the development of a coherent body of theory or data.

Perhaps the biggest problem of all, however, is the over-representation of urban black adolescent girls and white female (and some male) college students. As the balance of this chapter demonstrates, little if anything is known about, for example, the motivational issues surrounding poor contraceptive use in women or couples over age 35, even though their rates of unintended pregnancy are relatively high (Chapter 2). Although there is new interest in contraceptive use by men, the majority of relevant behavioral research is focused on their use of condoms and rarely on their support of or participation in their partner's use of various methods. As such, the picture of the psychology of contraceptive use provided by the available data is often incomplete.

UNDERLYING THEMES

Although not often explicitly stated, much of the research on the psychology of contraceptive use views efforts to avoid unintended pregnancy as being based on a "benefit:burden ratio"—the notion that sexually active individuals and couples carry within themselves a complicated equation balancing the benefits and burdens of becoming pregnant (or causing pregnancy) and having a child versus the benefits and burdens of not becoming pregnant (or causing pregnancy) (Furstenberg, 1980). At different stages of life, these factors are weighted differently: sometimes the scales tip in favor of pregnancy, sometimes against it. In the language of behavioral theories of fertility, contraceptive decisions are influenced by the perceived costs of a pregnancy and the perceived costs of obtaining and using different contraceptive methods (Bulatao and Lee, 1983). The higher the costs of an unintended pregnancy, the more likely couples are to use an effective method; conversely, the perception of low costs attached to an unintended pregnancy will reduce the likelihood of using an effective method. One important value of this perspective is its recognition that pregnancy and childbearing can be very rewarding experiences and that, in addition, using contraception can be an intrusive, complicated undertaking requiring considerable skill and knowledge; it may be expensive as well.

Luker (1975) was one of the first to articulate this perspective in her theory of contraceptive risk taking, which argued that both pregnancy and pregnancy prevention have pluses and minuses and that it is the net effect of how each of these variables is valued, by the individual and couple, that determines ultimate outcome (i.e., use of contraception or the occurrence of unintended pregnancy). Zabin (1994) has referred to this as the "personal calculus of choice." And Miller (1986) has argued that a woman's contraceptive vigilance and her actual use of birth control on any given occasion frequently depend on where the internal balance lies among her positive and negative feelings toward getting pregnant and toward her contraceptive method. Other models that are consistent with this general approach and that have been variously applied to studies of contraceptive use include the health belief model (Rosenstock et al., 1988), the theory of reasoned action (Fishbein and Ajzen, 1980), and the theory of planned behavior (Ajzen, 1991). Related investigations of adolescent risk taking (of which unprotected intercourse is a good example) increasingly suggest that although some risky behaviors may seem totally irrational to adults, they derive from the adolescent's own weighing of the benefits and costs of various courses of action (Furby and Beyth-Marom, 1990).

The policy debate about welfare reform rests in large part on this benefit:burden notion. Those who advocate reducing or eliminating welfare benefits for unmarried women who conceive and bear children while on welfare suggest that without such measures there are no disincentives (or only weak disincentives) to avoid childbearing while receiving public assistance; furthermore, some suggest that welfare is actually a positive incentive for childbearing (Chapter 7) and that welfare reduces incentives for men to avoid causing pregnancy or, once a child is born, to participate in the child's support.

Closely related to this idea of the benefit:burden ratio is the importance of motivation in contraceptive use. In truth, using the reversible methods of contraception carefully to avoid pregnancy can be a complicated, challenging task that requires consistent dedication over an extended period of time, often from both partners; even a fleeting step off the straight and narrow can result in pregnancy. Absent the utmost contraceptive vigilance, the human organism is designed to reproduce under even adverse biological circumstances, including famine—an evolutionary inheritance that was designed for species survival. This theme of motivation to avoid unintended pregnancy—that it must be powerful if pregnancy is to be prevented—bubbles to the surface from widely different data sets and forms a common theme among disparate investigations.

Several studies have looked at contraceptive use from this motivational perspective, and their findings offer important insights into why some women become pregnant even when they do not intend to. Over a two-year period,

Zabin and colleagues (1993), for example, studied a sample of 313 inner-city girls 17 years of age and under to learn how their attitudes toward childbearing, contraception, and abortion and their beliefs about their partners' views of these same issues affected their use of contraception and their rates of both pregnancy and childbearing. Like many other students of adolescent pregnancy, the investigators were struck by the fact that although few girls say they want to be pregnant, many conceive nonetheless. They found that simple measures of intent—for example, did you plan to become pregnant?—fail to capture the complexity of motivations that surround the use of contraception or attitudes toward the desirability (or lack of desirability) of pregnancy. Zabin (1994:94–95) summarized this seminal work:

> We . . . explored the concept of "wantedness" in some depth and [found that] although few want to conceive, there is considerable ambivalence on that issue and, surprisingly, those who are ambivalent about childbearing are at just as high risk of having a child as those who positively desire to conceive. In this research we defined "wantedness" not by the single variable most surveys use: "Did you want to get pregnant," but by three variables [questions] that also tapped how they would feel if they became pregnant and whether they saw a pregnancy as problematic at this stage in their lives. Following this study group for two years, we compared childbearing rates of those whose answers to all three questions suggested that they unequivocally wanted to avoid pregnancy (47%), those who unequivocally wanted to conceive (only 5%), and those whose answers to the three questions suggested some ambivalence (48%). Rather than falling midway between the other two groups, *the ambivalent girls were just as likely to become mothers in the next two years as the few who unequivocally wanted to conceive* [emphasis added]. Furthermore, the same research showed that to use contraception and reduce the probability of childbearing, the same kind of unambivalent attitude had to support its use. . . . Ambivalence put these girls at risk; when engaging in coital activity, it is hard to avoid conception. The motivation for contraception is not easy to maintain, and negative attitudes toward it abound in the United States—not merely among teenagers. . . . Here one might legitimately ask: What kind of identity, what view of self, what view of the future, might provide strong enough motivation to stay the course?

The findings of Zabin and colleagues are highly consistent with the eloquent ethnographic writings of several authors regarding pregnancy among poor adolescents (Quint et al., 1994; Anderson, 1994; Musick, 1993; Dash, 1989). Anderson, for example, has written about differing male and female orientations to sex and childbearing as one explanation for unintended pregnancy among very poor inner-city adolescent girls in particular. He describes the important role for young men and boys that sexual activity itself may play in building and sustaining self-esteem and a sense of self-worth. He argues that, largely in response to profound poverty and absent opportunities, young men and boys may become absorbed into powerful peer groups that emphasize "sexual prowess as proof of manhood, with babies as evidence." The girls, by contrast, may engage in sex to secure the attentions of a young man, hoping that some better future will come from the liaison—that is, "the girls have a dream, the boys a desire" (Anderson, 1994:11). Although Anderson reports that "an overwhelming number [of the girls] are not trying to have babies," their hopes for attachment and closeness, as well as a generally positive orientation toward the rewards and sense of maturity and status that childbearing may bring, overpower short-term resolve to use contraception and avoid pregnancy. "With the dream of a mate, a girl may be indifferent to the possibility of pregnancy" (Anderson, 1994:9–10). He thus characterizes sexual conduct among this especially impoverished group as a contest, with the boys seeking conquest, status, and control over the girls, and the girls hoping that a sexual relationship will begin a journey into a secure, middle-class future with a house and husband. Given such differing orientations to sex and pregnancy, it is not surprising that contraceptive vigilance may be poor and that unintended pregnancy is a common occurrence.

Musick's observations, consistent with those of Anderson, focus especially on young girls in poverty. She describes a broad array of psychological, developmental, and situational factors that may interfere with careful contraceptive use. She argues that many young girls enter adolescence with unresolved issues of identity and security, limited vocational or professional aspirations (largely because of the absence of mentors and role models), and a personal history—often involving childhood sexual abuse—that leaves them powerless and vulnerable to early sexual activity and childbearing. Histories of dysfunctional relationships with largely absent fathers set the stage for unhealthy relationships with other males who may easily draw them into destructive sexual liaisons. She suggests that in order to understand adolescent pregnancy and childbearing, one must recognize the troubled childhoods and families that shape the development of girls who then go on to become teenage mothers. She notes, in particular, a puzzling phenomenon that has been observed by many who have worked in teenage pregnancy prevention programs: that, just on the brink of advancement and new opportunities, young adolescent girls are particularly likely to become pregnant. Such pregnancies, although usually not fully intended, are portrayed by Musick as a complex response to fear of major life changes, of differentiating oneself from peers and relatives, and of separation from the mother especially.

Like Zabin, Musick finds that although many adolescents are not motivated to become pregnant—i.e., they may not fully "intend" to become pregnant—they are insufficiently motivated to avoid pregnancy. As Maynard (1994:10) has observed, "most teens on welfare do use contraception (83 percent)—and most often they use a relatively effective method like the pill or an IUD (75 percent). However, most are also pregnant again within a relatively short time. . . . The clear implication is that many who are using 'effective' contraception are not using them 'effectively' A pregnant teenager captured the essence of this dynamic:

'I didn't plan it, and then again I kind of knew what was going to happen because I wasn't like really taking the pills like I was supposed to. I couldn't remember every day to take the pill. And I still don't' (Polit, 1992:69)."

Musick notes the enormous attraction and fulfillment that childbearing can offer to young women with few alternatives and little hope for personal economic betterment through the conventionally touted avenues of high school graduation and full-time employment. A baby offers the promise of unconditional love, a chance to feel needed and valued, and a feeling of accomplishment and achievement. Moreover, the urge and presumed benefits of having a child and being a mother are rarely countered by equally powerful forces to take a different life course.

This body of information is important to ponder in the context of public policy discussions regarding adolescent childbearing. It has been suggested that most teenage mothers get pregnant and bear children purposefully, perhaps to get on welfare, to get away from home, to hold onto a boyfriend, etc. Yet survey data show that more than 85 percent of births to unmarried women less than 20 years old are unintended at the time of conception (Chapter 2); in Zabin's small sample, described above, the figure is arguably higher. It is puzzling that these two images are so out of sync with each other—the belief that teenagers are having babies largely as the result of conscious choice, versus survey data saying that the vast majority of births to teenagers are unintended at conception. The explanation may be that, in some sense, both are right. On the one hand, few teenagers "intend" their pregnancy in the sense of actively planning and wanting a child as might a 30-year-old married couple. This strict definition of intended pregnancy is consistent with the survey data showing that few births to teenagers are the product of intended pregnancies. But that does not mean that they are fully unintended either. Zabin uses the term "ambivalence" to describe the underlying dynamic. Because the reasons to delay childbearing may not seem very persuasive to some adolescents, especially those who are poor, there may be appreciable ambivalence—even confusion—about pregnancy and contraception. These feelings are not consistent with the strong motivation required to use reversible methods carefully and consistently over an extended period of time. The result can often be pregnancy—not really intended, not really unintended, but caught somewhere in between.

This dynamic of ambivalence and related psychological issues is directly relevant to many of the measurement issues and caveats discussed in both Chapters 2 and 3 as well as in Appendix G. These various sections argue that "intendedness" is often more complicated than is suggested by such measures as those used in the National Survey of Family Growth (NSFG) or other investigations. Consistent with this view, the NSFG plans to use more elaborate measures of intendedness in the 1995 cycle, as detailed in Appendix C. Miller (1992), in particular, has directly addressed this issue of ambivalence by proposing a seven-point continuum of intendedness that helps to capture the complexities described by Zabin and others. This scale may be particularly useful in that it was developed on the basis of extensive interviews with both adolescents and adults and with both married and unmarried women.

The work of Zabin, Anderson, Musick, and others as well (see, for example, Klerman, 1993; Furstenberg, 1987) suggests that, particularly for low-income teens in urban settings, preventing unintended pregnancy will require strengthening the familial, social, educational, and employment environment of children and youth such that both boys and girls reach adolescence with a greater sense of self-worth and a vision of the future in which pregnancy and childbearing before schooling is completed and employment secured are seen as significantly less desirable than other life options. These investigators suggest that hopes and plans for a better adult life—and reason to believe that the plans are realistic—may provide critical energy for overcoming all the other obstacles to preventing pregnancy that this report and many others have detailed. Absent such countervailing forces, the motivation to be abstinent or use contraception carefully and consistently may be too weak to avoid conception; pregnancy, although not fully intended, will probably continue to characterize the adolescence of disadvantaged, poor girls.

Are these same forces at work among older men and women? Unfortunately, an equally rich body of research on motivation to use contraception and avoid pregnancy does not exist for older women, for couples, or for men, although there are some important exceptions (see, for example, Miller, 1986). It is reasonable to believe that motivational issues are powerful at all stages of reproductive life, not just adolescence, but the ethnographic and behavioral research available to help in understanding these other periods is thin.

SINGLE FACTOR INVESTIGATIONS

Many researchers have investigated the effect on contraceptive use of more specific issues than the broad motivational ones noted above. These include personality characteristics, feelings about sexuality and fertility and about specific contraceptive methods themselves, such behavioral factors as alcohol and substance abuse, family and peer interactions, and the quality of a couple's relationship. These are reviewed briefly in this section.

Personality Characteristics

The influence of specific personality characteristics on the use, nonuse, or poor use of contraception has been a particular focus of several investigators. In studying contraceptive use among adolescents, most of this research has focused on self-esteem, self-efficacy, and locus of control. Several studies have examined the association between self-esteem and events (e.g., sexual intercourse, nonuse of contraception, pregnancy) that lead to nonmarital childbearing. Herold et al. (1979), for example, found that high self-esteem was associated with more positive attitudes toward contraception and more effective contraceptive use among adolescent clients of family planning clinics. In another study, for both men and women, positive descriptions of one's self and body image were significantly associated with more consistent contraceptive use (McKinney et al., 1984). And both Neel et al. (1985) and Rosen and Ager (1981) found that a favorable self-concept, variously defined, was positively associated with contraceptive use. However, other studies on this issue, including prospective studies, have shown inconsistent results (see, for example, Plotnick, 1992; Plotnick and Butler, 1991; Durant et al., 1990; Burger and Inderbitzen, 1985).

The failure to find a consistent relationship between contraceptive behavior and self-esteem may stem from the possibility that the measure of self-esteem is too general to capture the direct effect that it has on contraceptive use. A more situation-specific concept of self-esteem—self-efficacy—has been used by many researchers with more consistent results. Self-efficacy refers to an individual's belief that he or she has the skills to control his or her own behavior to achieve the desired outcome or goal (Bandura, 1982, 1977). Hence, individuals with higher self-efficacy would be more likely to use contraception to avoid an unintended pregnancy. Several investigations of this notion support the importance of self-efficacy in the careful use of contraception (Heinrich, 1993; Brafford and Beck, 1991; Levinson, 1986).

Another body of work has explored the concept of "locus of control," that is, individuals' belief that they can control what happens to them. The evidence is mixed, however, on the relationship between contraceptive behavior and various measures of locus of control (see, for example, Sandler et al., 1992; Visher, 1986; McKinney et al., 1984; Lieberman, 1981), possibly because of the general nature of the measure. But even when a measure more specific to contraceptive use was studied in relationship to consistency of condom use among a sample of clients at a family planning clinic, no significant association was found (Jaccard et al., 1990).

Attitudes and Feelings About Sexuality and Fertility

Another set of factors studied in relationship to contraceptive use is feelings about sexuality generally, as well as the guilt, fear, or embarrassment that the subjects of sexuality and contraception (and even the process of obtaining contraception) may engender. Concerns about one's fertility have also been studied in relationship to contraceptive use.

The theory of sexual behavior sequence, for example, hypothesizes that an individual's emotional response to sexuality may influence and mediate the avoidance of or approach to contraception because using contraception is a behavior with important sexual overtones (Byrne, 1983). Consequently, the theory states, persons with negative feelings about sexuality may find it difficult to learn contraceptive information, may avoid public acquisition of contraceptives, and may therefore be inconsistent users of contraception. A test of this hypothesis among sexually active college men showed a moderate relationship between feelings about sexuality and contraception: those with more positive feelings were more likely to report condom use (Fisher, 1984). Similarly, Winter extended the psychological notion of self-concept to include one's evaluation of one's own sexuality and defined it as the "sexual self-concept"—an individual's evaluation of his or her own sexual thoughts, feelings, and actions. In an exploratory analysis among college students, positive sexual self-concept was found to be associated with frequency of contraceptive use, with use at most recent intercourse, and with choice of method. Students who had used prescription methods at last intercourse scored higher on the sexual self-concept than did students who had used nonprescription methods or no method at all (Winter, 1988).

Negative emotions about nonmarital sex, such as fear or guilt, may inhibit sexual intercourse. When these emotions are not strong enough to deter intercourse, however, there is strong evidence that they may actually reduce the individual's ability to use contraception (Strassberg and Mahoney, 1988; Gerrard, 1987, 1982; Burger and Inderbitzen, 1985; Mosher and Vonderheide, 1985; Gerrard et al., 1983; Herold and McNamee, 1982). For example, the reasons given by sexually active college women for not using contraception show a tendency for denial and guilt over their sexuality (Sawyer and Beck, 1988), and high levels of guilt about sexual issues further predispose adolescents to taking contraceptive risks (Morrison and Shaklee, 1990). Similarly, among 13- to 20-year-old sexually active single females attending family planning clinics, significant relationships were found between guilt over premarital sex and both consistency of contraceptive use and contraceptive method choice at last intercourse (Herold and Goodwin, 1981). "High-guilt" women were significantly more embarrassed attending the clinic and having an internal examination than "low-guilt" women. High-guilt women were also more likely to perceive barriers to obtaining birth control information and contraceptives. A similar relationship between guilt about premarital sexual activity and contraceptive use among never-married female college students was shown by Keller and Sack (1982). The findings of these various investigations support the hypothesis that acceptance of one's own sexuality is positively related to the consistent use of a reliable form of contraception. Furthermore, the hypothesized relationship seems to hold regardless of whether a female or a male contraceptive method is used.

Focus groups designed to learn more about how adolescents feel about obtaining contraception at clinics confirm the importance of shame, embarrassment, and fear related to the medical examinations; embarrassment about being sexually active; and concern about confidentiality (Silverman and Singh, 1986). Pelvic examinations are often required before securing such prescription-based methods as oral contraceptives or diaphragms. In some clinics, such examinations are also required before nonprescription contraceptive methods are supplied. Consequently, among adolescents, in addition to the fear that their families will find out, another important factor in delaying a visit to a family planning clinic can be the fear of medical examination (Zabin and Clark, 1981). As noted in Chapter 5, this finding has led some groups to experiment with providing the first several cycles of oral contraceptives to adolescents without first requiring a pelvic exam.

Similarly, one of the major reasons given by men for not using condoms is because of embarrassment involved in obtaining them. Among a sample of adult males between the ages of 20 and 39 interviewed in 1991, 27 percent stated that it was embarrassing to buy condoms, and 20 percent stated that discarding condoms was embarrassing (Grady et al., 1993). The television comedian Jerry Seinfeld captured the essence of the embarrassment factor in a recent monologue (Seinfeld, 1993):

> Which brings us to the condom. There's nothing wrong with the condom itself. The problem with condoms is still buying them. I think we should have like a secret signal with the druggist. You just walk into the drugstore, you go up to the counter, he looks at you and if you nod slowly, he puts them in the bag for you. That's it.
>
> You show up there, you put your little shaving cream, your little toothpaste at the counter.
>
> "How are you today?" (You nod.)
>
> "Not bad. Yourself?" (He puts them in.)
>
> "Oh, pretty good."
>
> And you've got them.

There is also a small but important body of data suggesting that fears of being infertile, as well as inaccurate assessments of the risk of pregnancy in a variety of circumstances, may limit the careful and consistent use of contraception. Perceived fertility has been found to affect contraceptive use, with those women who perceived themselves as less fertile being more likely not to use contraception (Rainey et al., 1993). Other studies, too, have found a lower perceived probability of pregnancy to be associated with less effective contraceptive use (Burger and Burns, 1988; Tsui et al., 1991), although this has not been found consistently (Whitley and Hern, 1991).

One final attitude toward sexuality merits mention—the capacity to plan for intercourse and for contraception. For many individuals, especially those who are young or who are in the early weeks and months of sexual activity, intercourse is often unplanned. And because contraceptive devices must be obtained before intercourse, lack of planning for the event is closely associated with either the failure to use any method of birth control at all or use of such poor methods as withdrawal. In a 1994 survey of more than 500 high school students, three-fourths of those who were sexually active said that their first sexual experience "just happened" (SIECUS/Roper poll, 1994), and a recent study of young adults aged 17–23 found that 79 percent of those who did not use contraception at first intercourse said that they "did not expect to have sex" (Winter, 1988). Despite such findings, National Survey of Family Growth data and smaller studies confirm that the use of contraception at first intercourse has risen appreciably in recent years, almost entirely because of greater reliance on condoms.

Lack of planning for intercourse may be partly due to a general disinclination to plan ahead on a wide variety of issues in daily life, and as such may be a basic personality trait. It may also be due to the well-recognized "swept away" phenomenon—the passion and desire that can accompany sexual contact and that are among the most powerful and often pleasurable human sensations. Indeed, some would say that satisfaction from sexual activity is enhanced by spontaneity and that deliberate planning for such activity (including securing contraception) detracts from the experience. However, failure to anticipate sexual intercourse and to secure contraception may also reflect guilt, ambivalence, or denial regarding sexual activity, as discussed above. It has been suggested that one consequence of the residual squeamishness in the United States about sex (Chapter 7) is that too many individuals begin their sexual careers with a high level of discomfort regarding sexual feelings and behavior, and that this discomfort in turn impedes planning for both intercourse and for using contraception (Haffner, 1994). It is also important to acknowledge, however, that some sexual encounters are nonconsensual; in these situations contraceptive use is obviously precluded (Chapter 7).

Attitudes and Feelings About Contraceptive Methods

The 1987 study by Silverman and colleagues noted in the introduction to this chapter underscores how opinions and feelings about contraceptive methods themselves can affect the use of contraception and therefore the risk of unintended pregnancy. A wide variety of studies confirm that attitudes toward contraception and feelings about specific methods are strong predictors of contraceptive behavior and patterns of contraceptive use (Balassone, 1989; Morrison, 1989; Grady et al., 1988; Miller, 1986; Tanfer and Rosenbaum, 1986; Houser and Beckman, 1978).

As noted briefly in Chapter 5, one reason women often give for not using contraceptives is that they are concerned about the side effects or health risks of contraception in general and of specific methods in particular (Zabin et al., 1991; Sawyer and Beck, 1988; Forrest and Henshaw, 1983). Overall, it appears that both nonuse and the use of less effective methods derive at least in part from method-related fears and dislikes and from a general negative feeling about contraception.

All barrier methods and other "ad hoc" methods (such as withdrawal) must be used at the time of intercourse, and they require a definite decision and some type of a specific action at each sexual intercourse, whereas methods such as the pill and the IUD are used independent of coital activity. Not suprisingly, when compared to women who use coitus-independent methods, women who rely on coitus-dependent methods have been found to be more likely to forget to use or fail to use their method, more likely to discontinue their method in favor of no method at all, and more likely to switch methods altogether. For example, among a nationally representative sample of 15- to 44-year-old married women, Grady et al. (1988) found that those who used coitus-dependent methods were more likely to discontinue contraceptive use or to switch to a different method than users of coitus-independent methods. User failure was also found to be higher among users of coitus-dependent methods than it was among pill or IUD users. The researchers speculate that differences in user satisfaction with different methods may underlie both method discontinuation and user failures (Grady et al., 1989, 1988). Miller (1986) also reports more discontinuation among women who were using coitus-dependent methods, regardless of women's marital status.

The effect of user–method interaction has gained new significance with the spread of HIV infection. The condom is the only reversible male method of contraception that also is a very effective prophylactic against sexually transmitted diseases (STDs), including HIV. With the increase in the incidence of STDs and the spread of HIV into the heterosexual population, a small but growing segment of the literature on contraceptive use has focused on the determinants of condom use and individuals' perceptions of the advantages and disadvantages of this method (Brafford and Beck, 1991; Kegeles et al., 1988;

Brown, 1984). Although the condom's effectiveness in reducing the risk of an unintended pregnancy as well as the risk of an STD is widely appreciated (Boyd and Wandersman, 1991; Bernard et al., 1989; Strader and Beamen, 1989), men generally report overwhelmingly negative views of condoms, focussing on such disadvantages as embarrassment in purchasing or using them (noted earlier), reduction in physical pleasure or sensation, and the intrusiveness of the method (Boyd and Wandersman, 1991; Brafford and Beck, 1991; Pleck et al., 1991; Bernard et al., 1989; Strader and Beamen, 1989).

Another very important but less commonly cited disadvantage of condom use is fear of breakage and slippage (Grady and Tanfer, 1994; Beaman and Strader, 1989; Consumers Union, 1989). In a nationally representative sample of 20- to 39-year-old men, three-fourths of the respondents agreed that condoms reduce sensation, 64 percent mentioned that condom users must be careful or the device may break, and 43 percent were concerned that a man must withdraw quickly when he is using a condom. Also mentioned were slippage (22 percent) and difficulty in putting it on (24 percent), with 13 percent indicating that condoms cost too much (Grady et al., 1993).

Substance Abuse, Peer Influences and Family Relationships

Two sets of factors that may affect the use of contraception have attracted some analysis: the effects of alcohol and/or drugs, and the effects of both family and peer relationships.

Alcohol and Substance Use

Nonuse or poor use of contraception may sometimes be linked to the use of alcohol or drugs. Nonconsensual sex, such as "date rape," may be linked to substance abuse as well (see Chapter 7 also). Consistent with this view, an exploratory study based on interviews with unmarried, young women drawn from a family planning clinic found a clear association between unplanned sex, alcohol consumption, and nonuse of contraception (Flanigan and Hitch, 1986). More than two-thirds of the respondents had their first sexual experience by age 17, and one-half of these women reported alcohol (43 percent) or drug (7 percent) use at the time of that first intercourse. For a majority of these women the first sexual intercourse was unplanned, more than one-half of these women used alcohol before intercourse, and more than 80 percent did not use a method of birth control. Similarly, a correlation between general substance use and poor contraceptive use among adolescents has also been documented (Ford and Norris, 1994; Mott and Haurin, 1988; Ensminger, 1987).

However, some studies suggest a more complicated picture (Flanigan et al., 1990; Harvey and Beckman, 1986; Donovan and Jessor, 1985; Zabin, 1984). For example, in one study that examined substance use and other factors associated with risky sexual behavior within a target group of urban, unmarried pregnant adolescents aged 17 and younger, cigarettes and alcohol in general, and alcohol and drug use during sex in particular, were found to be positively associated with risky sexual behavior, including the nonuse or poor use of contraception. The effect of substance use, however, disappeared when the confounding effects of family bonding, parental monitoring, commitment to conventional values, peer associations, self-esteem, and delinquent activities were controlled (Gillmore et al., 1992). Such findings suggest that both substance use and behaviors that increase the risk of pregnancy may be part of a more general syndrome of risk-taking behavior and troubled life circumstances.

Parents and Peers

The fear of their sexual activity being detected by their family and meeting with strong disapproval can be a potent barrier to teenagers' use of effective contraception (Zabin et al., 1991), and improving communication about sex and birth control between parents and their children has therefore often been cited as a means to encourage young people to use contraceptives more effectively. However, much of the research in this area suggests that parent–child communication is not as powerful an influence on adolescent contraceptive use as common sense would suggest.

Furstenberg and colleagues (1984) found, for example, that family communication about sex and birth control appeared to count for very little with regard to levels of contraceptive use among sexually active teenagers. Similarly, using data collected over a period of two years from teenagers and their mothers, Newcomer and Udry (1985) found that neither parental attitudes toward premarital sex nor parent–child communication about sex and contraception affects teenagers' subsequent sexual and contraceptive behavior. Not only were the teenagers often ignorant of their parents' attitudes toward sex-related issues but also they and their parents often contradicted one another in describing the kinds of sex-related conversations that they had had. In only two cases was a significant relationship found between communication and subsequent behavior: adolescents whose mothers reported that they had discussed sex with them were less likely to subsequently initiate coitus, and adolescents who reported that their mothers had discussed birth control with them were more likely to use effective contraceptives. However, the former association disappeared when it was the daughters who reported the communication, and the latter association disappeared when it was the mothers who reported it.

One other aspect of parent-child interaction that should be noted is the possibility that some pregnancies among young adolescents occur during intervals of inadequate adult supervision, such as the unstructured hours between school dismissal and the return of parents from work in the early evening. Unfortunately, there are no data available to judge the merits or magnitude of this explanation, although it is intuitively appealing. This issue of supervision is also addressed in Chapter 7, in the context of preventing nonconsensual sexual activity.

Peer influences on contraceptive use have also been studied (see, for example, Whitley, 1991). Using data obtained in the 1982 National Survey of Family Growth, Mosher and Horn (1988) found that among sexually active women aged 15–24, friends and parents were the main sources of referral for first family planning visits. More specifically, friends were the leading referral source for women who attended clinics, and parents were the leading referral source for those who went to private physicians. Despite the importance of confidentiality to many teenagers, women who made their first family planning visit before the age of 17 were more likely to be referred by their parents than were those whose first visit occurred when they were age 17 or older. Since the analysis by Mosher and Horn is confined to those who made a family planning visit, these findings do not necessarily contradict the findings of other research (reported above) showing a lack of communication about sex and birth control between parents and their daughters or the findings indicating that family communication about these matters count for very little in explaining contraceptive behavior among sexually active teenagers. More recent research by Laumann and colleagues (1994) confirms that peers exert a significant influence on both sexual activity and contraceptive use.

Partner and Couple Issues

Numerous studies support the notion that a woman's partner may have a major impact on her use or nonuse of a contraceptive method; this may be especially true for young adolescent girls, given their relatively greater reliance on male contraceptive methods, especially condoms and withdrawal. For example, partner encouragement to use contraception had a direct effect on the contraceptive behavior of a sample of female high school and college students (Herold and McNamee, 1982). And in a prospective study among a sample of adolescent family planning clinic patients who were followed for six months after they were prescribed oral contraceptives, women's perception of partner support was the best predictor of compliance. Similarly, perceived partner support was also a good predictor of condom use for disease prevention among adolescent users of oral contraceptives (Weisman et al., 1991). Pleck et al. (1991) reported that among adolescent males, the anticipation that a partner would appreciate the respondent's willingness to use condoms was significantly associated with consistency of condom use.

However, couples may often disagree on various aspects of contraceptive choice and practice. In a study of married couples, for example, Severy (1984) found that appreciable differences between the fertility values of husbands and wives occurred one-fourth of the time, and that one spouse's perceptions of the other's values were at variance one-half of the time. Miller (1986) showed that, among married women, dislike by the husband of the method being used was significantly associated with an increased incident of subsequent nonuse. More recently, Severy and Silver (1993) showed that in light of the substantial misperception of one spouse's attitudes and intentions by the other spouse, joint decision-making was indeed an important factor for effective contraceptive behavior.

Many studies confirm that the nature and quality of a couple's relationship affect contraceptive use (Miller, 1986), particularly the use of coitus-dependent methods, because they generally require partner cooperation and support. The length of the relationship, for example, has been confirmed as an important factor in the contraceptive behavior of unmarried couples (Foreit and Foreit, 1981). Cvetkovich and Grote (1981) found that contraceptive use was positively associated both with the duration of the relationship and with trust in the partner. The authors suggest that men in stable relationships are more likely to care about the well-being of their partners and to actively encourage contraceptive use. Similarly, in a study of sexually active adolescent couples, those with good communication patterns were found to be significantly more likely to practice effective contraception; the risk of an unintended pregnancy was highest among couples who felt that contraception had not been adequately discussed (Polit-O'Hara and Kahn, 1985). Many other studies confirm these general themes (O'Campo et al., 1993; Adler and Hendrick, 1991; Pleck et al., 1988; Sawyer and Beck, 1988; Burger and Inderbitzen, 1985; Sack et al., 1985; Foreit and Foreit, 1978).

Some investigators have explored the relative influence of partners versus peers on contraceptive use. Whitley (1991, 1990) examined the sources and effect of social support on contraceptive use in a small survey of sexually active female and male college students. Although friends and partners were identified as equally supportive, only partner support was found to be related to contraceptive use. Furthermore, the nature and the quality of the relationship between the partners was a major factor in contraceptive use; contraceptive use increased with the intimacy of the relationship. Students also reported more motivation to comply with the views of their partners than with their friends, and this was more so among women than it was among men. Young men were willing to use condoms when they were encouraged by their partner, despite widespread dislike of this method. The finding that parental support was not an important factor suggests that contraceptive use may best be promoted through the self-disclosure and open discussion young adults enjoy with peers, and that a desire to please one's sexual partner seems to outweigh advice provided by a best friend. The findings of Cohen and Rose (1984) also indicate that for adolescent males, like females, sexual partners are the primary direct social influence with regard to contraceptive use.

CONCLUSION

Personal attitudes and feelings, both within males and females individually and through their connections as couples, clearly exert a major influence on contraceptive use and therefore unintended pregnancy. The concepts of personal motivation, the "benefit:burden ratio," and ambivalence, in particular, provide an integrating framework for numerous investigations of more limited concepts such as self-efficacy. Partner influence, and particularly the depth and quality of a couple's relationship, is an important influence on contraceptive use and therefore unintended pregnancy, underscoring the need to include men and couples in research on unintended pregnancy, as well as in interventions to reduce such pregnancies.

Overall comfort with sexuality and an absence of shame, embarrassment, guilt, or fear about sexual issues appear to support the careful use of contraception among both men and women. Data are also persuasive that feelings about contraceptive devices themselves—both overall and with regard to specific methods—can influence the choice of methods and the success with which they are used. Although sometimes associated with unprotected sex, alcohol or substance abuse are often not isolated influences explaining poor contraceptive use (or nonuse), but may rather be part of more general patterns of problem behavior and risk-taking.

Unfortunately, the research that lies behind many of these observations rests largely on samples of low-income black urban teenagers and white college students, even though a large portion of unintended pregnancies occurs among other groups. Too few investigations include older women and men or couples, and the racial and ethnic diversity of the populations studied, taken as a whole, is very narrow. Thus, available research is limited in its ability to explain the personal and interpersonal issues that affect contraceptive use and the risk of an unintended pregnancy among all of the populations in whom unintended pregnancy occurs. Finally, the lack of common theory and measurement instruments across the many investigations noted in this chapter makes it difficult to pool results or to integrate them with other bodies of information, especially material reviewed earlier on contraceptive knowledge and access (Chapter 5).

REFERENCES

Adler N, Hendrick S. Relationships between contraceptive behavior and love attitudes, sex attitudes, and self-esteem. J Counseling Dev. 1991;70:302–308.

Anderson E. Sexuality, Poverty, and the Inner City. Menlo Park, CA: Henry J. Kaiser Family Foundation; 1994.

Ajzen I. The theory of planned behavior. Organ Behav Hum Decis Process. 1991;50: 179–211.

Balassone M. Risk of contraceptive discontinuation among adolescents. J Adolesc Health Care. 1989;10:527–533.

Bandura A. Self-efficacy mechanisms in human agency. Am Psychol. 1982;37:122–147.

Bandura A. Self-efficacy: Toward a unifying theory of behavioral change. Psychol Rev. 1977;84:191–215.

Beamen ML, Strader MK. STD patients' knowledge about AIDS and attitudes toward condom use. J Community Health Nurs. 1989;6:155–164.

Bernard J, Hebert Y, de Man A, Farrar D. Attitudes of French-Canadian university students toward use of condoms: A structural analysis. Psychol Rep. 1989;65: 851–854.

Boyd B, Wandersman A. Predicting undergraduate condom use with the Fishbein and Ajzen and the Triandis attitude-behavior models: Implications for public health interventions. J Appl Soc Psychol. 1991;21:1810–1830.

Brafford LJ, Beck KH. Development and validation of a condom self-efficacy scale for college students. J Am Coll Health. 1991;39:219–225.

Brown IS. Development of a scale to measure attitude toward the condom as a method of birth control. J Sex Res. 1984;20:255–263.

Bulatao RA, Lee RD. An overview of fertility determinants in developing countries. In Determinants of Fertility in Developing Countries. Vol. 2. Bulatao RA, Lee RD, eds. New York, NY: Academic Press; 1983.

Burger J, Inderbitzen H. Predicting contraceptive behavior among college students: The role of communication, knowledge, sexual anxiety, and self-esteem. Arch Sex Behav. 1985;14:343–350.

Burger JM, Burns L. The illusion of unique invulnerability and the use of effective contraception. Personality Soc Psychol Bull. 1988;14:264–270.

Byrne D. Sex without contraception. In Adolescents, Sex, and Contraception. Byrne D, Fisher WA, eds. Hillsdale, NJ: Lawrence Earlbaum Associates; 1983.

Cohen D, Rose R. Male adolescent birth control behavior: The importance of developmental factors and sex differences. J Youth Adolesc. 1984;13:239–252.

Consumers Union. Can you rely on condoms? Consumer Reports. 1989;March:135–142.

Cvetkovich G, Grote B. Psychosocial maturity and teenage contraceptive use: An investigation of decision-making and communication skills. Popul Environ. 1981;4:211–226.

Dash L. When Children Want Children. New York, NY: Penguin Books; 1989.

Donovan JE, Jessor R. Structure of problem behavior in adolescence and young adulthood. J Consult Clin Psychol. 1985;53:890–904.

Durant R, Sanders J Jr, Jay S, Levinson R. Adolescent contraceptive risk-taking behavior: A social psychological model of females' use of and compliance with birth control. Adv Adolesc Mental Health. 1990;4:87–106.

Ensminger ME. Adolescent sexual behavior as it relates to other transition behaviors in youth. In Risking the Future: Adolescent Sexuality, Pregnancy, and Childbearing. Vol. II. Hoffert SL, Hayes CD, eds. Washington, DC: National Academy Press; 1987.

Fishbein M, Ajzen I. Understanding Attitudes and Predicting Social Behavior. Englewood Cliffs, NJ: Prentice-Hall; 1980.

Fisher, W. Predicting contraceptive behavior among university men: The role of emotions and behavioral intentions. J Appl Soc Psychol. 1984;14:104–123.

Flanigan B, Hitch M. Alcohol use, sexual intercourse, and contraception: An exploratory study. J Alc Drug Educ. 1986;31:6–40.

Flanigan B, McLean A, Hall C, Propp V. Alcohol use as a situational influence on young women's pregnancy risk-taking behaviors. Adolescence. 1990;25:205–214.

Ford K, Norris A. Urban minority youth: Alcohol and marijuana use and exposure to unprotected intercourse. J Acquir Immune Defic Syndr. 1994;7:389–396.

Foreit JR, Foreit KG. Risk-taking and contraceptive behavior among unmarried college students. Popul Environ. 1981;4:174–188.

Foreit KG, Foreit JR. Correlates of contraceptive behavior among unmarried U.S. college students. Stud Fam Plann. 1978;9:169–174.

Forrest JD, Henshaw SK. What US women think and do about contraception. Fam Plann Perspect. 1983;15:157–166.

Furby L, Beyth-Marom R. Risk Taking in Adolescence: A Decision-Making Analysis. Washington, DC: Carnegie Council on Adolescent Development; 1990.

Furstenberg FF. Race differences in teenage sexuality, pregnancy and adolescent childbearing. Milbank Q. 1987;65:381–403.

Furstenberg FF. Burdens and benefits: The impact of early childbearing on the family. J Soc Issues. 1980;36:64–87.

Furstenberg FF, Herceg-Baron R, Shea J, Webb D. Family communication and teenagers' contraceptive use. Fam Plann Perspect. 1984;16:163–170.

Gerrard M. Sex, sex guilt and contraceptive use revisited: The 1980's. J Pers Soc Psychol. 1987;52:975.

Gerrard M. Sex, sex guilt and contraceptive use. J Pers Soc Psychol. 1982;42:153–158.

Gerrard M, McAnn L, Geiss BD. The antecedents and prevention of unwanted pregnancy. Issues Ment Health Nurs. 1983;5:85–101.

Gillmore M, Butler S, Lohr M, Gilchrist L. Substance use and other factors associated with risky sexual behavior among pregnant adolescents. Fam Plann Perspect. 1992;24:255–261, 268.

Grady WR, Hayward MD, Billy JOG, Florey FA. 1989. Contraceptive switching among currently married women in the United States. J Biosocial Sci Suppl. 1989;11: 117–132.

Grady WR, Hayward MD, Florey FA. Contraceptive discontinuation among married women in the United States. Stud Fam Plann. 1988;19:227–235.

Grady WR, Klepinger DH, Billy JOG, Tanfer K. Condom characteristics: The perceptions and preferences of men in the United States. Fam Plann Perspect. 1993; 25:67–73.

Grady WR, Tanfer K. Condom breakage and slippage among men in the United States. Fam Plann Perspect. 1994;26:107–112.

Haffner D. Sexuality Issues and Contraceptive Use. Paper prepared for the Committee on Unintended Pregnancy, Institute of Medicine. Washington, DC; 1994.

Harvey S, Beckman L. Alcohol consumption, female sexual behavior and contraceptive use. J Stud Alcohol. 1986;47:327–332.

Heinrich L. Contraceptive self-efficacy in college women. J Adolesc Health. 1993;14:269–276.

Herold ES, Goodwin MS. Premarital sexual guilt and contraceptive attitudes and behavior. Fam Relat. 1981;30:247–253.

Herold ES, Goodwin MS, Lero DS. Self-esteem, locus of control, and adolescent contraception. J Psych. 1979;101:83–88.

Herold ES, McNamee JE. An explanatory model of contraceptive use among young single women. J Sex Res. 1982;18:289–304.

Houser BB, Beckman LJ. Examination of contraceptive perceptions and usage among Los Angeles County women. Contraception. 1978;18:7–18.

Jaccard J, Helbig D, Wan CK, Gutman M, Kritz-Silverstein D. Individual differences in attitude-behavior consistency: The prediction of contraceptive behavior. J Appl Soc Psychol. 1990;20:575–617.

Kegeles SM, Adler NE, Irwin CE. Sexually active adolescents and condoms: Changes over one year in knowledge, attitudes, and use. Am J Public Health. 1988;78:460–463.

Keller J, Sack A. Sex guilt and the use of contraception among unmarried women. Contraception. 1982;25:387–393.

Klerman LV. Adolescent pregnancy and poverty: Controversies of the past and lessons for the future. J Adolesc Health. 1993;14:553–561.

Laumann EO, Gagnon JH, Michael RT, Michaels S. The Social Organization of Sexuality: Sexual Practices in the United States. Chicago, IL: University of Chicago Press; 1994.

Levinson RA. Contraceptive self-efficacy: A perspective on teenage girls' contraceptive behavior. J Sex Res. 1986;22:347–369.

Lieberman JJ. Locus of control as related to birth control knowledge, attitudes and practices. Adolescence. 1981;16:1–10.

Luker K. Taking Chances: Abortion and the Decision Not to Contracept. Berkeley, CA: University of California Press; 1975.

Maynard R. The Effectiveness of Interventions on Repeat Pregnancy and Childbearing. Paper prepared for the Institute of Medicine Committee on Unintended Pregnancy. Washington, DC; 1994.

McKinney K, Sprecher S, DeLamater J. Self images and contraceptive behavior. Basic Appl Soc Psychol. 1984;5:37–57.

Miller WB. An empirical study of the psychological antecedents and consequences of induced abortion. J Soc Issues. 1992;48:67–93.

Miller WB. Why some women fail to use their contraceptive method: A psychological investigation. Fam Plann Perspect. 1986;18:27–32.

Morrison DM. Predicting contraceptive efficacy: A discriminant analysis of three groups of adolescent women. J Appl Soc Psychol. 1989;19:1431–1452.

Morrison DM, Shaklee H. Poor contraceptive use in the teenage years: Situational and developmental interpretations. Adv Adolesc Mental Health. 1990;4:51–69.

Mosher D, Vonderheide S. Contributions of sex guilt and masturbation guilt to women's contraceptive attitudes and use. J Sex Res. 1985;21:24–39.

Mosher W, Horn M. First family planning visits by young women. Fam Plann Perspect. 1988;20:33–40.

Mott FL, Haurin RJ. Linkages between sexual activity and alcohol and drug use among American adolescents. Fam Plann Perspect. 1988;20:128–136.

Musick JS. Young, Poor and Pregnant. New Haven, CT: Yale University Press; 1993.

Neel E, Jay S, Litt I. The relationship of self-concept and autonomy to oral contraceptive compliance among adolescent females. J Adolesc Health Care. 1985;6:445–447.

Newcomer SF, Udry JR. Parent-child communication and adolescent sexual behavior. Fam Plann Perspect. 1985;17:169–174.

O'Campo P, Faden R, Gielen A, Kass N, Anderson J. Contraceptive and sexual practices among single women with an unplanned pregnancy: Partner influences. Fam Plann Perspect. 1993;25:215–219.

Pleck JH, Sonenstein FL, Ku LC. Adolescent males' condom use: Relationships between perceived cost-benefits and consistency. J Marriage Fam. 1991;53:733–745.

Pleck JH, Sonenstein FL, Swain SO. Adolescent males' sexual behavior and contraceptive use: Implications for male responsibility. J Adolesc Res. 1988;3:275–284.

Plotnick RD. The effects of attitudes on teenage premarital pregnancy and its resolution. Am Sociol Rev. 1992;57:800–811.

Plotnick RD, Butler SS. Attitudes and adolescent nonmarital childbearing: Evidence from the National Longitudinal Survey of Youth. J Adolesc Res. 1991:6:470–492.

Polit DF. Barriers to Self-Sufficiency and Avenues to Success Among Teenage Mothers. Princeton, NJ: Mathematica Policy Research; 1992.

Polit-O'Hara D, Kahn J. Communication and contraceptive practices in adolescent couples. Adolescence. 1985;20:33–43.

Quint JC, Musick JS, Ladner JA. Lives of Promise, Lives of Pain: Young Mothers After New Chance. New York, NY: Manpower Development Research Corporation; 1994.

Rainey DY, Stevens-Simon C, Kaplan DW. Self-perception of infertility among female adolescents. Am J Dis Child. 1993;147:1053–1056.

Rosen R, Ager J. Self-concept and contraception: Pre-conception decision-making. Popul Environ. 1981;4:11–23.

Rosenstock IM, Strecher VJ, Becker MH. Social learning theory and the health belief model. Health Educ Q. 1988;15:175–183.

Sack AR, Billingham RE, Howard RD. Premarital contraceptive use: A discriminant analysis approach. Arch Sex Behav. 1985;14:165–182.

Sandler AD, Watson TE, Levine MD. A study of the cognitive aspects of sexual decision making in adolescent females. J Dev Behav Pediatr. 1992;12:203–207.

Sawyer R, Beck K. Predicting pregnancy and contraceptive usage among college women. Health Educ. 1988;19:42–47.

Seinfeld J. Seinlanguage. New York, NY: Bantam, Doubleday and Dell; 1993.

Severy LJ. Couples' contraceptive behavior: Decision analysis in fertility. Address delivered at the Annual Meeting of the American Psychological Association, August 28, 1984, Toronto, Ontario, Canada.

Severy LJ, Silver SE. Two reasonable people: Joint decision-making in contraceptive choice and use. In Advances in Population Psychosocial Perspectives. Vol. 1. Severy LJ, ed. London: Jessica Kingsley Publishers; 1993.

SIECUS/Roper Poll, 1994. Cited in Haffner D., Sexuality Issues and Contraceptive Use. Paper prepared for the Institute of Medicine Committee on Unintended Pregnancy. Washington, DC; 1994.

Silverman J, Singh S. Barriers to the use of contraception in four US cities: Results from focus groups. Unpublished report; 1986.

Silverman J, Torres A, Forrest JD. Barriers to contraceptive services. Fam Plann Perspect. 1987;19:94–102.

Strader MK, Beamen ML. College students' knowledge about AIDS and attitude toward condom use. Public Health Nurs. 1989;6:62–66.

Strassberg D, Mahoney J. Correlates of the contraceptive behavior of adolescents/young adults. J Sex Res. 1988;25:531–536.

Tanfer K, Cubbins L, Brewster K. Determinants of contraceptive choice among single women in the United States. Fam Plann Perspect. 1992;24:155–173.

Tanfer K, Rosenbaum E. Contraceptive perceptions and method choice among young single women in the United States. Stud Fam Plann. 1986;17:269–277.

Tsui AO, de Silva SV, Marinshaw R. Pregnancy avoidance and coital behavior. Demography. 1991;28:101–117.

Visher S. The relationship of locus of control and contraception use in the adolescent population. J Adolesc Health Care. 1986;7:183–186.

Weisman CS, Plichta S, Nathanson CA, Chase GA, Ensminger ME, Robinson JC. Adolescent women's contraceptive decision-making. J Health Soc Behav. 1991;32: 130–144.

Whitley B Jr. Social support and college student contraceptive use. J Psychol Hum Sexuality. 1991;4:47–55.

Whitley B Jr. College student contraceptive use: A multivariate analysis. J Sex Res. 1990;27:305–313.

Whitley B Jr, Hern AL. Perceptions of vulnerability to pregnancy and the use of effective contraception. Pers Soc Psychol Bull. 1991;17:104–110.

Winter L. The role of sexual self-concept in the use of contraceptives. Fam Plann Perspect. 1988;20:123–127.

Zabin LS. Addressing adolescent sexual behavior and childbearing: Self esteem or social change. Women's Health Issues. 1994;4:93–97.

Zabin LS. The association between smoking and sexual behavior among teens in US contraceptive clinics. Am J Public Health. 1984;74:261–263.

Zabin LS, Astone NM, Emerson MR. Do adolescents want babies? The relationship between attitudes and behavior. J Res Adolesc. 1993;3:67–86.

Zabin LS, Clark SD Jr. Why they delay: A study of teenage family planning patients. Fam Plann Perspect. 1981;13:205–217.

Zabin L, Stark H, Emerson M. Reasons for delay in contraceptive clinic utilization: Adolescent clinic and nonclinic populations compared. J Adolesc Health Care. 1991;12:225–232.

7

Socioeconomic and Cultural Influences on Contraceptive Use

Contraceptive knowledge and access (Chapter 5) are undoubtedly shaped by the surrounding socioeconomic and cultural environment, as are personal attitudes and feelings about contraception (Chapter 6). This observation is consistent with a number of studies—often called areal research—showing that various community attributes, as distinct from individual characteristics, are associated with the likelihood of using contraception (see, for example, Mosher and McNally, 1991; Singh, 1986; Tanfer and Horn, 1985). It is also consistent with data suggesting that the more favorable rates reported by numerous Western European and other industrialized countries on such maternal and child health measures as infant mortality partly reflect the more generous policies and supports that these countries often provide pregnant women and young families (Miller, 1993). Accordingly, this chapter discusses several socioeconomic and cultural factors that, in varying ways, may affect contraceptive use and therefore unintended pregnancy: the large and increasing diversity of the U.S. population (including ethnic, cultural, and religious diversity), conflicting views of sexuality and how such views might influence the use of contraception, economic issues, the roles that racism and violence play in various aspects of reproductive life, selected aspects of gender bias that relate to unintended pregnancy, and how organized opposition to abortion might affect access to contraception.

It is not always clear what the precise relationship is between these factors and the risk of unintended pregnancy. Nonetheless, in the aggregate, they help to form the environment in which individual decisions about contraception and sexual activity occur. Consideration of them must be part of any serious inquiry into the reasons that lie behind high rates of unintended pregnancy in the United States.

DIVERSITY IN U.S. CULTURE

The large and increasing diversity of the U.S. population is unmistakably one of its strengths, celebrated throughout the country with flair and enthusiasm. It is also a factor that makes understanding the determinants of unintended pregnancy more difficult. For example, even the concept of unintended pregnancy may be alien to some groups whose views of pregnancy and childbearing may be based more on fatalism or other value systems than the notion that these events can or should be carefully planned by such artificial means as contraception. Appreciable diversity can also complicate the task of designing culturally competent intervention programs that respect differences in feelings and values regarding unintended pregnancy, contraception, and related topics. This section briefly explores several aspects of diversity: cultural, ethnic, religious, and political.

Cultural and Ethnic Diversity

The United States is already a diverse mix of cultural, racial, and ethnic groups, and will be even more so in future years. The Bureau of the Census estimates that by the year 2050, non-Hispanic whites will constitute 56 percent of the U.S. population, versus 76 percent in 1990; people of Hispanic origin will be 20 percent of the population in 2050, versus 9 percent in 1990; and the proportion of blacks will grow from 12 to 14 percent over the same interval (Day, 1993). Similarly, some projections suggest that non-white individuals will be the majority in as many as 53 of America's largest cities only 5 years from now, by the year 2000 (Nestor, 1991). The full impact of such diversity is not just a promise for the future, however. School districts in some sections of the country already report that their enrolled children represent many different language groups. One school in suburban Virginia claims that there are more than 36 language groups represented in its student population.

Even the terms used to describe the growing diversity of the United States—Asian/Pacific Islander, Middle Eastern, or Hispanic/Latino—fail to capture the full complexity. For example, Asian/Pacific Islanders include Laotians, Cambodians, Vietnamese, Hawaiians, Filipinos, Samoans, Guamanians, Japanese, Chinese, Koreans, and others as well. Moreover, in assessing ethnic, racial, and cultural diversity, it is important to distinguish recent immigrants, such as the majority of Southeast Asians now in the United

States, from native-born Americans such as the vast majority of black Americans.

This cultural and ethnic diversity is reflected in widely varying knowledge about and attitudes toward contraception and fertility control. For example, some immigrants arrive in the United States from countries whose systems of family planning services are arguably better organized than those here and whose range of available contraceptive methods is broader. Some bring with them rich traditions of folk medicine (such as reliance on herbal medicines and various folk remedies and use of neighborhood practitioners rather than doctors for health care) that do not always blend easily with U.S. approaches to medicine in general or contraception in particular. Some contraceptive methods available in the United States may be unfamiliar to recent immigrants, and the health care system that one must negotiate in the United States to obtain the more effective methods is certainly different, and often more complicated and inaccessible, than systems in the immigrants' countries of origin. Contraception especially may be associated with images and practices that limit its acceptability. For example, in Thailand, condom use is associated with a vigorous prostitution industry in that country, which may mean that efforts in the United States to encourage greater condom use might be resisted by recent Thai immigrants (Healthy Mothers, Healthy Babies Coalition, 1993). For illegal immigrants, the task of securing contraception may be further complicated because of their general inability to use such programs as Medicaid to help finance primary health care, including contraceptive services.

Religious and Political Diversity

As fundamental human behaviors, sexuality and family formation represent legitimate areas of concern for most organized religions. Thus, the moral or ethical principles expounded by religious leaders include such issues as the appropriate age of onset of sexual activity, the regulation of non-marital sexual activity, contraception and abortion, appropriate partners, rituals for recognition of marital unions, and responsibilities and obligations for child rearing. As a country historically considered a refuge for those experiencing religious persecution, the United States is characterized by a large number of religious groups quite heterogeneous as to their principles and practices and the historical antecedents of their beliefs.

Despite the sometimes quite ancient lineage of these principles and prescriptions, the current entanglement of religious and political groups over issues of sexuality and contraception in the United States reflects a relatively recent effort of religious groups to adapt to events coming to prominence largely in this century (D'Antonio, 1994). As discussed elsewhere in this report, these events include the development of effective and reliable means of contraception, wider access to safe abortion, a broader and often conflicting array of sources of information on sexual behavior and mores including the media and sexuality education provided in public schools, and an overt recognition of and pressure to accept sexual activities and alternate family configurations not consonant with traditional religious teachings.

In addressing the current overlap of religious doctrine and political ideology, it is helpful to consider several separate dimensions, including the appropriate locus for transmission of information and values regarding sexual behavior and family function, the use of contraception both within and outside of marriage, the increased public visibility and wider availability of abortion, the extent to which individuals adhere to the official positions of their religions, and the use of political strategies to assert religious and philosophical positions.

Most organized religions transmit values through an alliance with the family, both through formal instruction during or in conjunction with religious services and through modeling of behavior by the family. This traditional mode of transmission has been complicated by the availability of alternative sources of information, especially media.

In response to persistently high rates of teenage pregnancy, and more recently the spread of HIV, efforts have been undertaken to provide information and more appropriate models of behavior through the schools. Although most organized religions support such efforts, some individuals perceive the information and values to run counter to their own religious principles. They view these efforts as encouraging premature sexual activity and sexual activity outside the bounds of formally approved unions. Hence, such efforts are perceived as undermining traditional family values.

In contrast to issues surrounding the transmission of values that generally involves custom rather than formal principles, many organized religions have formal principles dealing with contraception and abortion. Most religions encourage responsible procreation within the confines of marital unions. Most did not, however, have strong moral or ethical traditions regarding contraception and abortion until this century, and there is only a very limited scriptural background on these issues. In Judeo-Christian traditions, only one Biblical passage can be construed as dealing with contraception (and that interpretation is controversial), and the Koran does not have any clear-cut teaching on this topic. Thus, most religious traditions prior to this century reflected the teachings of religious scholars, often in response to specific questions, events, or heresies. Until this century, most Christian scholars condemned contraception and abortion, with more variability within the Jewish and Islamic traditions (D'Antonio, 1994).

In the 1930s, however, this situation changed when the mainline Protestant churches in the United States began to approve contraceptive use by married couples and then later to accept abortion. As is well known, the Roman Catholic Church formally forbids the use of any contraceptive techniques other than "natural family planning" or the rhythm method, and any use of abortion for any reason. Other conservative religious groups also proscribe contraception and abortion, including the Lubavitcher Hasidic sect, the Church of Latter Day Saints, and several conservative fundamentalist and evangelical groups (Carlson, 1994; D'Antonio, 1994).

Regardless of the formal religious positions on sexual activity and control of fertility, substantial variation in practice occurs among those belonging to specific religious groups. The most dramatic example is the disparity between the position of the Catholic Church and most of its American members regarding contraceptive use. Despite the Church's clear stand against artificial means of birth control, most Catholic women and couples in the United States use a wide variety of contraceptive methods; 75 percent of white Catholic couples practice contraception, and among those couples, 63 percent use sterilization or oral contraceptives (Goldscheider and Mosher, 1991). Not surprisingly, the major predictor of personal practice is the degree of "religiosity," that is, the degree to which religion is seen as important and to which individuals observe other aspects of their religion (D'Antonio, 1994).

The considerable diversity of opinion among organized religions and the considerable diversity of personal practice among the membership of these religions, do not, by themselves, explain the vehemence of the current political debate on abortion and family values. The major change over the past decade has been the emphasis on conservative forms of family values and a coalescence of Catholics and the conservative elements within many Protestant denominations into politically active groups. Although certainly initiated among Roman Catholics, this movement now includes a large number of conservative Protestants who share a common vision of a threat to traditional family values. Furthermore, although the National Conference of Catholic Bishops has certainly played a seminal role in bringing its resources to political activity, evangelical Protestant groups such as the Moral Majority are equally committed and also bring substantial resources (Carlson, 1994).

Even though people and financing are important elements in attaining political power, another element also contributes to the current political climate. Blendon and colleagues (1993) report that the majority of Americans support the availability of abortion, but they do so conditionally and do not consider it their most important political issue. By contrast, those who strongly oppose abortion view it as a top priority and often vote for candidates on the basis of their expressed positions on abortion. In exploring this phenomenon more carefully, Blendon and colleagues (1993) found that there is no evidence that groups who strongly support abortion vote with the same single-issue orientation as do those who strongly oppose abortion. They also found that the tendency to view political issues through the lens of abortion is directly related to an individual's participation in his or her religion (or to their degree of "religiosity"). One noteworthy aspect of the continuing opposition to abortion is that some of those who strongly oppose abortion are increasingly engaged in aggressive and organized political activity at all levels of government with abortion as their major, but no longer their sole, focus. This issue is addressed directly later in this chapter under the heading "Opposition to Abortion." The expansion of opposition to abortion into opposition to other aspects of reproductive health, especially contraception and family planning, is a puzzling and distressing development, inasmuch as contraception helps to reduce the need for abortion by reducing the occurrence of unintended pregnancies in the first place.

In summary, the availability of effective contraception and abortion and the broader range of sexual behavior considered acceptable in many groups in the United States present a challenge to those espousing traditional family values. Although the majority of Americans profess relatively tolerant attitudes, there is no single shared ethic about what constitutes appropriate family structures or sexual behavior. In response to what is perceived as a threatening liberalization of sexual behavior, conservative elements of many religious denominations have joined in a common cause to protect what are defined as traditional values. The political controversy, in contrast to the moral controversy, reflects the fact that these groups are willing to use the resources of their religious groups for campaigning and lobbying, and they represent single-issue constituencies voting solely on the issues of abortion and family values. Participation in such political activity is less a function of formal religious affiliation than of degree of attachment to religion or religiosity (D'Antonio, 1994).[1]

CONFLICTING VIEWS ABOUT SEXUALITY

A particularly provocative explanation for the patterns of contraceptive misuse and nonuse (and therefore unintended pregnancy) seen in the United States is that American culture embraces conflicting views and attitudes toward sexual behavior, and that this underlying inconsistency impedes discussion about, and careful use of, contraception (Reiss, 1991). As Rhode (1993–1994:657) has said so bluntly, "Few if any societies exhibit a more perverse combination of permissiveness and prudishness in their treatment of sexual issues." This reluctance—this "prudishness," it is suggested—makes it difficult to disseminate clear, accurate information about contraception, which in turn may limit contraceptive use. Advocates of this perspective cite a wide variety of data, noted below, to support this point of view.

The first is that the Victorian ideal of coitus only within marriage and with only one partner lingers in the American consciousness, despite the fact that

---

[1]Appendix B presents additional historical perspectives on the interaction of religion and contraception.

patterns of sexual activity now bear little if any resemblance to that bygone era. As noted earlier, the age of first intercourse has steadily dropped, and the image of virginity until the time of marriage—often a fiction in part—is now significantly out of line with current American practices. For example, among women who turned age 20 between 1985 and 1987, almost three-fourths (73 percent) had had intercourse before marriage and before turning age 20 (The Alan Guttmacher Institute, 1994). But even in the face of large numbers of people having nonmarital sex at all ages and with more than one partner, there is still appreciable support for virginity if one is not married (Haffner, 1994). In a study undertaken by Klassen and colleagues (1989), for example, half of the adult respondents reported that they disapproved of adult women having nonmarital sex with a partner they love, and 41 percent disapproved of men doing so.

There are other examples of the mismatch between image and reality as well. Sexual activity in late adolescence has become increasingly common in recent years (Laumann et al., 1944). In the late 1960s, for example, about 55 percent of boys and 35 percent of girls had had intercourse by the age of 18; by the late 1980s, these figures had increased to 73 percent for boys and 56 percent for girls (The Alan Guttmacher Institute, 1994). Nonetheless, a majority of adults disapprove of unmarried teenagers having sexual intercourse (Haffner, 1994). Moreover, although three-fourths of adults believe that unmarried teenagers should have access to contraception, and almost all would want their children to use contraception if the children were sexually involved (Gallup Organization, 1985; Timberlake and Carpenter, 1990), only a third of parents who have talked about sex with their children say that they have included any discussion about contraception (Klassen et al., 1989). Such data suggest that opinions and feelings about sexual behavior may not fit comfortably with contemporary reality (particularly as regards adolescents)—a dynamic that may well limit the ability of individuals and communities to communicate clearly about numerous sexual topics, including ways to reduce unintended pregnancy.

The Media

Observers of the print and electronic media are especially persuasive in suggesting that mixed messages regarding sex and contraception dominate these pervasive forms of communication, and that the prudishness that Rhode (1993–1994) has referred to impedes clear communication about contraception especially. On the one hand, popular American media (network programming, music videos, advertising, etc.) are filled with sexual material; on the other hand, there is a noted absence of equal attention to contraception, responsible personal behavior, and values in sexual expression. The United States has, in effect, a media culture that glorifies sexual activity (especially illicit, romantic sex between unmarried people), but is squeamish about contraception. McAnarney and Hendee (1989:78) note, "The print and electronic media are filled with seductive messages, yet [Americans] are given little support or assistance in understanding sexual feelings, defining responsible sexual behavior, and learning respect for themselves and for others."

That the media are saturated with sexual material is incontestable. A 1991 study of sexual behaviors on network prime time television (i.e., ABC, CBS, NBC, and Fox) found an average of 10 instances of "sexual behavior" per hour (Lowry and Shidler, 1993). Given that a full 98 percent of American households have a television, many more than one, and that 71 percent of U.S. households are tuned in to a network television program during prime time, the exposure level is clearly very high (Brown and Steele, 1994). Although the overall prevalence of sexual material had declined slightly since a similar study was conducted 4 years earlier, in 1987, decreases in portrayals of prostitution and physical suggestiveness (displays of the body without touching) were almost offset by increases in portrayals of heterosexual intercourse (e.g., mentions or allusions to intercourse, as well as suggestive or actual images). Such portrayals on television increased by 84 percent between 1987 and 1991, from 1.8 to 3.3 behaviors per hour (Lowry and Shidler, 1993). Moreover, the promotional messages for other prime-time programs that surround regular programming include even higher rates of sexual behavior. Lowry and Shidler conclude that the networks "clearly are using sex as bait in promos to attempt to increase their ratings." When the sexual behavior in promos is added, the rate of sexual behaviors per hour increases from about 10 to more than 15 (Lowry and Shidler, 1993:635).

With regard to cable television, videocassettes, music rock videos, and movies, the picture is similar. For example, "adult programming" (i.e., X-rated content designed specifically to portray explicit sexual behavior) is cable television's fastest growing segment (Kaplan, 1992). With the advent of a fiber optic infrastructure, a projected 500 channels are expected to include even more such programming. The videocassette recorder (VCR) also provides greater access to sexually explicit material. In 1993 two of the most frequently purchased videos featured Playboy centerfold Jessica Hahn and the "Playmate of the Year" (Billboard Magazine, 1994). Moreover, according to recent content analyses, sex is more frequent and more explicit in movies than in any other medium. Virtually every R-rated film contains at least one nude scene, and some favorites, such as *Fast Times at Ridgemont High* and *Porky's*, contain as many as 15 instances of sexual intercourse in less than 2 hours (Greenberg et al., 1993). Despite the R-rating that supposedly restricts viewing to people over 18 unless accompanied by an adult, two-thirds of a sample of high school students in Michigan reported that they were allowed to rent or watch any VCR movie they wanted, and the movies they most frequently viewed were R-rated (Buerkel-Rothfuss et al., 1993).

Such sexual enticement is not balanced by or accompanied by clear messages about avoiding unintended pregnancy or sexually transmitted diseases (STDs) or about managing sexual activity in a safe, caring, and healthy manner. For example, few television programs ever mention the adverse consequences that may result from having sex—rates of mention of pregnancy or disease declined to about one per 4 hours of programming between 1987 and 1991. Thus, a typical viewer would see about 25 instances of sexual behavior for every 1 instance of preventive behavior or comment. Even then, the message may not be constructive—all of the references to STDs coded in the Lowry and Shidler study, for example, were in a joking context (Lowry and Shidler, 1993).

The issue of contraceptive advertising on television brings the mixed message issue into sharp relief. Despite the high level of sexual activity in television programming, as just described, the major national networks have adopted the position that contraceptive advertising will not be accepted, although there is more receptivity on cable and independent stations, and some local affiliates as well, mainly to messages about condoms. Lebow (1994) reports, for example, that ABC feels that in catering to a mass audience, contraceptive advertising would be controversial and offend the moral and ethical tastes of a good part of its audience, and the Fox network says that it will possibly accept condom advertisements only if they are designed to prevent disease; messages about preventing unintended pregnancy remain off limits. Similar views constrain the airing of public service announcements (PSAs) that offer general information about contraception, although there were some brief periods of receptivity to selected PSAs developed by the Planned Parenthood Federation of America and the American College of Obstetricians and Gynecologists. By contrast, the print media have been more accepting of contraceptive advertising. Advertisements for birth control now routinely appear in many magazines and some, though not all, newspapers (Lipman, 1986). Interestingly, public opinion appears to favor contraceptive advertising through the media. A Roper organization survey in 1991 found that two-thirds of Americans age 18 or older supported the airing of contraceptive advertisements (Lebow, 1994).[2]

---

[2]It is important to note that television advertising of such prescription-based methods as oral contraceptives faces restrictions from the Food and Drug Administration, which requires that complete listings of risks and side effects accompany any advertisement—a requirement that is not practical for television in particular. Recently, the American College of Obstetricians and Gynecologists, the American Academy of Pediatrics, the American Medical Association, and others have urged that new policies and guidelines be developed to allow direct advertising to consumers of these effective methods.

Commercial advertisers may be limited in their ability—and sometimes their willingness—to promote contraception directly, but they often use sexual appeals to sell their products. A study of 4,294 network television commercials found that 1 of every 3.8 commercials includes some type of attractiveness-based message (Downs and Harrison, 1985). Although most advertisements do not directly model sexual intercourse, they help set the stage for sexual behavior by promoting the importance of beautiful bodies and products that enhance attractiveness to the opposite sex.

In sum, all forms of mass media, from prime-time television to music videos, magazines, advertising, and the news media, include vivid portrayals of sexual behavior. Sexual activity is frequent and most often engaged in by unmarried partners who rarely appear to use contraception, yet rarely get pregnant.

Does exposure to such content contribute to early or unprotected sexual intercourse with multiple partners and high rates of unintended pregnancies among both adolescents and adults? At this point, more is known about what is in the media and how much people are exposed to it, than is known about how the media's content is interpreted or how it affects sexual behavior. According to classic social scientific methods, an ideal test of the effect of sexual content in the media would involve either randomized assignment to different media diets or longitudinal surveys. Such studies would establish whether media exposure or the specific behaviors of interest came first. Unfortunately, the perceived sensitivity of sex as a topic and a focus on adolescents and television to the exclusion of other age groups and other media have restricted the kind of research that has been done. Only a handful of studies has attempted to link exposure to such measures as audience beliefs, attitudes, or subsequent behavior. Moreover, a number of factors, such as gender, cultural background, developmental stage, and prior sexual experience, influence what media are attended to and how images are interpreted. It is reasonable to expect, for example, that individuals who are more sexually active and people who are anticipating having sex will see media content about sexuality as more relevant and thus seek it out. The most likely scenario is that the media's influence is cyclical—individuals who are interested in sex begin to notice sexual messages in the media, may be influenced by and act on them, and then may attend to such messages more in the future (Brown, 1993).

In a comprehensive review of the literature in this area covering both correlational studies as well as experimental studies, Brown and Steele (1994:16) concluded that "the few existing studies consistently point to a relationship between exposure to sexual content and sexual beliefs, attitudes, and behaviors." For example, studies of adolescents have found that heavy television viewing is predictive of negative attitudes toward remaining a virgin. Two studies have found correlations between watching high doses of "sexy" television and early initiation of sexual intercourse (Brown and Newcomer, 1991; Peterson et al., 1991).

There probably are useful lessons to be learned from reviewing the large literature on the role of the media in violent behavior. Violence and sex have been used throughout the short history of television, and for a longer time in other media, to attract attention and arouse viewers, keeping them interested enough so that they will attend to the advertising. Both violence and sex are frequently and positively portrayed. Further studies of the impact of the media on sexual behavior may well find patterns of effects similar to those established for violence. More than 1,000 studies have consistently found small positive relationships between exposure to violent content in the visual media (primarily television and movies) and subsequent aggressive and antisocial behavior (Comstock and Strasburger, 1993). Both the 1972 Surgeon General's Report and a 1982 report from the National Institute of Mental Health concluded that exposure to violence in the media can increase aggressive behavior in young people (Brown and Steele, 1994).

International Comparisons

Cross-national comparisons give added weight to the idea that America's conflicted views and values regarding sexuality contribute to unintended pregnancy. Noting, for example, that in Denmark the proportion of pregnancies estimated to be unintended is far lower than that in the United States, David and colleagues (1990:3) have commented:

> In Denmark, as in other Nordic countries, the approach to sex is pragmatic, not moralistic. Most Danes deem sexuality as a natural and normal component of a healthy life, similar to eating and sleeping, for which individuals must assume personal responsibility through effective contraception to prevent unintended pregnancies. Sexuality and contraception are openly discussed in the media and the location of contraceptive counselling centers is advertised. Information is provided to children at an early age. There is an entrenched national consensus to limit childbearing to wanted pregnancies.

A different set of investigators (Jones et al., 1986) expressed a similar view after studying the factors associated with varying patterns of teenage fertility in the United States and several other industrialized countries. One of their conclusions was that, compared with several other countries with lower rates of teenage childbearing, the United States is far less open about sexuality in general. The authors refer to the "underlying puritanical values" in the United States as limiting effective, easy communication about the importance of using contraception unless pregnancy is actively sought, how specific methods work and what their benefits and risks are, and where to obtain them.

The picture that these various data sets present is troubling: a country that has left its Victorian, perhaps puritanical, past far behind but is not comfortable with present day sexual practices; and a popular culture that, paradoxically, glorifies sexual expression—especially illicit romantic sex between perfectly formed, unmarried young people—but cannot accompany this fascination with plentiful messages of health promotion and disease prevention, including the use of contraception to avoid unintended pregnancy.

ECONOMIC INFLUENCES ON FERTILITY

A large and rich body of research has probed the relationship of various economic factors to fertility. Although other sections of this report address some of these issues, such as financial barriers to contraception (Chapter 5) and publicly financed family planning programs (Chapter 8), several additional topics merit highlighting. Federal and state legislators are particularly interested in the impact on fertility of such welfare programs as Aid to Families with Dependent Children (AFDC), but this section will first note a broader range of economic factors in the United States in order to provide a perspective on the welfare issue. It examines whether fertility is influenced by (1) nationwide trends in prosperity, (2) present or future individual or family financial status, (3) whether a woman is employed, and (4) whether the woman or the family receives welfare.

In trying to understand the influence of economic factors on fertility, a number of analysts have focused on the Depression especially. A glance at fertility rates over time indicates clearly that the rates declined during the Great Depression, suggesting that economic stress may decrease childbearing especially. However, since fertility rates were already declining before the Depression, most analysts believe that although the Depression may have increased this trend and made it longer, the Depression itself was not responsible for most of the decline. The Depression was closely followed by World War II, which disrupted family formation, so the decline continued, despite greater economic prosperity. Fertility rates rose sharply after the end of the war, creating the Baby Boom, and then continued their pre-Depression decline, despite the continued post-war economic expansion (Klerman, 1994).

In terms of present financial status, conventional economic theory suggests that fertility should increase with family income if children are a valued commodity. This theory is not supported by trends in the United States and other industrialized nations. There are several reasons for this. Infant and child mortality has declined markedly such that it is no longer necessary to have many children in order to ensure that a few live to adulthood. Moreover, although children may still be valued, they no longer add to family income by working in the fields or in factories. They are not an economic asset; in fact they are a major liability. Thus, particularly for families in the middle- and high-income brackets with high, and expensive, expectations for their children, larger incomes might be associated with lower rates of fertility. The empirical evidence in this area, as in the others presented in this section, is mixed.

In terms of future financial status, a major question is why adolescents have children despite the fact that early childbearing is associated with limited income later in life. Early childbearing may occur because adolescents vaguely realize what researchers are now confirming, that is, that the association is probably not entirely causal (Chapter 3). An adolescent's future financial situation may be bleak even if she delays childbearing because women who become pregnant as adolescents are more likely than those who do not to come from poor families, and growing up in a poor family is probably the major reason why many women who begin childbearing in their teens are poor as adults. The magnitude of the independent contribution of a teenage birth to a girl's financial status as an adult is controversial, but it is probably less than her family's initial economic status (Hoffman et al., 1993). Adolescents may not wish to forego their present enjoyment of children for the limited possibility that their financial status may be brighter if they wait. This may explain why even programs that suggest life options other than early parenthood often fail to prevent first pregnancies among adolescents and why programs that provide job skills training and that assist with employment for those who are already mothers seldom succeed in having a long-term impact on subsequent fertility (Maynard, 1994). The influences of poor neighborhoods, inadequate schools, and broken families, themselves caused in part by economic trends, may be too strong to be overcome by short-term programs, even those based on improving adolescents' future economic status. This issue is also addressed in Chapter 6.

For some women employment is an option, but for many it is a necessity. Among those for whom it is an option, choosing a career may lead to the postponement of childbearing, limiting of family size, or foregoing childbearing entirely. Women who work out of necessity may also try to limit the number of children they bear, since they would lose time from work at least immediately before and after the pregnancy and, in the child's early years, might need to pay for child care. There is some support for the theory that higher market wage opportunities for women reduce fertility (Schultz, 1994).

AFDC and Other Transfer Programs

A large literature has addressed the influence of the major income transfer programs in the United States (especially AFDC, Medicaid, and the Food Stamp program) on marriage, the labor supply, household structure, pregnancy and fertility of low-income women and households. Very little of this literature, however, has been concerned with the linkages between such programs and unintended pregnancy, which is the focus of this report.

Potential Influences

From a theoretical point of view, there are at least three kinds of program effects that deserve consideration, two of these effects being direct and the other somewhat indirect. First, it is at least conceivable that for some women the presence of AFDC, which provides a thin cushion of economic support in the event of a birth, may be seen as reducing the full costs of such a birth. In so doing, the program may thereby reduce the degree of contraceptive vigilance maintained by the woman and also reduce the likelihood of abortion in the event of an unintended pregnancy. In theory, any income support program could have such an effect, so long as program eligibility is defined in terms of family size relative to income and total benefits increase with family size. Thus, the Food Stamp program, in which roughly 1 in 10 Americans participates, might conceivably have an influence on contraceptive use and unintended pregnancy. The case of AFDC is somewhat more complicated, in that receipt of benefits is made conditional on family structure—that is, on the absence of a spouse—although in the 1980s many states implemented the so-called "AFDC-UP" version of the program, which allows benefits to be distributed even if an (unemployed) spouse is present.

A second potential influence comes about because of the specific financing provisions embedded in the Medicaid program and the close ties between Medicaid eligibility and participation in AFDC. Medicaid eligibility is an important avenue to free or highly subsidized contraceptive services for many poor women and in the past was also a source of financing for some abortions (see Jackson and Klerman, 1994). To the degree that contraceptive prices act as barriers to contraceptive access for poor women, the Medicaid program should improve contraceptive access and thereby reduce the risk of unintended pregnancy. To the degree that Medicaid and AFDC are tied, however, these contraceptive subsidies are implicitly conditioned on family structure as well as income, so that the implied change in risks of unintended pregnancy would be circumscribed and limited to female-headed households.

A third and somewhat indirect link is that, particularly in those states that do not implement AFDC-UP provisions, AFDC establishes a set of incentives that collectively discourage marriage and perhaps encourage marital dissolution. In particular, welfare rules and regulations that made receipt of benefits contingent on there being no man in the house may have had the effect of pushing men out of families. Unmarried women are less likely than married women to intend to become pregnant, other things being equal. Thus, by discouraging marriage, AFDC may, in effect, increase the number and percentage of women who are exposed to the risk of an unintended pregnancy, although there is very little scholarship on this issue.

Empirical Findings

As was noted above, unintended pregnancy has not emerged as a major theme or focus of research in the literature on AFDC and other income transfer programs. One exception to this is in the area of teenage childbearing, which is disproportionately the result of unintended pregnancy, and some of the recent literature on abortion is also relevant (Jackson and Klerman, 1994).

In Moffitt's (1992) recent and authoritative review, the literature on the effects of AFDC on marriage, marital dissolution, and female headship was divided into a set of studies pertaining to the period of the 1970s and earlier, and a more recent literature dealing with the experiences of the 1980s. The time period of a study is important, since the real value of AFDC benefits declined sharply after 1967 (Moffitt 1992:Figure 1) and by 1985 the level of real benefits had fallen below what was available in 1960. These declines in AFDC benefits were largely offset by expansions in the Food Stamp and Medicaid programs; for the former, at least, eligibility does not depend on the absence of a male spouse.

With respect to marriage and female headship, the earlier literature produced no clear consensus on either AFDC or total transfer program effects. The empirical findings from the 1970s displayed great diversity and inconsistency across studies (see Groenveld et al., 1983). According to Moffitt, stronger and somewhat more consistent program effects are often estimated for the 1980s, suggesting that income transfer programs do have a discernible effect on female headship (Ellwood and Bane, 1985) and remarriage (Duncan and Hoffman, 1990). Even these effects, however, are small in magnitude. Moffitt (1992:31) writes that "none of the studies finds effects sufficiently large to explain, for example, the increase in female headship in the late 1960s and early 1970s. If this result continues to hold up, research in this area would better direct itself toward a search for the other causes presumably generating the increases in female headship."

With regard to effects on childbearing (which is not separated into its intended and unintended components), the findings of the recent literature remain weak and inconsistent. Ellwood and Bane (1985) and Duncan and Hoffman (1990) find no significant effects. Plotnick (1990) and Lundberg and Plotnick (1990), by contrast, find significant positive influences of benefit levels on non-marital childbearing, but only for whites. In their preliminary work on teens, Jackson and Klerman (1994) report that AFDC benefit levels seem to exert a modest positive influence on non-marital fertility rates measured at the state level. The authors are concerned with the possibility that the apparent influence is not causal in nature but rather reflects other factors that could not be measured. Preliminary estimates also suggest that Medicaid funding for abortion—now provided by a few states without accompanying federal financing—does not appear to influence teen nonmarital fertility rates.

In summary, the empirical literature does not lend support to the popular perception that AFDC and other income transfer programs exert an important influence on non-marital fertility. The literature suggests that these programs may well affect female headship, however, although there are other factors, not yet well-understood, that appear to be much more important.

RACISM

As noted earlier in this report, the proportion of births derived from unintended pregnancies is higher among black Americans than among other racial groups, and there are also data suggesting that rates of unintended pregnancy are higher as well. There are undoubtedly many explanations for these observed differences. For example, to the extent that blacks are disproportionately poor, the problems of access to contraception and lack of health care that are associated with poverty fall particularly heavily on this group. Similarly, the greater risk of poor quality care faced by black women in two important components of women's health—hysterectomy (Kjerulff et al., 1993) and prenatal care (Kogan et al., 1994)—raises the possibility that in the field of contraceptive services, too, black women may be at risk of less than adequate care. Another set of factors that may help to account for the differences is based in the long and complicated relationship of black Americans to contraception and the birth control movement generally.

In summarizing this important history, Gamble and Houck (1994) have noted that from 1920 through 1945 the birth control movement was generally supported among blacks because it meshed with their political and social efforts to improve both the health and economic status of the black community. By allowing women to space their children, birth control was seen as leading to better maternal health, and better maternal health was seen as a way to decrease infant mortality. Furthermore, with fewer children families would have more resources to care for their offspring. Thus, birth control could be seen as a strategy to shed the burden of poverty that kept black people at the bottom of the social strata. Black proponents of birth control believed that birth control translated directly into material improvement in terms of housing conditions, food, clothing, and educational opportunities. Similarly, Rodrique wrote (1991:26, 48): "The black community in general had a . . . broad, political agenda for contraceptive use. Afro-Americans saw birth control as one means to attain improved health, and having secured that, equal rights and social justice." A controlled birth rate would be a "step toward independence and greater power" and would allow more resources to be used for the advancement of the entire group.

This is not to say that all members of the black community supported birth control efforts at that time; in 1925, for example, Dean Kelly Miller of Howard University expressed concern that black women were having fewer children and feared that the result would be race suicide (Rogers, 1925). During this time, concerns began to develop that have continued to influence the attitudes of many black Americans toward birth control programs:

> The question of who is to control the programs and whose objectives are they to meet clearly surfaced during this period. . . . Historical analysis . . . illuminates the importance of seeking assistance from institutions that African Americans had established themselves. African Americans may perceive their needs in a different fashion than other segments of society may view them and may shape activities accordingly [Gamble and Houck, 1994:18].

Two additional issues surfaced in the postwar period. These issues, like the control and participation issue noted directly above, produced a more complicated picture of the relationship of the black community to contraception: the divisive entanglement of race, welfare, and birth control; and the issue of contraception as racial genocide. These issues remain current and painful, as the contemporary discussion of welfare reform in particular makes clear.

Race, Welfare, and Birth Control

Gamble and Houck (1994) observe that taxpayer resistance to welfare expenditures grew after World War II. The disproportionate number of blacks who received public assistance may have been the primary factor for the opposition. In response to public demands, several state legislators introduced bills throughout the 1950s and 1960s to institute punitive sterilization for unwed mothers on welfare. Black women were frequently the targets of the legislation. For example, in 1958 Mississippi State Representative David H. Glass sponsored the bill "An Act to Discourage Immorality of Unmarried Females by Providing for Sterilization of the Unwed Mother Under Conditions of the Act; and for Related Purposes." Glass did not conceal the impetus behind the proposed legislation. He asserted,

> During the calendar year 1957, there were born out of wedlock in Mississippi, more than seven thousand Negro children. . . . The Negro woman because of child welfare assistance [is] making it a business, in some cases, of giving birth

> to illegitimate children. . . . The purpose of my bill was to try to stop, slow down, such traffic at its source [Solinger, 1992:41].

Glass's bill was not enacted. However, the sentiment that it represented did not die with it, as evidenced by legislative initiatives with similar intent in other states (all of which were unsuccessful).

The entanglement between welfare and contraception continued after the introduction of oral contraceptives in the 1960s. In 1960, for example, the welfare and health departments of Mecklenburg County, North Carolina, launched a joint program to provide contraceptive services to women on public assistance. Four years later, the county welfare director concluded that the program had proven to be extremely cost-effective. He reported that for every $1 spent on a package of birth control pills the county saved $25 in welfare costs; he further estimated that the county had saved $250,000 in Aid to Dependent Children grants (Shepherd, 1964). Other localities moved to initiate programs with the hopes of duplicating the Mecklenburg County results. Despite some opposition from religious organizations, most notably the Catholic Church, by 1967, 33 states provided contraceptive services for women on welfare (Harting et al., 1969; Morrison, 1965; Shepherd, 1964).

Black Americans called attention to the potential for coercion in the implementation of the contraceptive programs. Although rules mandated that participation in government-subsidized family planning programs should be voluntary, stories soon surfaced about case workers who had informed women that their public assistance depended on their use of birth control. Critics argued that the specter of governmental coercion made birth control appear to be an obligation for poor women rather than a matter of personal choice.

The entanglement of contraception in matters of welfare policy continued with the development of Norplant (Rosenfield et al., 1991). Since the 1990 U.S. Food and Drug Administration approval of Norplant, legislation promoting its use has been proposed in several state legislatures as a way to decrease welfare costs and to combat poverty. In February 1990, for example, Kansas State Representative Kerry Patrick proposed legislation to pay welfare mothers $500 to use Norplant. Insertion would also be covered by the state, plus the women would receive free annual checkups and $50 for each year that they kept the implant. Kerry proclaimed that "the creation of this program has the potential to save the taxpayers millions of their hard-earned dollars" (Rees, 1991:16). Similarly, in Louisiana, State Representative David Duke proposed legislation that would offer women on welfare $100 a year to use Norplant (Rees, 1991). During the first 6 months of 1993, legislation introduced in seven states would have established incentives for welfare recipients to use Norplant or would have mandated decreased welfare benefits for women who refused to use it. None of these bills passed, but activities to link birth control with state welfare policies continue (Lewin, 1991).

Members of the black community, including health activists, social scientists, and ethicists have harshly criticized these efforts (see, for example, Scott, 1992). They have pointed out the potential coercion inherent in these efforts. In addition, they have decried efforts to narrowly define the causes of poverty. As one observer has noted, "The solution to poverty is not combating fertility. It's creating opportunities" (Rodriguez, 1991).

Genocide

As suggested by the welfare–contraception entanglement, probing the black community's views on genocide is also central to understanding its attitudes toward birth control. Although members of the black community expressed some concerns about birth control and race suicide during the 1930s and 1940s, development of governmental family planning programs in the 1960s and 1970s fueled renewed concerns about the links between birth control and genocide. Black Americans responded to such programs with suspicion, ambivalence, skepticism, and, at times, open hostility. Some black people contended that they were targets of a government policy that was "more concerned about stopping babies than stopping poverty." The objectives of the initiatives, they argued, appeared to be to control the number of poor and minority people rather than to attack their social and economic conditions. Blacks pointed out that other antipoverty measures such as education, housing, comprehensive health care, and employment did not receive the vigorous support from politicians that family planning did. As Malveaux stated (1993:34): "Genocide is often used as a code word for many inequities related to race and reproductive rights—the use of Norplant . . . forced on poor black women; the unavailability of basic health care for many low-income and working people in our community; [and] the apparent disinterest of pro-choice activists in a broader range of social issues that affect the black community."

A history of coercive sterilization practices against poor women and black women also fueled distrust. In 1968 Douglas Stewart, director of Planned Parenthood's Office of Community Relations, acknowledged the impact of these abuses on black women's acceptance of family planning. He stated,

> Many Negro women have told our workers, "There are two kinds of pills—one for white women and one for us . . . and the one for us causes sterilization." This is a very real fear for some women. Perhaps it's because many of them are from the South where black people have heard instances of unwarranted sterilization by white clinic workers whose attitude seems to be "Let's get the Negro before he's born" (cited in Smith, 1968).

In the 1970s numerous reports of sterilization abuses against women of color surfaced. In the 1974 *Relf* case (*Relf* v *Weinberger*), a federal district court found that an estimated 100,000 to 150,000 poor women were sterilized annually under federally-funded programs. Some of these women had been coerced into consenting to the procedure by threats that failure to do so would result in the termination of welfare payments. This historical legacy of distrust profoundly affected black Americans' attitudes toward family planning. Many viewed the increased availability of oral contraceptives not solely as a matter of individual choice but also as a reflection of a government policy to decrease their numbers.

Some black men, many associated with nationalist organizations, have voiced strong opposition to government-sponsored family planning programs, although many black women have not agreed, seeing birth control more as a survival mechanism than as a genocidal tool. The words of Congresswoman Shirley Chisholm (1970:114) reflect this view:

> To label family planning and legal abortion programs "genocide" is male rhetoric, for male ears. It falls flat to female listeners and to thoughtful male ones. Women know, and so do many men, that two or three children who are wanted, prepared for, reared amid love and stability, and educated to the limit of their ability will mean more for the future of the black and brown races from which they come than any number of neglected, hungry, ill-housed and ill-clothed youngsters.

However, black women were not blind to the incongruity of the government plan to make contraceptives free and accessible to black communities that lacked basic health care. Black women acknowledged that they had to be vigilant in their acceptance of the government programs.

Vocal allegations of genocide diminished by the mid-1970s, but they have resurfaced in the 1990s. Continuing economic and social problems in portions of the black community, ongoing racism, and the growth of black nationalism have played roles in the resurgence. Charges of genocide have been raised in connection with AIDS, needle exchange programs, and reproductive health issues (see, for example, Cary, 1992; Thomas and Quinn, 1991; Bates, 1990). Turner (1993) underscores why it is important not to dismiss concerns about contraception as genocide. She argues that examining these feelings reveals a great deal about the viewpoints of black Americans. She contends that these views are based in and grow out of deeply felt beliefs held by many minority members that white Americans have historically been and continue to be ambivalent and perhaps hostile to their well-being.

Gamble and Houck (1994:31) conclude: "Historical analysis makes clear why issues surrounding birth control can touch . . . such high voltage sensitivity among black people. They provoke fears of genocide; they prompt concerns about who should make decisions and control the direction of the African-

American community; [and] they expose the perniciousness and tenacity of racial stereotypes." The precise extent to which historical wounds and current injustices affect contraceptive use, misuse, and failure among black Americans is unknown, but there clearly is reason to see a connection—one that is rarely acknowledged candidly in discussions about differing patterns of contraceptive use and unintended pregnancy.

VIOLENCE

Violence against women—rape and sexual abuse in particular—may also be associated in several ways with unintended pregnancy, especially among adolescents. Violence against women is increasingly evident and has recently captured the nation's attention as a major public health problem. Current estimates are that as many as 4,000 women die each year from domestic violence (i.e., violence that occurs between partners in an ongoing relationship), and some 4 million are beaten annually by boyfriends or husbands (National Women's Health Resource Center, 1991). The American College of Obstetricians and Gynecologists estimates that one-fourth of American women will be abused by a current or former partner in their lifetime (American College of Obstetricians and Gynecologists, 1989). In addition, various studies estimate that between 4 and 17 percent of women experience violence during pregnancy (Centers for Disease Control and Prevention, 1994). Interestingly, a recent analysis of 1990–1991 data from the Pregnancy Risk Assessment Monitoring System found rates of physical violence against women within the 12 months preceding childbirth to be significantly higher among women with unintended pregnancies than among those with intended ones (Centers for Disease Control and Prevention, 1994).

The incidence of rape appears to be very high, though estimates vary widely. The U.S. Department of Justice suggests that there were between 100,000 and 130,000 rapes in 1990 (National Research Council, 1993); other estimates are substantially higher after attempts are made to correct for underreporting, showing that perhaps as many as 700,000 to 1 million rapes occur annually (Sorenson and Saftlas, 1994; National Victim Center, 1992). Some of this violence against women, including date rape and other forms of nonconsensual sex, has been attributed to the presence of alcohol or substance abuse. Recent data underscore the special vulnerability of very young girls to rape and other forms of nonconsensual sexual contact. A 1992 study from the U.S. Department of Justice found that, in a survey of 11 states and the District of Columbia, half of the women and girls who had been raped were under the age of 18 and 16 percent were under the age of 12 (Bureau of Justice Statistics, 1994).

These data on the rape of girls and young women are consistent with the analysis of Moore and colleagues (1989) of the 1987 National Survey of Children, which found that 7 percent of all respondents (men and women aged 18–22) reported that they had experienced at least one episode of nonvoluntary sexual intercourse. There were, however, important race and gender differences; for example, white women were more likely than black women to report nonvoluntary intercourse before the age of 20 (13 versus 8 percent). That study also demonstrated that if nonvoluntary intercourse were eliminated from the sample studied, the age of first intercourse would be appreciably different. At age 14, for example, almost 7 percent of white women reported that they had had intercourse; if, however, one restricts the variable to the first *voluntary* intercourse, the figure drops to 2.3 percent; for black women, the comparable figures are 9.0 and 6.2 percent. Moore and colleagues (1989) conclude that forced sexual activity is one of the factors contributing to pregnancy among younger adolescents especially, inasmuch as the use of contraception in these circumstances is an unreasonable expectation. "If the prevention of pregnancy . . . is difficult for adults, the obstacles to rational, prophylactic behavior among children and adolescents exposed to nonvoluntary sex seem almost insurmountable" (Moore et al., 1989:114).

Other research confirms the prevalence of nonvoluntary sexual activity. Small and Kerns (1993) reported that in a medium-sized city in the Southwest, 21 percent of a large sample of girls (1,149 girls in grades 7, 9, and 11) reported that they had experienced unwanted sexual contact in the preceding year; for the girls in the 11th grade, about half of this unwanted sexual contact was intercourse, whereas for the younger women, unwanted intercourse represented between 25 and 30 percent of the unwanted sexual contacts.

These various data suggest the need for more careful supervision of young adolescent girls especially. Even without knowing what proportion of pregnancies among young adolescents occur during intervals of inadequate supervision, as noted in Chapter 6, it is reasonable to believe that more adequate adult monitoring of adolescents' safety and whereabouts could decrease these alarming figures on nonconsensual sexual activity.

A growing body of research suggests a particularly important connection between unintended pregnancy and sexual abuse. At least three studies have shown that a history of childhood sexual abuse among teenage mothers is common, and given that the majority of pregnancies among teenagers are unintended (Chapter 2), a link between the two is plausible (Boyer and Fine, 1992; Butler and Burton, 1990; Gershenson et al., 1989). Researchers have hypothesized that pregnancy is more likely among those with a history of sexual abuse because sexual victimization can be associated with lower self-esteem, sexual maladjustment, and feelings of powerlessness and hopelessness—feelings that might in turn impede careful use of contraception once sexual activity has begun (Musick, 1993). Boyer and Fine (1992), for example, found strong histories of abuse in their 1988–1992 study of 535 teenage girls who were pregnant or had already given birth; almost 66 percent reported that they had been the subject of sexual abuse. Forty-four percent had been raped, with 30 percent raped two to three times; the average age of first rape was 13.3, with the rapist's average age being 22.6. Of the adolescents who had been raped, 11 percent said that pregnancy had resulted. In comparing those who were pregnant or parenting and had been abused with those who were pregnant or parenting but had not been abused, the abused group was more likely to report use of alcohol or drugs or to have had a partner who used alcohol or drugs at first intercourse as well as at the time that pregnancy occurred (which in turn may interfere with vigilant contraceptive use or be a marker of risk-taking generally; see Chapter 6). The abused group was also more likely to report that they had not wanted to have intercourse at the time that pregnancy occurred, and the mean age of first intercourse was younger than that for the nonabused group (mean age, 13.2 versus 14.5). However, the reported use of contraception at the time that pregnancy occurred was similar in the two groups. The investigators concluded that the link between sexual victimization and adolescent pregnancy is important and underappreciated and deserves additional research.

These data highlight an additional component of the sexual abuse picture—the evidence that an appreciable portion of the sexual relationships and resulting pregnancies of young adolescent girls are with older males, not peers. For example, using 1988 data from the NSFG and The Alan Guttmacher Institute, Glei (1994) has estimated that among girls who were mothers by the age of 15, 39 percent of the fathers were ages 20–29; for girls who had given birth to a child by age 17, the comparable figure was 53 percent. Although there are no data to measure what portion of such relationships include sexual coercion or violence, the significant age difference suggests an unequal power balance between the parties, which in turn could set the stage for less than voluntary sexual activity. As was recently said at a public meeting on teen pregnancy, "can you really call an unsupervised outing between a 13-year-old girl and a 24-year-old man a 'date'?"

GENDER BIAS

At least two forms of gender bias have been suggested as contributing to the high proportion of pregnancies that are unintended. The first is that the apparent tolerance for unintended pregnancy in the United States reflects a subtle but powerful underlying attitude that women are expected to have children and that therefore whether a pregnancy is wanted or intended is not particularly important. The second is that the prevailing policy and program emphasis on women as the key figures in contraceptive decision making unjustly and unwisely excludes boys and men.

With regard to the first aspect of gender bias, contemporary feminists argue that there is a systematic undervaluing of women and a lack of attention to their needs, especially in the health sector (Rodriguez-Trias, 1992). They further suggest that the lack of concern generally over unintended pregnancy—and, in particular, the failure to make contraceptive services and information easily available—is but another example of women's second-class status, joining such other public health injustices as the slow-to-surface outrage against violence directed at women (see above), the over-representation of women in the uninsured and underinsured populations (Institute of Medicine, 1992), the failure to include women in selected types of clinical research (Institute of Medicine, 1994), the fragmentation of health services for women (Rosenthal, 1993), their poor receipt of preventive care (Wall Street Journal, 1993), and similar issues described by leaders of the women's health movement (see, for example, Hafner-Eaton, 1993; Zimmerman, 1987). Indeed, many leaders of the women's health movement began their public advocacy around issues of reproductive rights (J. Norsigian, pers. com., 1994), and many of the core issues of that movement remain centered on reproduction—access to contraception and abortion, development of better and safer contraceptive devices, and reducing unintended pregnancy.

Feminists assert that if women cannot control their fertility due to prevailing public policies and attitudes, they cannot control their lives, and moreover, that many of the problems surrounding contraception, abortion, and reproduction are attributable to patriarchal and paternalistic attitudes and policies in this country and elsewhere, based on a male wish and ability to control women. They suggest that the continued occurrence of unintended pregnancy and other reproductive health problems can be traced to the controlling ideologies and practices of male-dominated religions, federal and state laws and regulations, and prevailing cultural traditions that keep women in subservient, relatively powerless roles. This view holds that because men neither become pregnant nor bear children, they are less interested in or sensitive to the many burdens that pregnancy (especially unintended pregnancy) can impose, and therefore are slow to take remedial action. This perspective is consistent with deliberations at the recent United Nations Conference on Population and Development in Cairo—a meeting that focused crisply on the pivotal role that women's status plays in overall social and economic well-being (United Nations, 1994).

The second view—that men have largely been excluded from the family planning movement—is an old observation that has recently received renewed attention. In 1968, for example, Chilman cautioned against organizing family planning education and programs that focus only on women, noting that the limited research available at the time suggested deep male interest in issues of family size and contraception. More recently, an increasing number of meetings, programs, and research have begun to probe the complicated relationship of men to contraception, pregnancy, and parenthood (Edwards, 1994). Some of this increased attention to men undoubtedly derives from the explosion of STDs, including HIV and AIDS, and the fact that one of the best means of preventing the transmission of STDs is through the male use of condoms. Another factor is the recent increase in nonmarital childbearing and the deepening concern over the number of children in the United States, especially black children, who will spend significant portions of their childhood and adolescence in households without fathers. The passage of the Family Support Act of 1988 also focused attention on men and family formation by developing new procedures to establish paternity and to collect child support payments from fathers, regardless of marital status, through the Child Support Enforcement Program. Current welfare reform proposals put even greater emphasis on establishing paternity. Heightened attention to gender bias in many aspects of American life may also be contributing to the increasing interest in the male role in family planning.

Research has also focused attention on men, particularly the accumulating evidence that contraceptive use by women is affected by partner communication and attitudes, as detailed in Chapter 6. Sonenstein and Pleck (1994) have concluded that males are relatively more involved in females' decisions to use female methods than is often realized. As early as 1978, Thompson and Spanier's multivariate analysis in a college sample found that of all the variables examined, male encouragement to use a method of contraception was the strongest predictor of female use of a method.

As a general matter, however, males are at the fringes of the nation's complex system of family planning services, in part because many of the most effective methods of contraception are used by females, and also because of the simple biological fact that pregnancy occurs in women, not men, and therefore women have the greatest self-interest in managing contraception. Very few males turn to family planning clinics or health personnel for contraceptive supplies. In the 1991 follow-up interviews for the National Survey of Adolescent Males, for example, only 3 percent of all 17- to 21-year-old males—but 9 percent of black males—indicated that they had obtained the last condom they used from a clinic or a physician (Sonenstein and Pleck, 1994).

These low rates of clinic participation by males conform with evidence provided by a recent survey of 421 publicly funded family planning clinics. Eighty-seven percent of these clinics' administrators reported serving no male clients (31 percent) or fewer than 10 percent male clients (56 percent) (Burt et al., 1994). Across all the clinics, the average proportion of male clients served was approximately 6 percent. Similarly, it is estimated that 2 percent of Title X program clients in 1991 and 2 percent of Medicaid family planning recipients in 1990 were male (Ku, 1993). Since Medicaid eligibility is based primarily on participation in AFDC or recent program expansions to low-income pregnant women, it is not surprising that few males receive family planning services through Medicaid. However, there is nothing in Title X law that forbids the use of these funds for men (Danielson, 1988).

Even though most family planning clinics report serving few male clients, they do not ignore condoms. Virtually all of the clinics surveyed by Burt et al. (1994)—99.6 percent—reported that they provide condoms, but it was more often for supplementary protection, not as the primary method. In fact, a recent survey revealed that three-fourths of family planning clinic workers say that they encourage most or all of their clients to use condoms regardless of the primary method chosen for contraception. Although many try, however, only one-fifth think that they are successful with most or all of their clients. Some family planning clinics also do outreach to male clients. Thirty percent of the clinics are reported by their administrators to have recruiting efforts targeted to males (Burt et al., 1994).

These various data sets portray a family planning system that for the most part does not serve male clients, although condoms are made available to the female clients. Because various data suggest that men believe contraception is a joint responsibility, future efforts to involve men may well be successful. For example, in the 1988 National Survey of Adolescent Males (aged 15–19), 97 percent of the young men responding agreed that "before a young man has sexual intercourse with someone, he should know or ask whether she is using contraception," and 95 percent agreed that "if a young man does not want to have a child, he should not have intercourse without contraception" (Sonenstein and Pleck, 1994).

OPPOSITION TO ABORTION

The Supreme Court ruling in 1973 that declared abortion legal in all 50 states and the District of Columbia spawned a vigorous movement to restrict access to and the legality of abortion in the United States. Variously labeled the "anti-abortion" or "right-to-life" movement, this force has had a marked presence in local, state, and national political campaigns, including the last few presidential elections, in family planning service programs and funding, and in the process by which funds are appropriated for research and for reproductive health services generally. The movement exists despite the fact that a majority of Americans continue to support the availability of safe, legal abortion, albeit with a variety of restrictions (Blendon et al., 1993), as noted earlier in this chapter. Organized opposition to abortion has led to legislative restrictions in numerous states on access to abortion (National Abortion and Reproductive Rights Action League, 1994), along with efforts to maintain blockades and other barriers at facilities where abortions are performed. In addition, some of those who oppose abortion now extend their opposition to other issues as well, such as school-based sex education, and are increasingly active at the local level, where they may seek to influence the composition of school boards and to control the content of curricula regarding human sexuality. The increasing stridency and polarization of public debate over abortion, sex education, and other related topics has created an atmosphere that endangers political and public financial support for sex education, family planning, and the provision of legal abortions.

The growing intensity even endangers the lives and resources of those providing these services, as the increasingly vehement rhetoric may be seen as a signal to action by those prone to violence. In particular, the movement has been associated with systematic and increasing harassment of abortion facilities and their personnel, including several murders. The National Abortion Federation (1993) reported that between 1977 and 1993, there were more than 6,000 incidents of clinic disruptions, 589 blockades against family planning and abortion clinics, and almost 1,500 acts of violence against abortion providers. Abortion facilities that are not based in hospitals are more likely to be harassed than those that are based in hospitals, as are facilities that perform relatively higher volumes of abortion. More than half of the providers who perform more than 400 abortions annually report that they have been picketed at least 20 times annually as well (Henshaw, 1991).

The relationship of abortion opposition to unintended pregnancy centers on three issues: first, because some facilities that provide abortions also dispense contraceptive services and supplies, any restriction on access to abortion facilities may also limit access to contraception; second, the number of unintended pregnancies resolved by abortion rather than childbearing may be affected; and three, the general climate of controversy created around the issue of abortion may spill over into other areas of reproductive services and education, confusing clients about what services are actually available and with what restrictions, affecting the morale and performance of those who work in the family planning field, and encouraging an atmosphere of high emotion on all issues of reproductive and sexual health, not just abortion.

With regard to the first issue, data show that only about 85 of the 4,000 contraceptive clinics that receive funding from the federal Title X program perform abortions (using funds other than Title X funds); and about half of these 85 are in hospitals (L. Kaeser, pers. com., 1994). Looked at from the opposite side, however, it is also apparent that many abortion facilities also are a main source of contraceptive services as well. Depending on how one defines a "nonhospital abortion facility," in 1989 somewhere between 83 and 94 percent of such facilities also provided contraceptive care to nonabortion patients. These facilities also offer many other services, including screening and treatment for STDs, general gynecologic care, and infertility services (Henshaw, 1991). To the extent that these facilities and their clients are harassed because of the facilities' abortion activities, access to contraceptive services is compromised, which in turn may contribute to the incidence of unintended pregnancy. Crossing a picket line to obtain an abortion is undoubtedly stressful; crossing the same picket line for a contraceptive visit—or even worrying that obtaining contraception could require confronting protesters—might be enough to avoid making the trip altogether and cause a couple to rely instead on less effective, nonprescription methods of birth control.

With regard to the second issue—that the ratio between unintended pregnancies resolved by abortion rather than childbearing may be affected by opposition to abortion—there are some data to suggest a possible connection. Recently, the number of abortions performed in the United States has begun to decline; in 1992, 1.5 million abortions occurred versus 1.6 million in 1990 (Henshaw and Van Vort, 1994), and a decreasing proportion of all pregnancies, including unintended pregnancies, are now being resolved by abortion (Henshaw and Van Vort, 1994; Henshaw et al., 1991) (see also Chapter 2). It is possible that at least one reason for such trends is the discomfort and fear among both patients and providers caused by the harassment described above. Other factors that may help to explain the decreasing number of abortions include a changing age structure in the population, with more women in the older age groups among whom abortion is less common, and less punitive attitudes towards nonmarital childbearing (Henshaw and Van Vort, 1994).

An additional factor that is probably contributing to the decrease is the decline in the number of facilities that perform abortions. Between 1978 and 1992, for example, the number of counties that reported the presence of at least one abortion provider declined by more than 30 percent, such that by 1992 more than 80 percent of all counties in the United States and more than half of all metropolitan counties had no abortion provider at all. Similarly, it is estimated that over the last decade and more, the number of clinics, hospitals, and physician offices that perform abortions has declined by approximately 65 a year (Henshaw and Van Vort, 1994). Again, this may reflect fear among providers, some of whom are understandably reluctant to work at an clinic that provides abortion services. The decline in the number of abortion providers may also reflect the limited training in the procedure that many physicians now receive, particularly as compared to several years ago. Goldstein (1995:A11) recently reported that "in 1975, two years after *Roe*, all but 7 percent of U.S. medical schools offered training in abortion to obstetrics residents, and 26 percent required it. By 1992, one third were not given any training, even when residents requested it, and 12 percent included it as a requirement." Similarly, Westoff and colleagues (1993) report that most programs training family practice physicians as well as obstetrician-gynecologists do not require competency in this procedure. Although the Accreditation Council for Graduate Medical Education recently revised its requirements for obstetrics-gynecology residency programs to insist that training in abortion be provided (with a few narrowly defined exceptions for religious or moral objections), these new requirements will not take effect until 1996, and their impact on abortion availability may not be apparent for several more years after that.

The third issue—that the general climate of controversy created around the issue of abortion may spill over into other areas of reproductive services and education—is less easily documented, although field reports suggest that this is the case. Some of the more vocal opposition to sex education provided in the schools, for example, is reported to be from anti-abortion groups (Haffner, 1994). Furthermore, Zero Population Growth (1993) reports that "the majority of anti-abortion organizations are also opposed to the use of and access to contraception." In part, this is probably due to the fact that some of these groups are loosely affiliated with, or closely tied philosophically to, the Catholic Church, which has taken a strong stand against all forms of contraception except periodic abstinence. The recent bombings of four contraceptive clinics that perform no abortions at all (located in Pennsylvania, Minnesota, Ohio, and Vermont) suggest that the high level of conflict that surrounds abortion may indeed place those who provide other related services at risk of violence and harassment (C. Glazer, pers. com., 1994).

It is also important to note that opposition to abortion, sometimes accompanied by opposition to organized family planning programs as well, has also affected a surprisingly wide variety of basic statistical and research functions related to unintended pregnancy. For example, some state and local systems to collect information on the number of abortions being performed (as well as on their possible complications) have been curtailed. That is, because some object to abortion, fewer abortion-related data are collected—a development that has affected the federal abortion surveillance system operated by the CDC, which relies on these state and local estimates in compiling its own aggregate statistics. Similarly, some systems to collect information on publicly supported family planning programs were shelved for years; research sponsored by such public agencies as the National Institutes of Health has been scrutinized and occasionally reshaped quite directly by abortion opponents; and efforts to increase public information and education about such lethal problems as HIV/AIDS have been stymied as well. The net result of such ideologically-driven developments has been to create a climate in which it has been increasingly difficult to take action to reduce unintended pregnancy, inasmuch as this particular problem can easily get entangled in the "culture wars" of recent years about abortion, contraception, and sexual behavior—wars that appear to be ongoing.

CONCLUSION

Many of the factors that may influence contraceptive use and therefore unintended pregnancy touch some of the most controversial and important issues facing contemporary U.S. society. The large number and great complexity of these forces—cultural values regarding sexuality, racism, violence against women, gender bias, the content of the media, and others as well—suggest that no single or simple remedy is likely to solve the unintended pregnancy problem. Research has not probed how some of the issues noted earlier in this report—contraceptive knowledge and access, as well as personal and interpersonal factors—are affected by the larger social phenomena outlined in this chapter. Nonetheless, it is reasonable to conclude that achieving major reductions in unintended pregnancy will require that socioeconomic and cultural issues be engaged.

REFERENCES

Acs G. The impact of AFDC on young women's childbearing decisions. Discussion Paper No. 1011-93: Madison, WI: Institute for Research on Poverty; 1993.

The Alan Guttmacher Institute. Sex and America's Teenagers. New York, NY; 1994.

American College of Obstetricians and Gynecologists. The Abused Woman. ACOG Patient Education Pamphlet No. 83. Washington, DC; 1989.

American Medical Association. Graduate Medical Education Directory, 1994–1995. Chicago, IL: American Health Information Management Association; 1994:91.

Bates KG. Is it genocide? Essence. September 1990:76–78, 118.

Billboard Magazine. Top video sales. January 8, 1994.

Blendon RJ, Benson JM, Donelan K. The public and the controversy over abortion. JAMA. 1993;270:2871–2875.

Boyer D, Fine D. Sexual abuse as a factor in adolescent pregnancy and child maltreatment. Fam Plann Perspect. 1992;24:4–19.

Brown JD. Theoretical overview. In Media, Sex and the Adolescent. Greenberg BS, Brown D, Buerkel-Rothfuss N, eds. Cresskill, NJ: Hampton Press; 1993.

Brown JD, Newcomer SF. Television viewing and adolescents' sexual behavior. J Homosex. 1991;21:77–91.

Brown JD, Steele JR. Sex, pregnancy and the mass media. Paper prepared for the Committee on Unintended Pregnancy, Institute of Medicine. Washington, DC; 1994.

Buerkel-Rothfuss NL, Strouse IS, Pettey G, Shatzer, M. Adolescents' and young adults' exposure to sexually oriented and sexually explicit media. In Media, Sex and the Adolescent. Greenberg BS, Brown JD, Buerkel-Rothfuss NL, eds. Cresskill, NJ: Hampton Press; 1993.

Bureau of Justice Statistics. Child Rape Victims, 1992. Publication No. NCJ-147001. Washington, DC: U.S. Department of Justice; 1994.

Burt MA, Aron LY, Schack L. Family planning clinics: Current status and recent changes in services, clients, staffing and income sources. In Publicly Supported Family Planning in the United States. Washington, DC: The Urban Institute and Child Trends, Inc.; 1994.

Butler J, Burton L. Rethinking teenage childbearing: Is sexual abuse a missing link? Fam Relat. 1990;39:73–80.

Carlson AC. The views of theologically and socially conservative American groups on contraception, family planning and related issues. Paper prepared for the Committee on Unintended Pregnancy, Institute of Medicine. Washington, DC; 1994.

Cary L. Why it's not just paranoia. Newsweek. April 6, 1992:23.

Centers for Disease Control and Prevention. Physical violence during twelve months preceding childbirth—Alaska, Maine, Oklahoma, and West Virginia, 1990–1991. MMWR. 1994;43:132–137.

Chilman CS. Fertility and poverty in the United States: Some implications for family planning programs, evaluation and research. J Marriage Fam. 1968;30:207–227.

Chisholm S. Unbought and Unbossed. New York: Hodge Taylor Associates; 1970, quoted in Ross LJ. African American Women and Abortion: A Neglected History. J Health Care Poor Underserved. 1992;3:282.

Comstock G, Strasburger V. Media violence: Q & A. In Adolescents and the Media. Strasburger VC, Comstock GA, eds. Philadelphia, PA: Hanley & Belfus; 1993.

Danielson R. Title X and family planning services for men. Fam Plann Perspect. 1988; 20:234–237.

D'Antonio WV. Human sexuality, contraception and abortion: Policies, attitudes and practices among major American religious groups. Paper prepared for the Committee on Unintended Pregnancy, Institute of Medicine. Washington, DC; 1994.

David HA, Morgall JM, Osler M, et al. United States and Denmark: Different approaches to health care and family planning. Stud Fam Plann. 1990;21:1–19.

Day JC. Population Projections of the United States by Age, Sex, Race and Hispanic Origin: 1993 to 2050. Bureau of the Census, Economics and Statistics Division. Washington, DC: U.S. Department of Commerce; 1993.

Downs AC, Harrison SK. Embarrassing age spots or just plain ugly? Physical attractiveness stereotyping as an instrument of sexism on American television commercials. Sex Roles. 1985;13:9–19.

Duncan G, Hoffman S. Welfare benefits, economic opportunities, and out-of-wedlock births among black teenage girls. Demography. 1990;27:519–535.

Edwards SA. The role of men in contraceptive decision-making: Current knowledge and future implications. Fam Plann Perspect. 1994;26:77–82.

Ellwood D, Bane M. The impact of AFDC on family structure and living arrangements. In Research In Labor Economics, Volume 7. Ehrenberg R, ed. Greenwich, CT: JAI Press; 1985.

Gallup Organization. Attitudes Towards Contraception. Princeton, NJ. March 1985.

Gamble VN, Houck JA. A high voltage sensitivity: A history of African Americans and birth control. Paper prepared for the Committee on Unintended Pregnancy, Institute of Medicine. Washington, DC; 1994.

Gershenson HP, Musick JS, Ruch-Ross HS, Magee V, Rubino KK, Rosenberg D. The prevalence of coercive sexual experience among teenage mothers. J Interpersonal Violence. 1989;4:204–219.

Glei D. Age of Mother by Age of Father, 1988. Unpublished data from Sex and America's Teenagers, 1994, by The Alan Guttmacher Institute; retabulated by Child Trends, Inc., Washington, DC; 1994.

Goldscheider C, Mosher WD. Patterns of contraceptive use in the United States: The importance of religious factors. Stud Fam Plan. 1991;22:102–115.

Goldstein A. U.S. abortion services drop: Fewer doctors performing procedure. Washington Post. January 22, 1995.

Greenberg BS, Siemicki M, Dorfman S, et al. Sex content in R-rated films viewed by adolescents. In Media, Sex and the Adolescent. Greenberg BS, Brown JD, Buerkel-Rothfuss NL, eds. Cresskill, NJ: Hampton Press; 1993.

Groenveld L, Hannan M, Tuma N. Final Report of the Seattle-Denver Income Maintenance Experiment, Volume 1: Design and Results. Menlo Park, CA: SRI International; 1983.

Haffner D. Sexuality issues and contraceptive use. Paper prepared for the Committee on Unintended Pregnancy, Institute of Medicine. Washington, DC; 1994.

Hafner-Eaton C. Will the phoenix rise, and where should she go? Am Behav Sci. 1993; 36 841–856.

Harting D, Stableford S, Eliot JW, Corsa L Jr. Family planning policies and activities of state health and welfare departments. Public Health Rep. 1969;84:127–128.

Healthy Mothers, Healthy Babies Coalition. Unity Through Diversity: A Report of the Healthy Mothers, Healthy Babies Coalition, Communities of Color Leadership Round Table. Washington, DC; August 1993.

Henshaw SK. The accessibility of abortion services in the United States. Fam Plann Perspect. 1991;23:246–263.

Henshaw SK, Koonin LM, Smith JC. Characteristics of US women having abortions. Fam Plann Perspect. 1991;23:75.

Henshaw SK, Van Vort J. Abortion Services in the United States, 1991 and 1992. Fam Plann Perspect. 1994;26:100–112.

Hoffman SD, Foster EM, Furstenberg FF Jr. Reevaluating the costs of teenage childbearing. Demography. 1993;30:1–13.

Institute of Medicine. Women and Health Research: Ethical and Legal Issues of Including Women in Clinical Studies. Washington, DC: National Academy Press; 1994.

Institute of Medicine. Including Children and Pregnant Women in Health Care Reform. Washington, DC: National Academy Press; 1992.

Jackson C, Klerman J. Welfare, abortion and teenage fertility. Paper presented at the 1994 Annual Meetings of the Population Association of America. 1994.

Jones EF, Forrest JD, Goldman N. Teenage Pregnancy in Industrialized Countries. New Haven, CT: Yale University Press; 1986.

Kaplan, M. You get what you pay for: Everything you ever wanted to know about cable sex. US, August 1992.

Kjerulff K, Guzinski GM, Langenberg PW, et al. Hysterectomy and race. Obstet Gynecol. 1993;82:757–764.

Klassen AD, Williams CI, Levitt EE. Sex and Morality in the US. Middletown, CT: Wesleyan University Press; 1989.

Klerman JA. Economic Perspectives on Unintended Pregnancy. Paper prepared for the Committee on Unintended Pregnancy, Institute of Medicine. Washington, DC; 1994.

Kogan MD, Kotelchuck M, Alexander GR, et al. Racial disparities in reported prenatal care advice from health care providers. Am J Public Health. 1994;84:82–88.

Ku L. Financing of family planning services. In Publicly Supported Family Planning in the United States. Washington, DC: The Urban Institute and Child Trends, Inc.; 1993.

Laumann EO, Gagnon JH, Michael RT, Michaels S. The Social Organization of Sexuality: Sexual Practices in the United States. Chicago, IL: University of Chicago Press; 1994.

Lebow MA. Contraceptive advertising in the United States. Paper prepared for the Committee on Unintended Pregnancy, Institute of Medicine. Washington, DC; 1994. Slightly revised version published as Lebow MA. Contraceptive advertising in the United States. Womens Health Issues. 1994;4:196–208.

Lewin T. A plan to pay welfare mothers for birth control. New York Times, February 9, 1991.

Lipman J. Controversial product isn't an easy subject for ad copywriters. Wall Street Journal. December 8, 1986:1.

Lowry DT, Shidler JA. Prime time TV portrayals of sex, safe sex and AIDS: A longitudinal analysis. Journalism Q. 1993;70:628–637.

Lundberg S, Plotnick R. Testing the opportunity cost hypothesis of adolescent premarital childbearing. Paper presented at the 1990 Annual Meetings of the Population Association of America. 1990.

Malveaux J. Black Americans' abortion ambivalence. Emerge. 1993;February:34.

Maynard R. The effectiveness of interventions on repeat pregnancy and childbearing. Paper prepared for the Committee on Unintended Pregnancy, Institute of Medicine. Washington, DC; 1994.

McAnarney ER, Hendee WR. The prevention of adolescent pregnancy. JAMA. 1989; 262:78–82.

Miller CA. Maternal and infant care: Comparisons between Western Europe and the United States. Int J Health Serv. 1993;23:655–664.

Moffitt R. Incentive effects of the U.S. welfare system: A review. J Econ Lit. 1992;30: 1–61.

Moore KA, Nord CW, Peterson JL. Nonvoluntary sexual activity among adolescents. Fam Plann Perspect. 1989;21:110–114.

Morrison JL. Illegitimacy, sterilization, and racism: A North Carolina case history. Soc Sci Rev. 1965:39:10.

Mosher W, McNally J. Contraceptive use at first premarital intercourse: United States, 1965–1988. Fam Plann Perspect. 1991;23:108–116.

Musick JS. Young Poor and Pregnant; The Psychology of Teenage Motherhood. New Haven, CT: Yale University Press; 1993.

National Abortion Federation. Incidents of Violence and Disruption Against Abortion Providers. Washington, DC; September 21, 1993.

National Abortion and Reproductive Rights Action League. 1994 Update to Who Decides? A State by State Review of Abortion Rights. Washington, DC; 1994.

National Research Council. Understanding and Preventing Violence. Washington, DC: National Academy Press; 1993.

National Victim Center, Crime Victims Research and Treatment Center. Rape in America, at a Glance. Arlington, VA; April 23, 1992.

National Women's Health Resource Center. Violence Against Women. Conference Report. Washington, DC; 1991.

Nestor LG. Managing cultural diversity in volunteer organizations. Vol Action Leadership. Winter 1991:1821.

Peterson JL, Moore KA, Furstenberg FF. Television viewing and early initiation of sexual intercourse: Is there a link? J Homosex. 1991;21:93–118.

Plotnick R. Welfare and out-of-wedlock childbearing: Evidence from the 1980s. J Marr and Fam. 1990;52:735–46.

Rees M. Shot in the arm. The New Republic. December 9, 1991:16.

Reiss IL. Sexual Pluralism: Ending America's Sexual Crisis. SIECUS Report, February/March 1991:5–9.

Rhode DL. Adolescent pregnancy and public policy. Polit Sci Q. 1993–1994;108:657–669.

Rodriguez R. Scholars decry the Norplant controversy that refuses to die. Black Issues in Higher Educ. April 11, 1991:15,17.

Rodriguez-Trias H. Women's health, women's rights, women's lives. Am J Public Health. 1992;82:663–664.

Rodrique JM. The Afro-American Community and the Birth Control Movement, 1918–1942. P.11. Ph.D. Dissertation. University of Massachusetts; 1991.

Rogers JA. The critic. The Messenger. April 1925:164.

Rosenfield A, Feringa B, Iden S. Long-Term Contraceptives and the Threat of Coercion. Paper presented at Dimensions of New Contraceptive Technologies: Norplant and Low-Income Women. New York, NY: Kaiser Family Foundation; 1991.

Rosenthal E. Does fragmented medicine harm the health of women? New York Times, October 13, 1993.

Schultz TP. Marital status and fertility in the United States: Welfare and labor market effects. J Hum Resourc. 1994;29:637–669.

Scott JR. Norplant and women of color. In Norplant and Poor Women. Samuels S, Smith M, eds. Menlo Park, CA: Henry J. Kaiser Family Foundation; 1992.

Shepherd J. Birth control and the poor: A solution. Look Magazine. April 17, 1964:67.

Singh S. Adolescent pregnancy in the United States: An interstate analysis. Fam Plann Perspect. 1986;8:10–20.

Small SA, Kerns D. Unwanted sexual activity among peers during early and middle adolescence: Incidence and risk factors. J Marriage Fam. 1993;55:941–952.

Smith M. Birth control and the Negro woman. Ebony. March 23, 1968:36.

Solinger R. Wake Up Little Susie: Single Pregnancy and Race Before Roe v. Wade. New York, NY: Routledge; 1992.

Sonenstein FL, Pleck JH. The male role in family planning: What do we know? Paper prepared for the Committee on Unintended Pregnancy, Institute of Medicine. Washington, DC; 1994.

Sorenson SB, Saftlas AF. Violence and women's health: The role of epidemiology. Ann Epidemiol. 1994;4:140–145.

Tanfer K, Horn M. Contraceptive use, pregnancy and fertility patterns among single American women in their 20s. Fam Plann Perspect. 1985;17:10–19.

Thomas SB, Quinn SC. The Tuskegee Syphilis Study, 1932 to 1972: Implications for HIV education and AIDS risk education programs in the black community. Am J Public Health. 1991;81:1498–1504.

Thompson L, Spanier GB. Influence of parents, peers, and partners on contraceptive use of college men and women. J Marriage Fam. 1978;40:481–492.

Timberlake CA, Carpenter WD. Sexuality attitudes of black Americans. Fam Relat. 1990;39:87–91.

Turner PA. I Heard It Through the Grapevine: Rumor in African-American Culture. Berkeley, CA: University of California Press; 1993.

United Nations. Program of Action: Report from the International Conference on Population and Development. New York, NY: United Nations; 1994.

Wall Street Journal. Many women aren't getting preventive care. Wall Street Journal. July 15, 1993.

Westoff C, Marks F, Rosenfield A. Residency training in contraception, sterilization and abortion. Obstet Gynecol. 1993;81:311–314.

Zero Population Growth. The Hidden Agenda: Anti-Abortion . . . Anti-Family Planning. Washington, DC; 1993.

Zimmerman MK. The Women's Health Movement: A Critique of Medical Enterprise and the Position of Women. In Analyzing Gender: A Handbook of Social Science Research. Hess BB, Ferree MM, eds. Newbury Park, CA: Sage Publications; 1987.

8

Programs to Reduce Unintended Pregnancy

Included in the committee's charge was the mandate to "describe the range of programs that have been organized in the last 10 years or so to reduce the incidence of unintended pregnancy and, to the extent possible, comment on the effectiveness of various approaches." This chapter addresses that charge by examining two types of programs: major national programs that help to finance contraceptive services (e.g., Medicaid and the Title X program) and a variety of community-based programs that have been evaluated. The chapter includes commentary on the possible economic effects of these programs, given the deep policy interest in this issue.

NATIONAL PROGRAMS

Although there is no national program whose primary mission is to reduce unintended pregnancy per se, several activities funded at the federal and state levels have great relevance to unintended pregnancy inasmuch as they help to finance contraceptive services. Approximately $622 million in public funds was spent on contraceptive services in 1990 (Gold and Daley, 1991). Many of these funds flowed through several large, national programs: Medicaid and the Title X Family Planning Program serve the greatest number of women, but the Maternal and Child Health Services Block Grant, the Social Services Block

Grant, community health centers, and migrant and rural health centers also help to provide reproductive health services in various ways.[1]

Title X of the Public Health Service Act was first authorized in 1970 and serves as the backbone of family planning services for many women in the United States. Title X authorizes project grants to public and private nonprofit organizations for the provision of family planning services to all who need and want them, including sexually active adolescents, but with a priority given to low-income persons. The program is buttressed by a training program for clinic personnel and has some community-based education activities as well. Federal monies are provided directly to state and local family planning providers, and state matching funds are not required. In 1990, more than 4,000 family planning clinics received $118 million in Title X support (Ku, 1993). During the 1980s, federal funding fell dramatically and the clinics became more dependent on state, local, and private resources (Gold and Daley, 1991). These family planning clinics served approximately 4.5 million women in 1991, an increase from 3.8 million women in 1981. The majority of family planning clinic clients are low-income women, and approximately one-third are adolescents. The average proportion of male clients served in family planning clinics is approximately 6 percent (Burt et al., 1994).

Medicaid is a national, publicly supported program that provides a unique 90 percent federal matching rate to state expenditures for the family planning care of women enrolled in the Medicaid program. Most public dollars spent on family planning are through the Medicaid program; federal and state expenditures in 1990 were approximately $270 million, serving an estimated 1.7 million clients, of whom 2 percent were men (Gold and Daley, 1991; Ku, 1993). In part because of the expansion in eligibility for pregnant and postpartum women, but primarily because of a rise in the number of people enrolled in Aid to Families with Dependent Children (AFDC), and therefore also in Medicaid, more women began using Medicaid to support contraceptive services in the mid- to late 1980s compared with the number in the 1970s and the early 1980s (Ku, 1993).

The impact of Title X and Medicaid, the two largest public programs, on unintended pregnancy has not been clearly defined, although a number of studies have tried to assess the effect of "publicly supported family planning programs" (which typically include the Title X and Medicaid programs) on various fertility

---

[1]Another national program relevant to unintended pregnancy is the contraceptive research and development activities of the National Institute of Child Health and Human Development. The Institute of Medicine (1990) report *Developing New Contraceptives*, commented extensively on that research program; additional analysis is currently under way through another Institute of Medicine study (Applications of Biotechnology to Contraceptive Research and Development: New Opportunities for Public/Private Sector Collaboration) focused on how to best stimulate research in this important area.

measures, usually pregnancy and birth rates.[2] Two major approaches have been used. In essence, the first approach posits a certain level of effect of family planning programs on fertility, and then, with that assumption in hand, goes on to analyze the effects of publicly funded family planning services on various other outcomes, such as overall welfare expenditures. For example, Forrest and Singh (1990b) hypothesized four possible patterns of contraceptive use that might result from a reduction in public support of family planning programs; each pattern produced a different level of unintended pregnancy, among other things. They concluded that had public sources of contraceptive services been unavailable in the late 1970s, low-income women would have had between 1.2 million and 2.1 million unintended pregnancies, rather than the approximately 400,000 unintended pregnancies that did occur in 1982. Using the same underlying assumptions, they also computed various estimates of cost savings that flow from public investments in family planning, as discussed later in this chapter. Similarly, Levey and colleagues (1988) constructed a detailed algorithm that allows one to estimate the impact of varying expenditure levels for family planning services on other state outlays, such as AFDC, in Iowa.

The other type of research often relies on state or county data and tries to estimate more directly the actual effect of publicly funded family planning programs on selected fertility measures. One such study, completed in the 1970s, examined fertility levels across various geographic areas to assess the impact of family planning programs. The analysis concluded that "the U.S. family planning program has reduced the fertility of low-income women by helping them to prevent unwanted and mistimed births" (Cutright and Jaffe, 1976:100).

Two more recent studies focused on different but closely related outcomes and used the same general methodology. Grossman and Jacobowitz (1981) and Corman and Grossman (1985) clearly documented that organized family planning services reduced both infant and neonatal mortality rates. These gains were probably accomplished, in part, by reducing pregnancies among various groups that are at high risk of such mortality, such as low-income women or those with very short interpregnancy intervals. Because these groups also tend to be at high risk of unintended pregnancy, it is reasonable to suggest that the positive effects observed by these investigators were due in part to reducing unintended pregnancy.

Other studies using state level data have also been completed and, in the aggregate, suggest that publicly funded family planning programs affect some fertility measures more than others. For example, Moore and colleagues (1994)

---

[2]This section reviews studies that have assessed the impact of publicly funded family planning services on unintended pregnancy; some of these studies are reviewed again from the perspective of economic impact in a later section of this chapter labeled "The Fiscal Impact of Family Planning Funding."

reported that total public expenditures on contraceptive services (including Medicaid, Title X, and state funds) per woman at risk of unintended pregnancy had no apparent effect on adolescent pregnancy rates, but did seem to have a variable effect on birth rates, differing somewhat by race and age. Singh (1986) also found lower teenage birth rates in states with higher proportions of adolescents served in family planning clinics, but did not find an association with lower pregnancy rates. Similarly, Anderson and Cope (1987) found that publicly funded family planning programs in the United States could be linked to lower birthrates; this analysis did not assess effects on pregnancy rates. Olsen and Weed (1986) also concluded (using 1978 data) that overall enrollment in family planning clinics is associated with reduced teen birth rates, but suggested that such enrollment may also be associated with increased teen pregnancy rates. In a subsequent analysis, these same investigators (Weed and Olsen, 1986:190) seemed to soften their earlier finding by concluding that "greater family planning program involvement does not result in a reduction in teenage pregnancy rates." It is important to add, however, that all of these analyses have some unresolved methodological problems that suggest their conclusions should be viewed carefully. None of them, for example, has been able to control for varying levels of sexual activity, nor do they factor in such other dynamics as the growing use of condoms—widely available outside of organized clinic systems—to prevent pregnancy.[3]

One of the most recent such investigations is that of Meier and McFarlane (1994). They conducted a state-level analysis to measure the effectiveness of publicly funded family planning during the mid-1980s in influencing a variety of outcomes. The analysis focused on several indicators of effectiveness: the state-level abortion rate, the age-specific fertility rate for adolescents, the incidence of low birthweight and premature births, the proportion of pregnant women receiving late or no prenatal care, and the neonatal and infant mortality rates. The principal measure of public funding was the level of family planning

---

[3]As noted, these studies rely on state-level data, and this choice of analysis unit has both advantages and disadvantages. The disadvantage is that the outcome indicators of effectiveness are not directly linked to program activities or to the behavior of program clients. Viewed from another perspective, however, the use of state aggregates may be a potential strength. As is argued in Appendix G, the evaluation of any given program is greatly complicated when a number of programs coexist in the same geographic area. For instance, the information provided by one program may encourage a potential contraceptive user to seek out the services that are provided by a different program or by the private sector. These cross-program and spillover effects cannot be captured using program data alone; they require histories of program contacts and service utilization on the part of clients. A state-level analysis is implicitly concerned with the net effects of all publicly funded activities, and may therefore provide a truer picture than would emerge from consideration of any one program in isolation.

funding per capita, a measure that draws together all Title X funds as well as funds from other federal and state sources (see Gold and Macias, 1986; and Gold and Daley, 1991, for discussions of these funding sources). They also defined a second and somewhat problematic measure of public funding: the publicly funded abortion rate. This rate is the ratio of publicly funded abortions in a given year to the number of women aged 15–44 in that year. In addition, the investigators included a set of socioeconomic control variables, such as income per capita in the state, the proportion of the population that is black and Hispanic, and the proportion of the population that is Catholic.

In a pooled regression analysis, they found that increases in family planning funding were associated with a number of beneficial outcomes, such as a reduction in the incidence of low birthweight and reductions in neonatal and infant mortality levels. These effects were statistically significant and, when translated into totals, demographically important. They also found lower abortion rates, and because abortion is in almost all cases a response to an unintended pregnancy, this study suggests that increases in family planning funding reduced the number of unintended pregnancies. Curiously, there is no apparent association with adolescent fertility rates, nor do significant effects emerge with respect to the proportion of births that are premature or the proportion of women who receive inadequate prenatal care.

These conclusions from the analysis of Meier and McFarlane (1994) should be accepted with caution. The regression specification includes the publicly funded abortion rate as an explanatory variable, yet the total abortion rate, to which publicly funded abortions contribute, is treated as one of the dependent variables or effectiveness indicators. Without a reanalysis of these data, it is not possible to say whether their mixing of explanatory and dependent variables renders all conclusions suspect. It would not be surprising, however, if the net effect of the misspecification is to understate the full beneficial impacts of family planning funding.

Again, though, none of these studies focus specifically on Title X or Medicaid. This gap in the literature is puzzling and remarkable. It means, in particular, that the largest public sector funding efforts, Title X and Medicaid, have not been well evaluated in terms of their net effectiveness, including their precise impact on unintended pregnancy. At the same time, it is important to acknowledge how difficult it would be to design an evaluation of either program in the aggregate, although studying effects on unintended pregnancy in small areas is possible and should be done. In any event, these programs clearly help to finance contraceptive services for many women (and some men) and there is a strong suggestion that, as part of overall "publicly funded family planning services," they help to reduce fertility. It is unlikely that careful evaluation would find no net effect on unintended pregnancy.

LOCAL PROGRAMS

Assessing the effectiveness of local programs in reducing unintended pregnancy is also difficult, in part because of the sheer number of programs involved. There are, in fact, hundreds of smaller programs ongoing or recently completed in the United States that in some way address unintended pregnancy, and the committee made no attempt to investigate them all in great detail. Rather, the committee's focus was on those whose results have been carefully evaluated, a focus that considerably narrowed the task. In the subsections below, lessons learned from the evaluated programs are discussed. It is important, however, to begin this consideration of local programs with a clear acknowledgment that the existing array of programs at the local level—those that have been evaluated and those that have not—reflects a unique history and, in particular, the changing interests and ideologies of both public and private funding agencies.

Historical Perspective

There are few references to adolescent pregnancy in the scientific literature before 1960, although there are many references to births among unmarried women (often called "illegitimacy" at the time). In that era, most researchers and program planners appeared to believe that a child's being born to a married woman, rather than the age of the woman, was the major factor determining pregnancy outcomes and life prospects for mother and child.

In the 1960s, however, this began to change. Health, education, and social service practitioners became concerned about the consequences of adolescent pregnancies, and therefore developed programs to assist pregnant adolescents, largely those still under 19 years of age. The emphasis of these early programs was on reducing maternal and infant morbidity and mortality through adequate prenatal care; keeping pregnant adolescents in school during their pregnancies, often through the development of special schools, and returning them to school after delivery of their child; and ameliorating problems in the areas of interpersonal relations, housing, and financial status through the provision of social services. The programs also worked to prevent rapid repeat pregnancies among the participants. Perhaps the first such program was the Webster School, begun in 1963 in Washington, D.C., and funded by the Children's Bureau. Programs in Syracuse, New Haven, Baltimore, and other cities followed, some with federal support, but most with local or, later, state funds.

In 1972, Kantner and Zelnik began to publish their pioneering studies of adolescent sexuality, contraceptive use, and pregnancy; and other researchers began to analyze the epidemiology, risk factors, and outcomes of adolescent pregnancy. In 1971 and 1976, federal agencies developed proposals to address the problem of adolescent pregnancy, but no major initiative was undertaken until the publication in 1976 of The Alan Guttmacher Institute's report, *11 Million Teenagers: What Can Be Done About the Epidemic of Adolescent Pregnancies in the United States?* (The Alan Guttmacher Institute, 1976). A federal task force was then assembled, and its report to U.S. Department of Health, Education and Welfare Secretary Joseph Califano led to the establishment of the federal Office of Adolescent Pregnancy Prevention (OAPP). Shortly thereafter, in 1978, the Adolescent Health, Services, and Pregnancy Prevention and Care Act was passed. Although it included prevention language, the primary emphasis of this act was on demonstration projects that would provide "services to adolescents who are 17 years of age and under and are pregnant or who are parents." Several foundations became interested in this problem and supported demonstration programs largely directed at pregnant adolescents (Klerman, 1981).

The 1981 federal Omnibus Budget Reconciliation Act effectively terminated the original grant program, but OAPP survived and the Adolescent Family Life Act was passed. The act specified that grants should be made for demonstration projects for the provision of prevention services as well as for care services, and stressed the prevention of sexual activity among adolescents (i.e. abstinence) and adoption as an alternative for adolescent parents. Under the terms of the new legislation, grantees could not provide family planning services, other than counseling and referral, unless appropriate family planning services were not otherwise available in the community (Vinovskis, 1988).

The 1981 legislation allowed OAPP to support education programs whose aim was to prevent pregnancy. This was a relatively new role for the federal government since most sex education was assumed to be conducted in schools, by religious organizations, or by families, and the federal role in curriculum development had traditionally been advisory, with state and local governments taking the lead.

Between 1978 and 1984, the Center for Health Promotion and Education at the Centers for Disease Control (CDC) supported research on different aspects of sex education programs. This research was an attempt to understand the range of approaches being used around the nation and to determine their effectiveness. During this time, several not-for-profit, intermediary organizations, such as the Center for Population Options and the North Carolina Coalition on Adolescent Pregnancy,[4] were organized to advocate for attention to the problem of teenage pregnancy, to act as intermediaries between policymakers and local program

---

[4]Over time, some of these organizations have made name changes. For the sake of clarity, it should be noted that the Center for Health Promotion and Education is now the Division of Adolescent School Health at the CDC; the Center for Population Options is now Advocates for Youth; and the North Carolina Coalition on Adolescent Pregnancy is now the Adolescent Pregnancy Prevention Coalition of North Carolina.

leaders, to perform research and promote networking, and to provide technical assistance to local agencies.

Major foundations, notably The Ford Foundation and The Robert Wood Johnson Foundation, provided financial assistance to a variety of community organizations to work with schools to open school-based clinics. The possibility that a school-based health clinic could prevent adolescent pregnancy was first suggested by the results of the St. Paul program in 1980 (Edwards et al., 1980). Many local and state agencies followed this lead and organized such clinics. However, school systems, wary of controversy, usually stressed the need to improve adolescent health generally rather than to prevent pregnancy only.

Foundation investments in this field have varied over the years and across individual grant programs, but they, like the government, first stressed care for pregnant and parenting adolescents and then moved gradually to emphasize the prevention of pregnancy among teenagers. The Charles Stewart Mott Foundation, for example, established the Too Early Childbearing Network in 1978. Other large foundations, such as the Carnegie Corporation of New York, The Ford Foundation, and The William T. Grant Foundation, developed demonstration projects to ameliorate the effects of childbearing by adolescents (Klerman and Horwitz, 1992). A more recent move by foundations toward primary prevention programs is exemplified by the development of New Futures and Plain Talk: A Community Strategy for Reaching Sexually Active Youth by the Annie E. Casey Foundation and heavy reliance in the developmental phase of school-based adolescent health centers on the support of The Robert Wood Johnson Foundation.

In sum, the existing network of programs around the country reflects a unique history, particularly the early interest in caring for pregnant adolescents, followed by changing ideologies at the federal level. Reducing unintended pregnancy has rarely been a goal of these community-based, local programs, even though their stated goals, such as reducing repeat pregnancies, are often closely related to unintended pregnancy.

Program Search and Selection

As just noted, few programs at the local level have been explicitly designed to prevent unintended pregnancy. Accordingly, the committee considered those programs whose various outcome measures or stated goals are closely related to reducing unintended pregnancy: (1) raising the age of first intercourse, (2) improving contraceptive use (or, similarly, decreasing unprotected sexual activity), and (3) reducing pregnancy among adolescents, including rapid repeat pregnancy.

The committee further decided that to be considered "evaluated," a program must meet the following criteria: (1) the evaluation was completed since 1980;

(2) the evaluation was performed using an experimental or quasi-experimental design; (3) the evaluation measured behavioral outcomes (e.g., sexual activity or contraceptive use); and (4) the evaluation results were published in peer-reviewed journals.

With these criteria in mind, the committee conducted a national search to learn, in general, about local programs to reduce unintended pregnancy and, in particular, to identify programs whose results had been evaluated. Letters requesting information were sent to the directors of programs receiving Title X funds and the directors of maternal and child health agencies; federal and local government programs were contacted; foundation officers were queried; the primary investigators of several leading initiatives and the project directors of many smaller initiatives were approached; notices asking for program leads appeared in newsletters of the National Association of County Health Officials and the American Public Health Association and online through the Women's Health Network; and relevant literature was reviewed through MedLine, Social Science Index, Sociological Abstracts, Psychological Abstracts, Popline, and Family Resources databases, as well as the Health Promotion and Education Database from the CDC.

This search resulted in the identification of more than 200 programs that in some way address unintended pregnancy. In the aggregate, they represent a wide array of approaches, from school-based condom distribution programs, to classic family planning clinics; from innovative programs of community education to highly targeted interventions to prevent rapid repeat pregnancy among adolescents. Some are well-known and have received significant public attention, such as the "I Have a Future" program at Meharry Medical College and the Family Life and Sex Education Program of the Children's Aid Society in New York City. However, only 23 met the committee's evaluation criteria. These programs are a small and unique subset of the many programs now under way that deal with issues of sexual activity and contraceptive use. Nevertheless, because their effectiveness has been assessed carefully, they constitute the available body of knowledge regarding how to intervene effectively at the local level to reduce unintended pregnancy.[5] The 23 programs that met the committee's criteria are listed in the following subsection.[6]

---

[5]Numerous programs to protect against HIV-AIDS have also been organized and evaluated, and they provide additional perspectives on strategies to reduce unintended pregnancy (Kirby et al., 1994; Institute of Medicine, 1988).

[6]Results from New Chance and the Summer Training and Education Program have been published, but not in peer-reviewed journals. Nevertheless, they are included here because of their superior evaluation designs.

Evaluated Programs

Background information on each program listed below is presented at length in Appendix F, including descriptions of program implementation, objectives, evaluation methodology, results, and primary references.

A. Community of Caring: several sites around the country providing prenatal care for pregnant adolescents, with an emphasis on planning for future goals, including prevention of repeated pregnancy.

B. Condom Mailing Program: direct mail program for adolescent men designed to increase their knowledge about and access to condoms.

C. Elmira Nurse Home Visiting Program: comprehensive program of prenatal and infancy nurse home visitation for low-income women bearing their first child.

D. Facts and Feelings: home-based abstinence program using sex education videotapes to encourage discussion between parents and young adolescents about sexual issues.

E. Girls Incorporated Preventing Adolescent Pregnancy: nationwide sexuality education program divided into four age-appropriate components.

F. Group Cognitive Behavior Curriculum: school-based sexuality curriculum using group cognitive behavior theory to personalize accurate information about sexuality and contraception.

G. McCabe Center: alternative public school for pregnant students providing prenatal and postnatal education, with an emphasis on delaying rapid repeat pregnancy.

H. New Chance: national demonstration program offering comprehensive services for low-income parenting adolescents and young adults.

I. The Ounce of Prevention Fund's Parents Too Soon Program: statewide program for pregnant and parenting adolescents using home visiting and parent groups.

J. Postponing Sexual Involvement: school-based curriculum encouraging middle school students to delay initiation of sexual intercourse in combination with a human sexuality and contraception component.

K. Project Redirection: comprehensive demonstration program targeting pregnant and parenting adolescents age 17 or younger, including an employment-orientation component.

L. Project Taking Charge: school-based program combining abstinence-only sexuality education and vocational education.

M. Reducing the Risk: school-based curriculum (based on several interrelated theoretical approaches) encouraging avoidance of unprotected intercourse through abstinence or contraceptive use.

N. Reproductive Health Screening of Male Adolescents: hospital-based reproductive health counseling for adolescent boys, aged 15–18.

O. School/Community Program for Sexual Risk Reduction Among Teens: community-based program to delay initiation of sexual intercourse and improve use of contraceptives by sexually active adolescents.

P. Self Center: full reproductive health services as well as health education and counseling services provided through a school-linked clinic.

Q. Six School-Based Clinics: school-based clinics providing comprehensive health care to students located in six sites around the country.

R. St. Paul School-Based Health Clinics: one of the first school-based health clinic systems in the country providing comprehensive health care, including reproductive health care.

S. Success Express: school- and community-based program emphasizing abstinence for middle school students.

T. Summer Training and Education Program: summer school program combining work experience with educational skills and information about responsible sexual decision-making.

U. Teenage Parent Demonstration: large-scale field test of a change in welfare rules and services, increasing self-sufficiency through enhanced services.

V. Teen Outreach Project: school-based program involving students in community volunteer service, designed to reduce adolescent problem behaviors.

W. Teen Talk: sexuality education program based on the health belief model and social learning theory, designed to make adolescents aware of the seriousness of adolescent pregnancy and the probabilities of such a pregnancy happening to them.

In the remainder of this chapter, reference is often made to "effective" programs. Given the fact that the 23 programs had many different, albeit overlapping, goals, the actual nature of the effectiveness varies from program to program: that is, some were found to delay the age of first intercourse, some were found to improve contraceptive use, and so forth. For simplicity, the specific outcome measures are not always referred to extensively in the text; however, they are described in more detail in Appendix F, and many of the examples used to illustrate cross-cutting themes are careful to specify what effectiveness means for a given program.

It is important to emphasize that these programs are not necessarily effective in achieving their program goals. The committee's criteria asked only that the program be well evaluated, not that it be successful.

A Comment on Program Evaluation

The fact that only 23 evaluated programs surfaced for detailed review merits comment. The limited number should not be construed as an indication that program managers in the area of reproductive health are uninterested in learning the effectiveness of their efforts, but rather that many obstacles stand in the way of conducting strong program evaluation: (1) cost, (2) methodological difficulties, and (3) a social environment in which research on fertility-related topics may be seen as controversial.

Cost

Methodologically rigorous evaluations that incorporate random assignment or the development of a comparison group can be expensive; for example, it is often necessary to hire outside evaluators, especially for smaller programs with limited staff. Few programs have the additional funding readily available in their budgets for such an undertaking, and program staff may be reluctant to spend program dollars on research evaluations that would not immediately translate into the ability to provide more or higher-quality service. In some cases, evaluations are mandated by federal or state legislation, but additional funding is often not provided for in the legislation or is budgeted on an unrealistically low level. This leaves the option of using funds designated for program service, much to the distress of program staff. Sometimes additional funds for evaluation can be raised from, for example, local foundations, but success with such an approach is often limited. This perennial problem in finding or being provided with adequate evaluation financing sets the stage for a particularly distressing sequence of events: a program is put in place without adequate funds for evaluation, and then when it is unable to prove its effectiveness, it is criticized for not knowing what impact it has had.

Methodological Issues

Most programs target only a small number of people, generally a convenience sample such as students in a classroom or teen mothers receiving public support in a community program. The sample size is usually limited, and often there is a selection bias toward people who want to participate in the program. Small sample size makes it difficult to detect statistically significant differences between intervention and comparison groups. And comparison groups can be difficult to select, in some cases because clinically oriented programs often provide basic health services that might be unethical to withhold. Determining the intervention "dosage," or amount of time spent in a program, is also challenging and must be carefully tracked, because some participants attend all segments of the program and some attend only a few. Similarly, the fact that unintended pregnancy prevention programs often consist of many components makes it difficult to assess the relative effectiveness of each component. It may be that no single component is the most effective piece, but rather that it is the combination of components that is effective. In addition, longitudinal follow-up of participants is difficult in general, but is particularly challenging in reproductive health programs because of confidentiality issues.

Another problem faced in many program evaluations is that outcome measures are limited to self-reported sexual activity and contraceptive use. Such reports may be unreliable, but there are often no alternative outcome measures available, save the most conspicuous consequences such as sexually transmitted diseases (STDs) and pregnancy. Even these obvious outcome measures can be difficult to assess precisely. For example, although births can be verified through the vital registration system, there is no universal system for reporting abortions or miscarriages, a fact that leads, among other things, to chronic problems in documenting the actual number of abortions performed annually in the United States, as discussed in Chapter 2.

These considerations argue in favor of evaluating only a few large, multisite, model programs relying on experienced evaluators having resources sufficient for the task. Stahler and DuCette (1991) suggest that individual programs should focus attention on process evaluation (i.e., the careful collection of data on client characteristics and service utilization) and that third parties should undertake well-funded impact evaluations (i.e., outcomes and long-term follow-up) of various program models that target different subpopulations.

Social Environment

Evaluation of local programs has also been impeded by the prevailing societal environment. The past 10 or 15 years has not been an era hospitable to research that might be seen as sex-related and therefore controversial. For example, very little survey and ethnographic research on sexuality has been done in the past two decades. Not only is it controversial politically to conduct research on sex-related issues, but involving adolescents in such research, particularly without parental consent, can raise legal issues as well.

During the 1980s especially, the federal government severely curtailed systems of data collection that had been used to monitor a wide variety of programs related to fertility, such as the national family planning reporting system. The view seemed to be that because such programs were seen by some public officials as objectionable, it was best to down play or ignore them altogether by, among other things, collecting little information on their activities or effects. Thus, the fact that only 23 programs met the committee's evaluation criteria may reflect more the political climate within which pregnancy-related programs have recently operated than a disinclination among program leaders to evaluate their activities. In addition, during the 1980s, the withdrawal of much federal funding from all but abstinence-only programs may have had a chilling effect on program directors and researchers who might otherwise have been inclined to evaluate their programs.

CROSS-CUTTING THEMES

Several cross-cutting themes emerged from a review of the 23 programs, offering clues for future intervention programs as well as for supportive public policies.

1. Knowledge about how to reduce unintended pregnancy at the local level is very limited. Only 13 of the evaluated programs (programs B, C, E, F, G, I, J, M, N, O, P, V, and W) were even somewhat effective in changing sexual and/or contraceptive behaviors that increase the risk of unintended pregnancy. Thus, knowledge about how to reduce unintended pregnancy through local programs is still quite limited. It is also apparent that even among those programs that did report varying degrees of success, the magnitude of impact was sometimes small. Success in raising the age of first intercourse, for example, is typically measured in increments of months, not years, as was the case with the Self Center. Small effects can translate into a reduced risk of unintended pregnancy at the individual level if a delay in the age of first intercourse, for example, also has the effect of increasing contraceptive use once sexual activity begins; nonetheless, the overall demographic impact of such small changes is apt to be minor.

2. Because most of the evaluated programs target adolescents, especially young women, knowledge about how to reach adult women or men is exceedingly limited. Although the large national programs mentioned above (e.g., the Title X and Medicaid programs) do help adult women and a very few men to gain access to contraception, almost none of the 23 evaluated programs operating at the local level has a clear focus on adults (even though a few programs include some adult women who became pregnant as adolescents). This reflects the history of program funding and development presented earlier and mirrors ongoing public concern over adolescent pregnancy, despite the fact that adults also become pregnant (or cause pregnancy) unintentionally and with serious consequences (Chapters 2 and 3).

Too little is known about meeting the reproductive health and contraceptive needs of adult men in particular. The two evaluated programs that did target men concentrated exclusively on adolescents. The Condom Mailing Program, for example, used direct mail to increase adolescents' knowledge about and access to condoms (Kirby et al., 1989), and the Reproductive Health Screening of Male Adolescents program used a hospital-based sexuality education program to increase contraceptive use among adolescent boys (Danielson et al., 1990). In general, however, *adult* men are invisible in the 23 evaluated programs. It seems, in some sense, that programs do not know what to do with men, save to provide them with condoms. It is possible, however, that programs could be developed to educate men about their own and their partners' reproductive lives, that men could be encouraged to offer increased personal and financial support for their partners' use of contraception, and that they could be drawn into a wider variety of reproductive health programs. There is some evidence of new interest in programming for males, but it is too soon for evaluations of recent efforts to have been completed (Edwards, 1994).

Few of the 23 evaluated programs target couples, or address male–female decision-making about contraception and pregnancy, despite the fact that sexual and contraceptive decisions often occur within the context of a couple. Although some programs focused on adolescents do seem to address the interaction of the couple, the context is usually to support girls in resisting sexual advances and in saying no to precocious sexual activity. These are exceedingly important skills, but it might also be helpful for individuals and couples to learn about non-adversarial cooperation and communication about sexual and contraceptive issues.

3. There is insufficient evidence to determine whether abstinence-only programs have been effective in increasing the age of first sexual intercourse. Abstinence is frequently emphasized in programs for young adolescents, and it is an important option at all life stages. As noted earlier in the historical review, a number of local programs (such as programs D, L, and S) were funded in the 1980s to stress abstinence as the only means of avoiding unprotected intercourse. Many of these programs were funded by OAPP through the 1981 Adolescent Family Life Act and funding recipients were required to evaluate the effectiveness of abstinence-only programs. To date, these evaluations are too weak to provide evidence for or against the ability of abstinence-only programs to help adolescents delay the onset of sexual activity.

One example of this approach is Success Express, an abstinence-only, school-based program for sixth through eighth graders. This program used a curriculum focusing on family values and self-esteem, pubertal development and reproduction, communication strategies and interpersonal skills about "how to say no," examination of future goals, the effects of peer and media pressures, and complications of premarital sexual activity, adolescent pregnancy, and STDs. Although the evaluation was carefully developed by using a quasi-experimental design, post-test data were gathered immediately following the 6-week intervention; no follow-up data were collected at a later point. It is not surprising that such short-term results showed no significant difference in timing of first sexual intercourse between the intervention and control groups (Christopher and Roosa, 1990; Roosa and Christopher, 1990). The only significant finding was that boys in the intervention group were more likely to participate in precoital sexual behaviors than were boys in the comparison group.

Another abstinence-only, school-based program, Project Taking Charge, combined sex education and vocational training for low-income seventh-grade students. The program was designed to promote abstinence from sexual activity through promotion of communication between adolescents and their parents and planning for the future in the world of work. Basic sexual anatomy and sexual development were taught, but contraception was not a part of the curriculum. At both 6 weeks' and 6 months' post-intervention, the evaluation found no significant differences in the sexual behaviors of the intervention and comparison groups, although the results indicated that students in the intervention group may have delayed the initiation of sexual intercourse. However, the small sample size limits the generalizability of the results (Jorgensen, 1991; Jorgensen et al., 1993).

A home-based abstinence-only program, Facts and Feelings, distributed a videotape designed to encourage parents and their seventh and eighth graders to discuss sexual issues before the youths' initiation of sexual intercourse. The objective of the program was to encourage discussion about sexual issues between the parents and the adolescent, and the long-term goal was to reduce early adolescent sexual behavior. The videotape promoted abstinence and did not include contraceptive information. At the 1-year follow-up, similar rates of adolescent sexual activity were found in the intervention and control groups (Miller et al., 1993).[7]

In the aggregate, the evaluations of programs that encourage abstinence only (with no additional material on contraception) provide insufficient evidence to determine if the programs delayed the initiation of sexual intercourse or reduced the frequency of intercourse. More research is needed to understand the impact of these programs more precisely.

4. Sexuality education programs that provide information on both abstinence and contraceptive use neither encourage the onset of sexual intercourse nor increase the frequency of intercourse among adolescents. In fact, programs that provide both messages appear to be effective in delaying the onset of sexual intercourse and encouraging contraceptive use once sexual activity has begun, especially among younger adolescents.

---

[7]Although some abstinence-only program curricula include life planning and goal-setting exercises, many rely on shame and fear to encourage young people to abstain from sexual relations. The Sex Information and Education Council of the United States reviewed 11 curricula that used fear as a motivating factor. These programs typically omit critical information about sexuality and contain medical misinformation (Kantor, 1992/1993). None has been rigorously evaluated and are therefore not included in the 23 programs reviewed in this report.

Concern has been expressed that sexuality education leads to earlier sexual intercourse. Ten of the 23 evaluated programs (programs B, E, F, J, M, N, O, P, Q, and W) were sexuality education programs that taught students about the benefits of abstinence for young adolescents as well as the benefits of contraceptive use once sexual activity had begun. All of these programs reported that the onset of sexual intercourse was not higher for the intervention group, nor was the frequency of intercourse higher for the intervention group. In fact, 7 of the 10 intervention programs (programs B, J, M, N, O, P, and W) had outcomes that can decrease the risk of pregnancy, such as raising the age of onset of sexual intercourse, decreasing the mean number of acts of sexual intercourse, and increasing contraceptive use among those students who were already sexually active. The remaining three programs (programs E, F, and Q) had mixed results, but in no instance was the onset of sexual intercourse earlier for the intervention groups.

Although these programs have been criticized for sending confusing messages about sexual behavior to adolescents ("don't do it, but if you do, protect yourself"), program evaluations indicate that adolescents do not have difficulty absorbing this two-part message or sorting through the information to find the material most relevant to their own situations. In addition, a recent worldwide literature review concludes that there is no support for the notion that sexuality education encourages the initiation of sexual intercourse or increased sexual activity. Even in the face of different methodologies and study locales, the aggregate effect of sexuality education is in the direction of postponing first sexual intercourse and using contraception more effectively (Grunseit and Kippax, undated).

One of the best known evaluated programs in the United States that explicitly includes information on both abstinence and contraceptive use is Postponing Sexual Involvement: An Education Series for Young Teens. This program includes two components: one on postponing sexual involvement and one on human sexuality. The first component emphasizes that abstinence is the best choice for young adolescents, and the second component provides basic information on reproduction and contraception. This combination has been shown to be effective: fewer members of the intervention group than those not offered the combined course initiated sexual intercourse, and contraceptive use was higher among sexually active students in the intervention group than in the comparison group.

The Reducing the Risk program also illustrates the effectiveness of the dual message. This curriculum was based on several interrelated theoretical approaches and explicitly emphasized that adolescents should avoid unprotected intercourse, either through abstinence or by using contraception. Results indicated that significantly fewer students in the intervention group than in the comparison group became sexually active. Of the students who did report being sexually active, significantly fewer reported the practice of unprotected sex, either by delaying first intercourse or by increasing contraceptive use.

Not all programs offering dual messages have had such clear success, however. For example, Teen Talk, a school-based program that uses small group discussions as a key feature, had mixed results. The curriculum was designed to make adolescents aware of the seriousness of adolescent pregnancy and the probabilities of such a pregnancy happening to them, as well as the benefits of and barriers to abstinence and contraceptive use. The evaluation revealed that young men in the intervention group were significantly more likely to have abstained from sex than were young men in the control group. Young women in the intervention group, on the other hand, were no less likely to begin sexual activity than young women in the control group, and furthermore, among the participants who became sexually active following the program, the women in the control group were significantly more likely to have used contraception at last intercourse than those in the intervention group.

Sexuality education in school-based settings was considered carefully in a comprehensive review by Kirby and colleagues (1994). The researchers identified studies of school-based sexuality education and HIV-AIDS education programs and summarized the results; although they looked at a slightly different program universe than the 23 programs reviewed here, the overlap is considerable. Consistent with the analysis presented in this chapter, they learned that none of the programs that discussed both abstinence and contraception significantly hastened the onset of intercourse. Nor did the programs change the frequency of intercourse among those students who were sexually experienced prior to receiving the curriculum. Some programs also increased contraceptive use among students who were sexually inexperienced at the onset of the program. They conclude that, overall, effective programs:

- focus specifically on reducing sexual risk-taking behaviors that might lead to unintended pregnancy or HIV or STD infection;
- use social learning theories as a foundation for program development;[8]

[8]These theories include the Health Behavior Model, the Group Cognitive Behavior Theory, the Social Learning Theory, and the Social Inoculation Theory. These theories of behavior change, which have been used to design programs focused on such risky behaviors as smoking, have also been used to design programs to change sexual and contraceptive behavior. All such programs attempt to achieve change by addressing social influences, values, group norms, and building social skills, and not just by focusing on information and knowledge (Kirby et al., 1994).

- provide basic, accurate information about the risks of unprotected intercourse and methods of avoiding unprotected intercourse through experiential activities designed to personalize this information;
- include activities that address social or media influences on sexual behaviors;
- reinforce clear and appropriate standards to strengthen individual values and group norms against unprotected sex;
- provide modeling and practice of communication and negotiation skills; and
- provide training for program implementation.

5. Even though most of the evaluated programs encourage contraceptive use in some way, there is a notable reluctance to actually provide program participants with the contraceptive methods themselves or even to help participants gain access to contraceptive services at some other site. Only nine evaluated programs (programs B, E, H, K, O, P, Q, R, and U) make a clear effort in at least some of their sites to provide contraception or increase access to it. This reluctance is due, in part, to the preponderance of programs targeting adolescents and the ongoing public debate about the appropriateness of providing sexually active, unmarried adolescents with contraceptives.

Even among the evaluated programs working with adolescents who are pregnant or are already parents—a group well known to be at risk of rapid repeat, often unintended pregnancy—the direct provision of contraception is not universal. Only three of seven programs (programs H, K, and U) working with pregnant or parenting adolescents actually provide methods of contraception or direct access to contraception, and two of these three programs (programs H and K) did not provide contraception at all program sites.

The School/Community Program for Sexual Risk Reduction Among Teens reveals the importance of actual access to contraception. This school- and community-based program was designed to reduce high rates of adolescent pregnancy and was a collective effort of parents, teachers, students, clergy, and community leaders. Contraception was made accessible to the students through a school nurse, who provided counseling for the students, condoms for sexually active young men, and transportation to the county health department family planning clinic for sexually active young women. The first evaluation of the program's effectiveness noted that in the 2 years following initiation of the education program developed by the community consortium, pregnancy rates among adolescent girls in the intervention area dropped significantly (Vincent et al., 1987). A reanalysis of this program confirmed that the adolescent pregnancy rate did indeed decrease during the years covered by the earlier evaluation (1984–1986). However, the reanalysis found that in subsequent years (1987–1988), the adolescent pregnancy rate in the intervention area increased to levels that were not significantly different from the pre-program rates. The authors suggest that this increase probably occurred because, in these later years, there was a general decrease in the program's overall momentum and, in particular, the school-based clinic stopped providing students with contraceptive methods and no provision was made to help them gain access to contraception elsewhere in the community (Koo et al., 1994).

Although the provision of contraception in school-based and school-linked health clinics receives significant media and political attention, only 21 percent of the approximately 500 school-based health clinics around the country actually dispense contraception (Dryfoos, 1994); one study suggests that family planning programs are the weakest component of school-based adolescent health centers (National Research Council, 1993). Evaluations from the three school-based or school-linked programs that provide reproductive health services (programs P, Q, and R) indicate that such programs do not encourage the onset of intercourse, nor do they increase the frequency of intercourse. The evidence is mixed, however, on the capacities of these programs to decrease pregnancy rates.

The Self Center is an example of one school-linked program for adolescents that did appear to decrease pregnancy rates by providing full reproductive health services as well as health education and counseling services to adolescents. Most services were offered in a school-linked clinic located close to both a senior and a junior high school. The program stressed messages of abstinence for young adolescents and contraceptive use for sexually active adolescents. At the 3 year follow-up, significantly more students in schools linked to the clinics attended a clinic before beginning sexual intercourse or attended a clinic during the first months of sexual activity, a period during which unintended pregnancy is especially likely to occur. A significant delay in the initiation of sexual intercourse for young women in the intervention schools was noted; the median delay was 7 months. A significant increase in the use of contraception at last intercourse was noted among both adolescent women and men. A significant reduction in pregnancy rates among the older adolescents in the intervention schools relative to that among older adolescents in the control schools, and a small decrease in the pregnancy rates among younger adolescents in the intervention schools, was found, whereas the pregnancy rates in the control school increased dramatically. Zabin and colleagues (1986:124) suggest that "it was the accessibility of the staff and of the clinic, rather than any 'new' information about contraception, that encouraged the students to obtain service." By contrast, evaluation results have differed about whether or not the St. Paul School-Based Health Clinics reduced pregnancy rates, and the six school-based clinics reported mixed results on contraceptive use.

The impression gained from all 23 program evaluations considered as a whole is that too few include actual, tangible assistance in helping participants to obtain contraceptive supplies. Program personnel often talk about contraception, and also counsel program participants about the methods available. But such encouragement is not uniformly accompanied by actually providing individuals with contraceptive methods or by focused efforts to link them to a source of contraceptive services, such as a family planning clinic.

6. About half of the evaluated programs attempting to reduce rapid repeat pregnancy, especially among adolescents, have been successful. Much effort has been expended in developing programs to mitigate the negative consequences of childbearing among adolescents and to reduce rapid repeat childbearing during adolescence. In the 1970s, the primary objective of many of these programs was the healthy birth of a child, but more recently emphasis has been placed on the young mother's needs post-delivery. Programs have become increasingly comprehensive, with an emphasis on education, employment, the child's developmental needs, and reducing subsequent pregnancy.

Seven of the 23 evaluated programs (programs A, C, G, H, I, K, and U) attempted to reduce rapid repeat pregnancy, and they share a common emphasis on attaining educational goals and increasing employability. Only three programs (programs C, G, and I) succeeded in helping young mothers postpone rapid subsequent births, and, interestingly, two of these three programs (programs C and G) took a health-oriented approach, such as involving nurses in contraceptive counseling, as distinct from relying exclusively on employment counselors, for example, to encourage contraceptive use.

The Polly T. McCabe Center, an alternative school for pregnant adolescents, is an example of one of the successful efforts that included a health orientation in its postnatal care. The program provided case management by nurses and social workers for up to 4 months after delivery, and such care included follow-up counseling about contraceptive choices made at the hospital, to ensure that the young women felt comfortable with their contraceptive method and knew how to use it most effectively. At both 2 and 5 years, students in the intervention group were significantly less likely to have another child. The researchers note that "the most surprising finding in this study was that relatively brief postnatal intervention with new adolescent mothers significantly reduced their likelihood of subsequent childbearing over the next five years" (Seitz and Apfel, 1993:578). They suggest that the critical period is the second month following the birth of the first child, in that this typically marks the end of the postnatal recovery period and sexual activity often resumes.

Project Redirection, which did not have a health orientation, is an example of one of the four programs (of seven) that did not succeed in reducing rapid repeat pregnancy. This was one of the first major demonstration projects to include employment issues as part of the care and counseling offered to school-age pregnant and parenting adolescents. Young women in the program were offered a range of services and were supported by community women volunteering to act as mentors. Although the 1-year evaluation results indicated that adolescents in the intervention group were significantly less likely to have a repeat pregnancy, the 5-year evaluation results gave a less positive picture. These longer term results showed that although the intervention group had an equal number of pregnancies compared with the number in the comparison group, they had fewer abortions and thus more births. Polit (1989:169) notes that "the larger number of children born to Project Redirection participants could . . . reflect the failure of the family planning component. The approach taken by program staff in the Project Redirection sites was 'low-key,' one that reflected (at least in part) the discomfort of some staff members about discussing issues relating to sexuality. Such an approach appears to have been insufficient to motivate the participants to use effective contraceptives regularly."

New Chance is another example of a program that was not successful in reducing rapid repeat pregnancies among a sample of women who gave birth in adolescence. Program goals included increasing the economic self-sufficiency of adolescent mothers, helping them become effective parents, enhancing the development of their children, and delaying repeat pregnancies. Program participants reported both a higher pregnancy rate and a higher rate of abortion; therefore, comparable rates of repeat childbearing (approximately 25 percent) were found in both intervention and control groups (Quint, Polit, et al., 1994).

7. Little is known from the evaluated programs about how to influence sexual behavior or contraceptive use by changing the surrounding socioeconomic or cultural environment. The objective of most evaluated programs is to affect the actions of individuals by working directly with them rather than by changing the cultural milieu in which they live. No evaluated programs address the sociocultural environment in which sexual decision-making takes place; thus, nothing is known about how, or even whether, to try to influence the surrounding culture as one way of changing sexual and contraceptive behavior.

The analysis of the Summer Training and Education Program (STEP) elucidates this point. Program leaders have hypothesized that the failure to seek any major environmental change was one reason for the program's lack of success. STEP combined work experience for adolescents with educational skills and information about responsible sexual decision-making. The evaluation found that although students in STEP gained significant life skills, no significant differences in sexual behavior were noted between the intervention and comparison groups. Walker and Vilella-Velez (1992:64) suggest that this is because no influence was made on "schools, peers, neighborhoods, family, family income, and perceived and real future job opportunities . . . almost half of the adolescents who dropped out of STEP cited the need for income or other causes in their environment as their primary reason for dropping out of school."

A notable exception to the pervasive emphasis on individuals is The Media Project, part of the nonprofit organization Advocates for Youth. Although not included in the 23 evaluated programs, this is one activity that has attempted to change the almost constant barrage of sexually enticing messages presented by the media. To do so, program staff work with, for example, writers, directors, and producers of television soap operas and situation comedies, providing them with information about responsible sexual behavior, including contraceptive use. The Media Project has not been evaluated in any substantial way.

It may well be that community-based programs are not the right mechanism for attempting broad cultural change. These programs are often small, involving a few hundred people or less, and they last only a few years. Programs designed to change individual behaviors may never be able to achieve more than marginal success in a society whose health care system, available information and education, and overall socioeconomic and cultural environments do not uniformly support careful use of the best methods of contraception, as discussed in Chapters 5, 6, and 7.

THE FISCAL IMPACT OF FAMILY PLANNING FUNDING

Policymakers are understandably interested in the budgetary impact of public investments in family planning programs, both those that operate at the national level and those that work in states and communities. A series of studies has attempted to assess the net fiscal impact of family planning funding, typically by asking: How does an extra dollar of public funding for family planning affect all public outlays for other health and social services? (The techniques and concepts that are involved in establishing program cost-effectiveness are discussed at length in Appendix G).[9] Recent studies of fiscal consequences have been

[9]The literature on budgeting effects is sometimes described as being concerned with cost–benefit analysis or with program cost-effectiveness. Neither characterization is correct. The concept of cost-effectiveness is briefly commented on here.

A program is said to be cost-effective relative to another program, or relative to the current state of affairs, if it can be demonstrated to provide the same level of effectiveness at lower total social cost. In general, effectiveness must be described in a number of distinct dimensions, as in the analysis of Meier and McFarlane (1994). No rigorous assessment of cost-effectiveness has been undertaken for U.S. family planning programs.

The assessment of program cost-effectiveness is a demanding task, particularly so with respect to the data that are required to support a rigorous analysis. If these data are not available, evaluation can proceed only on an informal basis by invoking strong assumptions on the nature of the cost functions. Much of the cost-effectiveness literature in family planning has rested on two exceedingly strong yet rarely scrutinized assumptions: (1) that the multiple dimensions of output can somehow be collapsed into a single output indicator and (2) that average costs, defined as total costs divided by (composite) output, are constant over the range of output. If both conditions are met, then a single observation on average costs can provide a basis for program comparisons. But in the absence of supporting evidence—the committee found none in the literature—these strong assumptions are not well justified and may be misleading as a guide to policy.

undertaken by, among others, Levey and colleagues (1988), Forrest and Singh (1990a,b), Vincent and colleagues (1991), Fitzgibbons (1993), Olds and colleagues (1993), and Trussell and colleagues (1995). These studies conclude that public expenditures in support of family planning are more than offset by the savings that are produced in other health and social services spending. Depending on the study, these services include the Medicaid, AFDC, food stamp, and Women with Infants and Dependent Children (WIC) expenditures associated with pregnancy, the medical expenditures associated with abortion or childbirth, and the programs that support low-income mothers and their infants and children.

The results of Forrest and Singh (1990b) can serve as an illustration of the nature of the findings in general. According to the authors, "for every government dollar spent on family planning services, from $2.90 to $6.20 (an average of $4.40) is saved as a result of averting [short-term] expenditures on medical services, welfare and nutritional services" (Forrest and Singh, 1990b:6). The range of such estimates found in the literature is great, and the figures depend on details in the assumptions employed and the range of health and social services under consideration. Nevertheless, given the entitlement nature of many of the services in question, family planning efforts would seem to make good sense from the viewpoint of a taxpayer concerned with government budgets (Levey et al., 1988).

Before the assumptions and the data that support this conclusion are assessed, a brief preface is in order. The taxpayer's benefit–cost approach, however useful as a device for marshaling political support, is a specialized and, in some respects, rather peculiar metric for evaluation. It frames the evaluation issue very narrowly, being concerned only with the impact of one form of public expenditure on another form. There is no clear or necessary relationship between the claims that programs make on government budgets and their cost-effectiveness or social desirability. A program that, from the social point of view, is so cost-ineffective that it should not be undertaken may nevertheless reduce claims on government budgets. Conversely, a program that is socially beneficial may increase claims on budgets. Thus, the terms *benefit* and *cost* that appear in a taxpayer's benefit–cost analysis bear no obvious correspondence to social benefits and costs. Having issued this warning about the interpretation of taxpayer benefit–cost analyses, some of the common features of these studies and avenues for further work can be addressed.

Program Reactions to Funding Withdrawal

A common assumption in studies of fiscal effects is that the withdrawal of public funding would simply cause the clinics or programs in question to vanish.

Program clients would then need to seek out services elsewhere, and would usually receive services on less advantageous terms. This assumption requires some justification and clarification.

First, it envisions an extreme case, in that total funding withdrawal would be a sharp departure from the current state of affairs. If the aim is to predict net fiscal impacts, a safer approach is to predict the impact of a marginal withdrawal of funds, for example, a cutback of 10 percent.

Second, no attempt is generally made to predict the reactions of clinics and programs to the withdrawal or reduction of state or federal support. Yet, as the experience of the late 1980s shows (Donovan, 1991), programs faced with declines in external support tend to rely more on fees for service, and may also make adjustments in services they provide and their referral practices. To explore the full consequences, two issues need to be identified: (1) the types of changes in pricing and service delivery that are feasible and how likely the different program reactions may be and (2) how women will react to the new provider prices and characteristics. These issues require, at a minimum, consideration of the price-responsiveness of demand for contraceptive services and reproductive health services more generally.

Treatment of Mistimed and Unwanted Pregnancies

A recurrent theme in this report is the importance of distinguishing between pregnancies that are mistimed and those that are unwanted. The distinction surfaces here with respect to the fiscal implications of preventing unintended pregnancies. If the pregnancy that is prevented by contraception was unwanted, then its prevention certainly reduces all future claims on Medicaid, AFDC, and the like. If the pregnancy in question was mistimed, however, these claims on budgets may only be deferred into the future. In other words, prevention of a mistimed pregnancy may well reduce claims on this year's budget; it does not necessarily reduce claims on future budgets.

Two points are therefore at issue. The first is whether to discount claims on all future budgets attributable to prevention, perhaps expressing the net public sector savings in terms of present values. It may be that when pregnancies are properly timed the likelihood of claims on public programs is much reduced. Discounting is therefore not only a matter of present versus future budgets. It also has to do with individual poverty dynamics and the likelihood that a properly timed pregnancy will coincide with periods of (relatively) high income, that is, income high enough to reduce or eliminate claims on AFDC and other income-conditioned services. The second point concerns the budget period envisioned in the fiscal evaluation. If the fiscal impact question is posed as "do family planning expenditures in this fiscal year reduce claims on budgets in this year and the next?", then it may well be reasonable to aggregate mistimed and unwanted pregnancies in the analysis. If, on the other hand, the time period envisioned in the analysis is longer, then the distinction between unwanted and mistimed pregnancies should be maintained. If the distinction is not maintained and unwanted and mistimed pregnancies are treated alike, there is the potential for gross overstatement of the public sector savings owing to prevention.

Program Eligibility Versus Participation

In the United States, far fewer women (or families) than are eligible for them actually participate in public support programs such as AFDC, Medicaid, WIC, and related programs. Yet the fiscal analyses of family planning either assume full participation among all eligible people or assume that a given proportion of eligible women participate irrespective of other socioeconomic characteristics. The first assumption is naive and clearly overstates the potential public sector savings that can be secured by prevention. The second assumption is less severe, but a more refined and informative estimate of public sector savings could be made by taking the socioeconomic characteristics of family planning clients into account.

Incomplete Accounting for Public Revenue Effects

When a working woman becomes pregnant unintentionally, she may experience at least a short period of withdrawal from the labor market; likewise, a nonworking woman may be discouraged from working as a result of the pregnancy. These labor market consequences result in lower tax revenues, a factor that many studies on fiscal consequences do not consider. The revenue implications extend beyond the period of labor market withdrawal or nonparticipation. When they are out of the labor market, women fail to add to their total labor market experience; this has implications for future earnings and tax payments. If a pregnancy to an adolescent interrupts schooling, human capital formation is also affected, again with lifetime implications for earnings and revenues. These effects have not been taken into account in any systematic fashion in the literature on fiscal consequences.

In spite of these caveats, which suggest that the public sector benefits of family planning funding may well have been exaggerated in some studies, the weight of the evidence presented by the several studies cited earlier (i.e., Levey et al., 1988; Forrest and Singh, 1990a,b; Vincent at al., 1991; Fitzgibbons, 1993; Olds et al., 1993; and Trussell et al., 1995) is that public funding of family planning services is likely to reduce net claims on public budgets. The magnitude of such reductions is much in doubt and will remain in doubt until rigorous research can be directed to this topic.

CONCLUSION

It is clear that much effort and many resources at the local, state, and national levels have been applied to programs to affect sexual behavior and contraceptive use, with much attention focused on young women. Although no formal evaluations of the large programs that help to finance or directly provide contraceptive services (such as Title X and Medicaid) have been completed, the support that these programs furnish undoubtedly helps to increase access to contraception, and thereby helps individuals avoid unintended pregnancy. Evaluations of the long-term effects of these programs are sorely needed, but they will be difficult to design.

Although there are hundreds of programs at the community level that in some way address sexual or contraceptive behavior related to unintended pregnancy, few have been carefully evaluated, and knowledge is therefore very limited about how local programs can reduce unintended pregnancy. Those that have been evaluated illustrate several cross-cutting themes:

- because most of the evaluated programs target adolescents, especially adolescent girls, knowledge about how to reach adult women or men is exceedingly limited;
- there is insufficient evidence to determine whether abstinence-only programs have been effective in increasing the age at first intercourse;
- sexuality education programs that provide information on both abstinence and contraceptive use neither encourage the onset of sexual intercourse nor increase the frequency of intercourse among adolescents; in fact, programs that provide both messages appear to be effective in delaying the onset of sexual intercourse and encouraging contraceptive use, especially among younger adolescents;
- even though most of the evaluated programs encourage contraceptive use in some way, there is a notable reluctance to provide program participants with contraceptive methods themselves or to help participants gain access to contraceptive services at some other site;
- about half of the evaluated programs attempting to reduce rapid repeat pregnancy, especially among adolescents, have been successful; and
- little is known from the evaluated programs about how to influence sexual behavior or contraceptive use by changing the surrounding socioeconomic or cultural environment.

Finally, the weight of the evidence is that public funding of family planning services is likely to reduce net claims on public budgets. The magnitude of such reductions is much in doubt, and will remain in doubt until rigorous research can be directed to this topic.

REFERENCES[10]

The Alan Guttmacher Institute. 11 Million Teenagers: What Can Be Done About the Epidemic of Adolescent Pregnancies in the United States? New York, NY: The Alan Guttmacher Institute; 1976.

Allen JP, Philliber S, Hoggson N. School-based prevention of teen-age pregnancy and school dropout: Process evaluation of the national replication of the Teen Outreach Program. Am J Commun Psychol. 1990;18:505–524.

Anderson JE, Cope LG. The impact of family planning program activity on fertility. Fam Plann Perspect. 1987;19:152–157.

Barth RP, Leland N, Kirby D, Fetro JV. Enhancing social and cognitive skills. In Preventing Adolescent Pregnancy: Model Programs and Evaluations. Miller BC, Card JJ, Paikoff RL, Peterson JL, eds. Newbury Park, CA: Sage Publications; 1992.

Burt MR. Estimating the public costs of teenage childbearing. Fam Plann Perspect. 1986; 18:221–226.

Burt MR, Aron LY, Schack LR. Family planning clinics: Current status and recent changes in services, clients, staffing, and income sources. In Publicly Supported Family Planning in the United States. Washington, DC: The Urban Institute and Child Trends, Inc.; 1994.

The Center for Health Training. Male involvement in family planning: A bibliography of project descriptions and resources. Seattle, WA: The Center for Health Training; February 1988.

Christopher FS, Roosa MW. An evaluation of an adolescent pregnancy prevention programs: Is "just say no" enough? Fam Relat. 1990;39:68–72.

Corman H, Grossman M. Determinants of neonatal mortality rates in the US. J Health Econ. 1985;4:213–236.

Cutright P, Jaffe FS. Family planning program effects on the fertility of low-income US women. Fam Plann Perspect. 1976;8:100–110.

Danielson R, Marcy S, Plunkett A, Wiest W, Greenlick MR. Reproductive health counseling for young men: What does it do? Fam Plann Perspect. 1990;22:115–121.

Danielson R, McNally K, Swanson J, Plunkett A, Klausmeier W. Title X and family planning services for men. Fam Plann Perspect. 1988;20:234–237.

Donovan P. Family planning clinics: Facing higher costs and sicker patients. Fam Plann Perspect. 1991;23:198–203.

Dryfoos JG. Full-Service Schools: A Revolution in Health and Social Services for Children, Youth, and Families. San Francisco, CA: Jossey-Bass Publishers; 1994.

Dryfoos JG. School- and community-based pregnancy prevention programs. Adolesc Med. 1992;3:241–255.

Edwards L, Steinmann M, Hakanson E. Adolescent pregnancy prevention services in high school clinics. Fam Plann Perspect. 1980;12:6–15.

Edwards SR. The role of men in contraceptive decision-making: Current knowledge and future implications. Fam Plan Perspect. 1994;26:77–82.

---

[10]Works listed below but not cited in the text of Chapter 8 appear as references in Appendix F, a supplement to Chapter 8.

Eisen M, Zellman GL. A health beliefs field experiment. In Preventing Adolescent Pregnancy: Model Programs and Evaluations. Miller BC, Card JJ, Paikoff RL, Peterson JL, eds. Newbury Park, CA: Sage Publications; 1992.

Eisen M, Zellman GL, McAlister AL. Evaluating the impact of a theory-based sexuality and contraceptive education program. Fam Plann Perspect. 1990;22:261–271.

Fitzgibbons E. Benefit:cost analysis of family planning in Washington State. Unpublished Master's thesis. University of Washington; 1993.

Forrest JD, Singh S. The impact of public-sector expenditures for contraceptive services in California. Fam Plann Perspect. 1990a;22:161–168.

Forrest JD, Singh S. Public-sector savings resulting from expenditures for contraceptive services. Fam Plann Perspect. 1990b;22:6–15.

Gilchrist LD, Schinke SP. Coping with contraception: Cognitive and behavioral methods with adolescents. Cognit Ther Res. 1983;7:379–388.

Girls Incorporated. Truth, trust and technology: New research on preventing adolescent pregnancy. Indianapolis IN; Girls Incorporated; October 1991.

Gold R, Daley D. Public funding of contraceptive, sterilization, and abortion services, fiscal year 1990. Fam Plann Perspect. 1991;23:204–211.

Gold R, Macias J. Public funding of contraceptive, sterilization, and abortion services, fiscal year 1985. Fam Plann Perspect. 1986;18:259–264.

Grossman M, Jacobowitz S. Variations in infant mortality rates among counties of the United States: The roles of public policies and programs. Demography. 1981;18: 695–713.

Grunseit A, Kippax S. Effects of Sex Education on Young People's Sexual Behavior. World Health Organization. No date.

Hershey A, Rangarajan A. Implementing employment and training services for teenage parents. Princeton, NJ: Mathematica Policy Research, Inc.; 1993.

Howard M, McCabe JB. An information and skills approach for younger teens. In Preventing Adolescent Pregnancy: Model Programs and Evaluations. Miller BC, Card JJ, Paikoff RL, Peterson JL, eds. Newbury Park, CA: Sage Publications; 1992.

Howard M, McCabe JB. Helping teenagers postpone sexual involvement. Fam Plann Perspect. 1990;22:21–26.

Institute of Medicine. Developing New Contraceptives: Obstacles and Opportunities. Washington, DC: National Academy Press; 1990.

Institute of Medicine. Confronting AIDS: Update 1988. Washington, DC: National Academy Press; 1988.

Jorgensen SR. Project Taking Charge: An evaluation of an adolescent pregnancy prevention program. Fam Relat. 1991;40:373–380.

Jorgensen SR, Potts V, Camp B. Project Taking Charge: Six-month follow-up of a pregnancy prevention program for early adolescents. Family Relations. 1993;42:401–406.

Joyce TJ, Grossman M. Pregnancy wantedness and the early initiation of prenatal care. Demography. 1990;27:1–17.

Kantner JF, Zelnik M. Sexual experience of young unmarried women in the United States. Fam Plann Perspect. 1972;4:9–18.

Kantor LM. Scared chaste? Fear-based education curricula. SIECUS Report. New York, NY: Sex Information and Education Council of the US; 1992/1993;2:1–18.

Kirby D. School-based programs to reduce sexual risk-taking behaviors. J School Health. 1992;62:280–287.

Kirby D. Sexuality Education: An Evaluation of Programs and Their Effects. Santa Cruz, CA: Network Publications; 1984.

Kirby D, Barth RP, Leland N, Fetro JV. Reducing the risk: Impact of a new curriculum on sexual risk-taking. Fam Plann Perspect. 1991;23:253–263.

Kirby D, Harvey PD, Claussenius D, Novar M. A direct mailing to teenage males about condom use: Its impact on knowledge, attitudes and sexual behavior. Fam Plann Perspect. 1989;21:12–18.

Kirby D, Resnick MD, Downes B, et al. The effects of school-based health clinics in St. Paul on school-wide birthrates. Fam Plann Perspect. 1993;25:12–16.

Kirby D, Short L, Collins J, Rugg D, Kolbe L, Howard M, Miller B, Sonenstein F, Zabin LS. School-based programs to reduce sexual risk behaviors: A review of effectiveness. Public Health Rep. 1994;109:339–360.

Kirby D, Waszak C, Ziegler J. Six school-based clinics: Their reproductive health services and impact on sexual behavior. Fam Plann Perspect. 1991;23:6–16.

Klerman L. Programs for pregnant adolescent and young parents: Their development and assessment. In Teenage Parents and Their Offspring. Scott KG, Field T, Robertson E, eds. New York, NY: Grune and Stratton; 1981.

Klerman LV, Horwitz SM. Reducing the adverse consequences of adolescent pregnancy and parenting: The role of service programs. Adolesc Med. 1992;3:299–316.

Koo HP, Dunteman GH, George C, Green Y, Vincent M. Reducing adolescent pregnancy through a school- and community-based intervention: Denmark, South Carolina, revisited. Fam Plann Perspect. 1994;26:206–211, 217.

Ku L. Financing of family planning services. In Publicly Supported Family Planning in the United States. Washington, DC: The Urban Institute and Child Trends, Inc.; 1993.

Lee P. Failing to prevent unintended pregnancy is costly. Am J Public Health. Forthcoming.

Levey L, Nyman J, Haugaard J. A benefit-cost analysis of family planning services in Iowa. Eval Health Prof. 1988;11:403–424.

Manpower Demonstration Research Corporation. New Chance: A new initiative for adolescent mothers and their children. New York, NY: Manpower Demonstration Research Corporation; April 1993.

Maynard R, ed. Building self-sufficiency among welfare-dependent teenage parents: Lessons from the Teenage Parent Demonstration. Princeton, NJ: Mathematica Policy Research; June 1993.

Maynard R, Rangarajan A. Contraceptive use and repeat pregnancies among welfare-dependent teenage mothers. Fam Plann Perspect. 1994;26:198–205.

Meier K, McFarlane D. State family planning and abortion expenditures: Their effect on public health. Am J Public Health. 1994;84:1468–1472.

Miller BC, Dyk PH. Community of Caring effects of adolescent mothers: A program evaluation case study. Fam Relat. 1991;40:386–395.

Miller BC, Norton MC, Jenson GO, Lee TR, Christopherson C, King PK. Impact evaluation of Facts and Feelings: A home-based video sex education curriculum. Fam Relat. 1993;42:392–400.

Moore KA, Blumenthal C, Sugland BW, Hyatt B, Snyder NO, Morrison DR. State variation in rates of adolescent pregnancy and childbearing. Washington, DC: Child Trends, Inc.; 1994.

National Research Council. Losing Generations: Adolescents in High-Risk Settings. Washington, DC: National Academy Press; 1993.

National Research Council. Risking the Future: Adolescent Sexuality, Pregnancy, and Childbearing. Vol. I. Washington, DC: National Academy Press; 1987.

Nicholson HJ, Postrado LT. A comprehensive age-phased approach: Girls Incorporated. In Preventing Adolescent Pregnancy: Model Programs and Evaluations. Miller BC, Card JJ, Paikoff RL, Peterson JL, eds. Newbury Park, CA: Sage Publications; 1992.

Olds D, Henderson C, Tatelbaum R, Chamberlin R. Preventing child abuse and neglect: A randomized trial of nurse home visitation. Pediatrics. 1986;78:65–78.

Olds DL, Henderson CR, Phelps C, Kitzman H, Hanks C. Effects of prenatal and infancy nurse home visitation on government spending. Med Care. 1993;31:155–174.

Olds DL, Henderson CR, Tatelbaum R, Chamberlin R. Improving the life-course development of socially disadvantaged mothers: A randomized trial of nurse home visitation. Am J Public Health. 1988;78:1436–1455.

Olsen JA, Weed SE. Effects of family-planning programs for teenagers on adolescent birth and pregnancy rates. Fam Perspect. 1986;20:153–170.

O'Sullivan A, Jacobson B. A randomized trial of a health care program for first-time adolescent mothers and their infants. Nurs Res. 1992;41:210–215.

Philliber S, Allen JP. Life options and community service. In Preventing Adolescent Pregnancy: Model Programs and Evaluations. Miller BC, Card JJ, Paikoff RL, Peterson JL, eds. Newbury Park, CA: Sage Publications; 1992.

Polit DF. Effects of a comprehensive program for teenage parents: Five years after Project Redirection. Fam Plann Perspect. 1989;21:164–187.

Polit DF, Kahn JR. Project Redirection: Evaluation of a comprehensive program for disadvantaged teenage mothers. Fam Plann Perspect. 1985;17:150–155.

Polit DF, Quint JC, Riccio JA. The Challenge of Serving Teenage Mothers: Lessons from Project Redirection. New York, NY: Manpower Demonstration Research Corporation; October 1988.

Postrado LT, Nicholson HJ. Effectiveness in delaying the initiation of sexual intercourse of girls aged 12–14: Two components of the Girls Incorporated Preventing Adolescent Pregnancy Program. Youth Soc. 1992;23:356–379.

Quint J, Musick J, Ladner J. Lives of Promise, Lives of Pain. New York, NY: Manpower Demonstration Research Corporation; January 1994.

Quint JC, Fink BL, Rowser SL. Implementing a Comprehensive Program for Disadvantaged Young Mothers and Their Children. New York, NY: Manpower Demonstration Research Corporation; December 1991.

Quint JC, Polit DF, Bos H, Cave G. New Chance: Interim Findings on a Comprehensive Program for Disadvantaged Young Mothers and Their Children. New York, NY: Manpower Demonstration Research Corporation; September 1994.

Roosa MW, Christopher FS. A response to Thiel and McBride: Scientific criticism or obscurantism? Fam Relat. 1992;41:468–469.

Roosa MW, Christopher FS. Evaluation of an abstinence-only adolescent pregnancy prevention program: A replication. Fam Relat. 1990;39:363–367.

Ruch-Ross HS, Jones ED, Musick JS. Comparing outcomes in a statewide program for adolescent mothers with outcomes in a national sample. Fam Plann Perspect. 1992; 24:66–71, 96.

Schinke SP, Blythe BJ, Gilchrist LD. Cognitive-behavioral prevention of adolescent pregnancy. J Couns Psychol. 1981;28:451–454.

Schinke SP, Gilchrist LD, Small RW. Preventing unwanted adolescent pregnancy: A cognitive-behavioral approach. Amer J Orthopsychiatry. 1979;49:81–88.

Seitz V, Apfel N. Effects of a school for pregnant students on the incidence of low-birthweight deliveries. Child Develop. 1994;65:666–676.

Seitz V, Apfel NH. Adolescent mothers and repeated childbearing: Effects of a school-based intervention program. Amer J Orthopsychiatry. 1993;63:572–581.

Singh S. Adolescent pregnancy in the United States: An interstate analysis. Fam Plann Perspect. 1986;8:10–20.

Stahler GJ, DuCette JP. Evaluating adolescent pregnancy programs: Rethinking our priorities. Fam Plann Perspect. 1991;23:129–133.

Thiel KS, McBride D. Comments on an evaluation of an abstinence-only adolescent pregnancy prevention program. Fam Relat. 1992;41:465–467.

Torres A, Donovan P, Dittes N, Forrest JD. Public benefits and costs of government funding for abortion. Fam Plann Perspect. 1986;18:111–118.

Trussell J, Leveque JA, Koenig JD et al. The economic value of contraception: A comparison of 15 methods. Am J Public Health. 1995;85:494—503.

Vincent ML, Clearie AF, Schluchter MD. Reducing adolescent pregnancy through school and community-based education. JAMA. 1987;257:3382–3386.

Vincent ML, Lepro S, Baker, Garvey D. Projected public sector savings in a teen pregnancy prevention project. J Health Educ. 1991;22:208–212.

Vinovskis MA. An "Epidemic" of Adolescent Pregnancy? Some Historical and Policy Considerations. Oxford: Oxford University Press; 1988.

Walker G, Vilella-Velez F. Anatomy of a Demonstration: The Summer Training and Education Program (STEP) from Pilot through Replication and Postprogram Impacts. Philadelphia, PA: Public/Private Ventures; 1992.

Weed SE, Olsen JA. Effects of family-planning programs on teenage pregnancy—replication and extension. Fam Perspect. 1986;20:173–194.

Zabin LS, Hirsch MB. Evaluation of Pregnancy Prevention Programs in the School Context. Lexington, MA: Lexington Books; 1987.

Zabin LS, Hirsch MB, Smith EA, Streett R, Hardy JB. Evaluation of a pregnancy prevention program for urban teenagers. Fam Plann Perspect. 1986;18:119–126.

Zabin LS, Hirsch MB, Streett R, Emerson MR, Smith M, King TM. The Baltimore Pregnancy Prevention Program for Teenagers. I. How did it work? Fam Plann Perspect. 1988;20:182–192.

9

Conclusions and Recommendations

The facts in this report should be distressing to all Americans. In 1988, the latest year for which complete data are available, almost 60 percent of all pregnancies in this nation were unintended, a percentage higher than that found in several other Western democracies. Unintended pregnancy is not just a problem of teenagers or unmarried women or of poor women or minorities; it affects all segments of society. For example, currently married women and those well beyond adolescence report sobering percentages of unintended pregnancy: in 1987, about 50 percent of pregnancies among women aged 20–34 were unintended, 40 percent of pregnancies to married women were unintended, and more than three-fourths of pregnancies to women over age 40 were unintended. The percentage of pregnancies that are unintended is, however, even higher among some other groups. In 1988, for example, 82 percent of pregnancies among teenagers were unintended, as were 88 percent among never-married women.

During the 1970s and early 1980s, a decreasing proportion of births were unintended at the time of conception. Between 1982 and 1988, however, this trend reversed and the proportion of births that were unintended at the time of conception began increasing. This unfortunate trend appears to be continuing into the 1990s. In 1990, about 44 percent of all births were the result of unintended pregnancy; the proportion is close to 60 percent among women in poverty, 62 percent among black women, 73 percent among never-married women, and 86 percent among unmarried teenagers.

The consequences of these high levels of unintended pregnancy are serious, imposing appreciable burdens on children, women, men, and families. A woman with an unintended pregnancy is less likely to seek early prenatal care and is more likely to expose the fetus to harmful substances (such as tobacco or alcohol). The child of an unwanted conception especially (as distinct from a mistimed one) is at greater risk of being born at low birthweight, of dying in its first year of life, of being abused, and of not receiving sufficient resources for healthy development. The mother may be at greater risk of depression and of physical abuse herself, and her relationship with her partner is at greater risk of dissolution. Both mother and father may suffer economic hardship and may fail to achieve their educational and career goals. Such consequences undoubtedly impede the formation and maintenance of strong families.

In addition, an unintended pregnancy is associated with a higher probability that the child will be born to a mother who is adolescent, unmarried, or over age 40—demographic attributes that themselves have important socioeconomic and medical consequences for both children and adults. Pregnancy begun without planning and intent also means that individual women and couples are not able to take full advantage of the growing field of preconception risk identification and management, nor of the rapidly expanding knowledge base regarding human genetics.

Moreover, unintended pregnancy leads to approximately 1.5 million abortions in the United States annually, a ratio of about one abortion to every three live births. This ratio is two to four times higher than that in other Western democracies, in spite of the fact that access to abortion in those countries is often easier than in the United States. Reflecting the widespread occurrence of unintended pregnancy, abortions are obtained by women of all reproductive ages, by both married and unmarried women, and by women in all income categories; in 1992, for example, less than one-fourth of all abortions were obtained by teenagers (Centers for Disease Control and Prevention, 1994). Although abortion has few long-term negative consequences for women's health, resolving an unintended pregnancy by abortion can often be a sobering and emotionally difficult experience that no woman welcomes. In addition, the political and social tensions surrounding abortion in the United States continue to be a divisive force at the national, state, and local levels. Recently, these tensions have taken a violent turn, as exemplified by the murder of several individuals associated with clinics that perform abortions.

A NEW SOCIAL NORM

The committee has found that the extent and consequences of unintended pregnancy are poorly appreciated throughout the United States. Although considerable attention is now focused on teenage pregnancy and nonmarital childbearing, and controversy over abortion continues, the common link among all these issues—pregnancy that is unintended at the time of conception—is essentially invisible. As a consequence, most proposed remedies ignore the common underlying cause or address only one aspect of the problem and a few vulnerable groups (such as young unmarried women on welfare) are singled out for criticism.

The committee has concluded that reducing unintended pregnancy will require a new national understanding about the extent and consequences of this problem. Accordingly, the committee urges, first and foremost, that the nation adopt a new social norm:

- **All pregnancies should be intended; that is, they should be consciously and clearly desired at the time of conception.**

This goal has three important dimensions. First, it is directed to all Americans and does not target only one group. Second, it emphasizes personal choice and intent. And third, it speaks as much to *planning for* pregnancy as to *avoiding* unintended pregnancy. This last point is particularly significant. Bearing children and forming families are among the most meaningful and satisfying aspects of adult life, and it is in this context that encouraging intended pregnancy is so central. The data presented in this report clearly indicate that the lives of children and their families, including those now mired in persistent poverty and welfare dependence, would be strengthened considerably by an increase in the proportion of pregnancies that are purposefully undertaken and consciously desired.

- **To begin the long process of building national consensus around this norm, the committee recommends a multifaceted, long-term campaign to (1) educate the public about the major social and public health burdens of unintended pregnancy; and (2) stimulate a comprehensive set of activities at the national, state, and local levels to reduce such pregnancies.**

The campaign should emphasize the fact that reducing unintended pregnancy will ease many contemporary problems that are of great concern. Childbearing by both teenagers and unmarried women would decline, and abortion in particular would be reduced dramatically. At the same time, however, it is important to help the public understand that even if it were possible to eliminate all unintended pregnancies among both teenagers and unmarried women, there would continue to be large numbers of such pregnancies, because it is not only these groups who contribute to the pool. For example, of all births from 1986 to 1988 that were unintended at conception, only 21 percent were to teenagers.

The campaign should also target national leaders and major U.S. institutions, as well as individual men and women. The problem of unintended pregnancy is as much one of public policies and institutional practices as it is one of individual behavior, and therefore the campaign should not try to reduce unintended pregnancies only by actions focused on individuals or couples. Although individuals clearly need increased attention and services, reducing unintended pregnancy will require that influential organizations and their leaders—corporate officers, legislators, media owners, and others of similar stature—address this problem as well.

As noted above, the committee calls for a campaign that is both multifaceted and long-term, emphases that derive from the data presented in Chapters 4 through 7 showing that no single factor accounts for unintended pregnancy and that the underlying issues are very complex. In truth, there are many antecedents to the problem: socioeconomic, cultural, educational, organizational, and individual. Therefore, only a comprehensive effort will succeed in reducing unintended pregnancy, as has been the case for other national campaigns, such as those to reduce smoking, limit drunk driving, and increase the use of seat belts. Unintended pregnancy will not be reduced appreciably, the committee believes, unless more individuals and institutions make a major commitment to resolving this problem. Similarly, the campaign must be long-term. Past experience teaches that brief, intermittent efforts to address important social and public health challenges have very limited success.

The U.S. Department of Health and Human Services, through its National Health Promotion and Disease Prevention Objectives, has urged that the proportion of all pregnancies that are unintended be reduced to 30 percent by the year 2000 (U.S. Department of Health and Human Services, 1990). The committee endorses this goal, and stresses that it is a realistic one, already reached by other industrialized democracies. Achieving this goal would mean, in absolute numbers, that each year there would be more than 200,000 fewer births that were unwanted at the time of conception and about 800,000 fewer abortions annually as well.

THE CAMPAIGN TO REDUCE UNINTENDED PREGNANCY

What should the campaign emphasize? Should it stress contraceptive services? School-based information? Abstinence? Parent–child or male–female communication about contraception? Community norms regarding reproductive behavior? The specific skills required to use reversible methods? Or, to put these questions in a slightly different way, which factors best predict unintended pregnancy and should therefore be the main targets of action?

The information presented throughout this report, past experience in the public health sector with complex health and social issues, and common sense itself are all helpful in sorting through various options. The committee proposes a portfolio of activities to prevent unintended pregnancy that, like many public health campaigns, emphasizes basic information and preventive services accompanied by comprehensive program evaluation and research. It also addresses the important domain of personal feelings and relationships.

· The committee recommends that the campaign to prevent unintended pregnancy stress five core goals broadly applicable to men as well as women and to older individuals as well as teenagers:

1. improve knowledge about contraception, unintended pregnancy, and reproductive health in general;

2. increase access to contraception;

3. explicitly address the major roles that feelings, attitudes, and motivation play in using contraception and avoiding unintended pregnancy;

4. develop and scrupulously evaluate a variety of local programs to reduce unintended pregnancy; and

5. stimulate research to (a) develop new contraceptive methods for both women *and* men, (b) answer important questions about how best to organize contraceptive services, and (c) understand more fully the determinants and antecedents of unintended pregnancy.

Before describing these five goals in more detail, it is important to comment on one particular aspect of contemporary American life that may influence the course of the recommended campaign. Over the last decade and more, the age of first intercourse has been steadily dropping, whereas the age of first marriage has been steadily rising, such that there is now an increasing gap between the two events; moreover, there has also been a significant increase in nonmarital childbearing and cohabitation (Bumpass et al., 1991)—trends that are not unique to the United States and are, in fact, widely shared by many other countries. Nonetheless, such trends represent major social and cultural changes in the United States and stand in stark contrast to values that were widely shared, at least in theory, throughout much of this century, such as female celibacy before marriage and the unacceptability of young teenagers being sexually active, let alone "living together."

There are many signs that the United States is struggling to come to terms with these new trends and realities. Things are not the way they used to be, but this diverse nation cannot yet seem to agree on what the new rules should be, particularly in the area of sexual behavior. Most probably agree that human sexual expression is a normal and central part of both individual pleasure and species survival, yet the serious issues and repercussions arising from sexual relationships—unintended pregnancy and sexually transmitted diseased (STDs), in particular—remain difficult to discuss, and in many instances they are considered controversial. Some urge that we turn back the clock and try to restrict sexual activity to marriage; others espouse a new ethic of sexual activity that emphasizes personal freedom and pleasure, finding little that is worrisome even about childbearing out of wedlock; still others stake out positions somewhere between these first two, trying to make room for nonmarital sexual activity under certain circumstances, but frowning on nonmarital childbearing, for example.

Concern about this underlying disagreement led the committee to three observations. First, the polarizing arguments about sexual activity have obscured common goals that many share, such as the desirability of all children being born into welcoming families who have planned for them and celebrate their arrival. Focusing on this common ground might help to foster a less adversarial, more tolerant environment, and thus make it easier to discuss contraception candidly and to organize a coherent set of intervention programs that are widely understood and supported. It would be particularly helpful if more people understood that the United States does not differ appreciably from many other countries in its patterns of sexual activity, but it does report higher levels of unintended pregnancy.

Second, abstinence cannot be counted on as the major means to reduce unintended pregnancy. Most of the men and women at risk of unintended pregnancy are beyond adolescence and many are married (Chapter 2), and for this large majority, the primary prevention strategy should be increasing contraceptive use. However, the committee unequivocally supports abstinence as one of many methods available to prevent pregnancy. Furthermore, it urges that young teenagers be counseled and encouraged to resist precocious sexual involvement. Sexual intercourse should occur in the context of a major interpersonal commitment based on mutual consent and caring and on the exercise of personal responsibility, which includes taking steps to avoid both unintended pregnancy and STDs. In this context, it is important to add that the committee did not define the age or life stages at which sexual behavior is appropriate; such decisions are matters best left to family, religious bodies, and other social and moral institutions. This issue is at the heart, however, of the disagreement described above.

Third, it is critically important that officials at all levels of government and public life not misinterpret or over-react to opposition regarding the strategies to reduce unintended pregnancy that are articulated in this report. Although there are some who object, for example, to comprehensive, high-quality sex education in schools or to helping all sexually active individuals gain access to contraception, these are minority views in many communities and they should not be allowed to paralyze efforts to mount major public health campaigns, such as the one outlined here.

One other comment should be made. Even if all five of the campaign elements outlined above and discussed in detail below were put into place, some number of unintended pregnancies would continue to occur. This is because many contraceptive methods have appreciable failure rates even under the best circumstances, and the individuals who use them are not always as careful as is required for maximum efficacy. In addition, there will still probably be some couples who take the risk of using no contraception at all for a period of time, despite having no clear desire to become pregnant. For those women who become pregnant unintentionally, access to both high-quality prenatal care as well as to safe abortion is needed in order to present women and couples with a range of options for managing the pregnancy. Unfortunately, access to both services is limited, especially in some areas of the country (Institute of Medicine, 1988; Henshaw and Van Vort, 1994), a situation that requires focused attention, advocacy, and resolution. Restricted access to safe, legal abortion, in particular, is often associated with maternal mortality and morbidity, as was the case before the full legalization of abortion in the United States over two decades ago (Institute of Medicine, 1975). Recent reports from Romania further underscore the horrors that women face when they must live in an environment that fails to provide accessible, medically safe termination of pregnancy (The Lancet, 1995).

Campaign Goal 1: **Improve knowledge about contraception, unintended pregnancy, and reproductive health.**

The first focus of the campaign to reduce unintended pregnancy should be to increase knowledge about contraception, unintended pregnancy, and reproductive health generally. The evidence summarized in Chapter 5 indicates that individuals of all ages are poorly informed about these issues. The fact that many people mistakenly believe that childbearing is less risky medically than using oral contraceptives and that so few providers or consumers know about emergency contraception are sobering examples of this problem. Misinformation can impede the careful and consistent use of contraception, particularly because many reversible methods in particular require considerable skill to be used properly. Although knowledge alone is often insufficient to increase contraceptive vigilance, it can be viewed as a necessary precondition to other actions needed to reduce unintended pregnancy.

- **The committee recommends that the national campaign to reduce unintended pregnancy include a wide variety of strategies for educating and informing the American public about contraception, unintended pregnancy, and reproductive health in general. These activities should be directed to more than just adolescent girls, highlighting the common occurrence of unintended pregnancy among women age 20 and over, and especially among those over age 40 for whom an unintended pregnancy may carry particular medical risks. They must also include messages for boys and men, emphasizing their stake in avoiding unintended pregnancy, the contraceptive methods available to them, and how to support their partners' use of contraception, along with related material on their**

responsibility for the children they father and the importance of fathers in child development.

The specific inclusion of boys and men in this recommendation deserves special emphasis. As this report has noted repeatedly, males are too often excluded from reproductive health campaigns, even though they often exert great influence on their partners' use of contraception or are themselves active contraceptors. The need to engage males in reproductive health issues is also underscored by the material reviewed in Chapter 7 on violence and nonconsensual sex as contributors to unintended pregnancy. Comprehensive education about human sexuality should stress respect for girls and women and the essential role of consent and caring in human relationships, including sexual ones. The data also point to a need for more adult supervision of adolescents, especially young girls, in order to decrease opportunities for coercive or precocious sexual activity.

Parents, families, and both religious and community institutions should be major sources of information and education about reproductive health and family planning, especially for young people, and they should be supported in serving this important function. Schools also help to provide education and information on these topics. Although large majorities of Americans support family life and sex education in the schools, many communities have poor-quality programs or none at all. Sex education is mandated in 47 states, but only 3 states include coverage of contraception at both the junior and the senior high school levels, and condoms are mentioned only in five state curriculum guides (Chapter 5).

The topic of family life and sex education in the schools has been controversial in some communities; in particular, there is considerable concern that sexual activity may be increased by direct discussion of sexual behavior and contraceptive use. The available data suggest the contrary. In Chapters 5 and 8, for example, the point is made that many adolescents become sexually active before having had *any* formal family life or sex education. Data are also summarized suggesting that there is insufficient evidence to determine whether abstinence-only programs are effective. However, several studies have shown that sexual activity in young adolescents can be postponed and that use of contraception can be increased once sexual activity has begun by comprehensive education that includes several messages simultaneously: the value of abstinence at young ages especially, the importance of good communication between the sexes and with parents regarding a range of interpersonal topics including sexual behavior and contraception, skills for resisting pressure to be sexually active, and the proper use of contraception once sexual activity has begun.

- **The committee recommends that all U.S. school systems develop comprehensive, age-appropriate programs of family life and**

sex education that build on the emerging body of data regarding more effective content, timing, and teacher training for these courses. State laws and policies should be revised, where necessary, to allow and encourage such instruction.

One component of such courses should stress the magnitude and consequences of unintended pregnancies, and how both males and females can avoid such pregnancies over a lifetime (e.g., through reversible contraception and sterilization, as well as abstinence). Instruction on contraception should include specific information on where to obtain contraceptives, how much they cost, and where to receive subsidized care if expense is a problem. Care should be taken to discuss all available forms of contraception, including emergency contraception as well as such longer-acting, coitus-independent methods as intrauterine devices and hormonal implants and injections. Instruction should include specific material on the details and mechanics of contraceptive use, emphasizing the fact that using many forms of contraception carefully and consistently requires specific skills. Material should also explain the value of using a condom and a female contraceptive method simultaneously to reduce the risk of both unintended pregnancy and contracting an STD.

The committee was impressed by the material suggesting that one of the main information and education sources in the nation—the media—is not helping in the task of conveying accurate, balanced information regarding contraception and sexual behavior, and too often highlights the risks rather than the benefits of contraception. Moreover, the electronic media especially continue to emphasize enticing, romantic, and "swept away" sexual encounters among unmarried couples. Only rarely do they present sexual activity in a manner that supports responsibility, respect, caring and consent, and protection against both unintended pregnancy and STDs. Many television executives decline to advertise contraceptive products because they fear controversy; at the same time, they air advertisements that routinely use sexual innuendo to help sell consumer products and programs that are peppered with sexual activity of all types.

- **The committee recommends that the electronic and print media help to educate all Americans about contraception, unintended pregnancy, and related topics of reproductive health. The media should present accurate material on the risks and benefits (including the non-contraceptive benefits) of contraception and should broaden messages about preventing STDs to include preventing unintended pregnancy as well. Media producers, advertisers, story writers, and others should also review carefully the overall amount and content of the sexual activity portrayed in the media and balance current entertainment programming so that sexual activity is preceded by a mutual understanding of both partners regarding its possible**

consequences and is accompanied by contraception when appropriate. Similarly, advertising of contraceptive products and public service announcements regarding unintended pregnancy and contraception should be more plentiful.

There is reason to be optimistic about enlisting the help of the media to reinforce messages about preventing unintended pregnancy. Over the last decade and more, programming has increasingly avoided the portrayal of smoking or drinking as glamorous, high-status activities, and seat belt use by actors in many movies and on television has increased significantly. In enlisting the help of the media in preventing unintended pregnancy, it will be important to ensure that any media-based social marketing efforts are theory-based, long-term, and carefully evaluated.

Campaign Goal 2: **Increase access to contraception.**

The second focus of the campaign to prevent unintended pregnancy should stress increasing access to contraception, especially the more effective methods that require contact with a health care professional. The committee was persuaded that one of the reasons for such high rates of unintended pregnancy in the United States is that, through a combination of financial and structural factors, the health care system in the United States makes access to prescription-based methods of contraception a complicated, sometimes expensive proposition. Private health insurance often does not cover contraceptive costs; the various restrictions on Medicaid eligibility make it an unreliable source of steady financing for contraception except for very poor women who already have a child; and the net decline in public investment in family planning services (especially those services supported by Title X of the Public Health Service Act), in the face of higher costs and sicker patients, may have decreased access to care for those who depend on publicly-financed services. Condoms, the most accessible form of contraception, provide valuable protection against STDs but must be accompanied by other contraceptive methods (preferably those that require a prescription) to afford maximum protection against unintended pregnancy. Unfortunately, other accessible nonprescription methods such as foam and other spermicides neither prevent the transmission of STDs nor offer the best protection against unintended pregnancy.

The two recommendations that follow take different approaches to increasing access to contraception: reducing financial barriers and broadening the pool of health professionals and institutions that promote pregnancy planning. These reflect the committee's conclusion that financial barriers may limit access to prescription-based methods of contraception, especially for low-income women, and that, overall, there are too few health professionals who actively promote contraception and pregnancy planning (Chapter 5). As is the case for the first recommended campaign goal—increasing knowledge—the committee views access to contraception as a basic first step toward reducing unintended pregnancy—a necessary precondition, and a fundamental requirement.

· The committee recommends that financial barriers to contraception be reduced by: (1) increasing the proportion of all health insurance policies that cover contraceptive services and supplies, including both male and female sterilization, with no copayments or other cost-sharing requirements, as for other selected preventive health services; (2) extending Medicaid coverage for all postpartum women for 2 years following childbirth for contraceptive services, including sterilization;[1] and (3) continuing to provide public funding—federal, state and local—for comprehensive contraceptive services, especially for those low-income women and adolescents who face major financial barriers in securing such care.

The first part of this recommendation addresses the need for contraceptive services to be covered more adequately by health insurance, as is increasingly the case for such other preventive interventions as immunizations. Mandates at the federal or state level would accomplish this goal quickly; it may also be possible to move in the needed direction by educating and encouraging all purchasers of health insurance to select policies that offer comprehensive coverage of contraceptive services and supplies.

The second and third elements in the recommendation above speak to the major role that such public financing programs as Title X and Medicaid have played in helping millions of people secure contraception, especially those who are young or poor. The Title X program in particular also has a long history of offering general health care to many low-income women, over and above family planning services, because in some communities, there are few alternative providers of primary care. Moreover, the clinical guidelines developed by the program, especially its protocols for annual visits, have helped to set a standard of care for both public and private gynecologic services. The program also laid the foundation for payment to county public health clinics as providers of direct services to the poor.

Although evaluation research has not yet defined the precise effects of either Medicaid or Title X on unintended pregnancy, those studies that have been completed on the effects of publicly-funded family planning services (which

---

[1]Currently, women who are enrolled in Medicaid through some avenue other than Aid to Families with Dependent Children (AFDC) are typically covered for only 60 days postpartum.

typically include both Medicaid and Title X funding) generally show a positive impact on a wide variety of fertility-related outcomes, including reduced adolescent birth rates. Moreover, there is no question that these programs help to finance contraceptive services for many women (and some men), the principal means by which unintended pregnancy is prevented. Whatever the current antagonism to Medicaid and Title X, including suggestions that both be either severely reduced or even eliminated, the important role that they have performed in supporting contraceptive care and related services must be recognized. It is essential that such public investment be maintained as part of the overall effort to help men and women avoid unintended pregnancy and achieve their reproductive goals.

One strength of the Title X program, in particular, is that because it is a federally administered program, states are prohibited from imposing restrictions on services at the local level that may limit access to contraception (such as not allowing minors to receive contraceptive care in clinics supported in whole or in part by Title X). If Congress decides to fold the Title X program into a block grant to the states, federal requirements and oversight of the program should continue to ensure maximum access to services at the local level. In addition, foundations and government should fund high-quality evaluations of public programs that help to support contraceptive services, Title X and Medicaid especially. Without better data regarding their impact on unintended pregnancy or other related outcomes, they remain particularly vulnerable to attack, and it is difficult to know how best to strengthen them.

- **To increase access to contraception, the committee also recommends that the campaign to reduce unintended pregnancy broaden the range and scope of health professionals and institutions that promote and provide contraception.**

Three steps will help meet this goal. First, medical educators should revise, where necessary, the training curricula of a wide variety of health professionals (physicians, nurses, and others) to increase their competence in reproductive health and contraceptive counseling for both males and females and, when appropriate, in actually providing contraceptive methods. Pediatricians in particular should include pregnancy planning and interconceptional care in their routine scope of practice to increase the proportion of pregnancies that are intended (e.g., counseling parents of infants and young children about the benefits of pregnancy planning and spacing for themselves and their young families). Second, administrators should increase the coordination, sometimes even co-location, between basic family planning services and many other health and social programs that typically serve individuals at high risk of unintended pregnancy, such as STD clinics, homeless centers, drug treatment programs, WIC offices (that is, offices that provide services financed by the Special

Supplemental Food Program for Women, Infants and Children), and well-child and immunization clinics. Third, those who provide social work, employment training, educational counseling, and other social services should be taught (in their initial training as well as through in-service programs) about the importance of talking with their clients regarding the benefits of pregnancy planning and how to do so.

· *Campaign Goal 3:* **Explicitly address the major roles that feelings, attitudes, and motivation play in using contraception and avoiding unintended pregnancy.**

Although increasing knowledge about and access to contraception (Campaign Goals 1 and 2) are important first steps, they are not enough. The data presented in Chapter 6 suggest that (1) personal and interpersonal factors exert a profound effect on whether and how well contraception is used, (2) using contraception carefully to avoid pregnancy requires strong, consistent motivation, and (3) such motivation is often based on the perception that pregnancy and childbearing, at a given point in time, are less attractive than other alternatives. In truth, avoiding unintended pregnancy is hard to do; it requires steady dedication over time, often from both partners, and specific skills. A significant portion of the unintended pregnancy experienced by low-income adolescents especially may be due to weak or inconsistent motivation to use contraception. Although pregnancy may not be fully intended in this population, there may be insufficient incentives to practice contraception scrupulously; pregnancy is the common result. This dynamic has been observed primarily among adolescents, but it is undoubtedly seen among older individuals as well. Being pregnant and having a child often bring significant psychological and social rewards, and there must be good reason to forego them.

These realities pose a great challenge to service providers and educators. For example, those who teach about contraception as well as those who provide it may well need to spend as much time on issues of personal feelings and interpersonal relationships as on the mechanics of contraceptive use. Accordingly, the third element of the campaign to reduce unintended pregnancy should emphasize the importance of motivation in using contraception and avoiding unintended pregnancy and the potent role that social environment can play in shaping such motivation at all ages.

> · **In order to increase the careful and consistent use of contraception, the committee recommends that contraceptive services be sufficiently well funded (through adequate reimbursement rates, increased public-sector support, or both) to include extensive counseling—of both partners, whenever possible—about the skills**

and commitment needed to use contraception successfully. Similarly, school curricula and programs that train health and social services professionals in reproductive health should include ample material about the skills that contraception requires and about the influence of personal factors on successful contraceptive use, along with more conventional information about reproductive physiology and contraceptive technology.

The influence of motivation in pregnancy prevention also underscores the importance of longer-acting, coitus-independent methods of contraception (e.g., hormonal implants and injections and, when appropriate, intrauterine devices) because they require only minimal attention once the method is established. Although few women and couples rely on these methods (Chapter 4), their long-term potential for reducing unintended pregnancy is great. When offered with careful counseling and meticulous attention to informed consent, these methods constitute an important component of the contraceptive choices available in this country. They do not, however, protect against the transmission of STDs, which requires that condoms be used also, as noted throughout this report. Earlier recommendations offered specific suggestions for increasing knowledge about and access to contraception; all of these efforts, including augmented provider training, should give special attention to longer-acting, coitus-independent methods.

On a broader level, policy leaders need to confront the likelihood that, particularly for those most impoverished, achieving major reductions in unintended pregnancies may well require that other more compelling alternatives to pregnancy and childbearing be available. These alternatives include better schools, realistic expectations that a high school diploma will lead to an adequate income, and jobs that are available and satisfying. Put another way, increasing knowledge about contraception and improving access to it as well may not be enough to achieve major reductions in unintended pregnancy when the surrounding environment offers few incentives to postpone childbearing. This comment is not meant to suggest that unless poverty is eliminated unintended pregnancy cannot be reduced. The point is rather that, in the poorest communities especially, only small reductions in unintended pregnancy will likely be achieved by the usual prescription of "more education, information and services." In this context, it is important to note that research findings do not support the popular notion that welfare payments (i.e., AFDC) and other income transfer programs exert an important influence on non-marital childbearing.

Although the committee has no simple recommendation about how to reduce poverty or its corrosive effects on human behavior, it does offer a modest suggestion.

· **The committee recommends that, in all of its activities, the campaign to reduce unintended pregnancy should stress the importance of personal motivation and feelings in careful contraceptive use and should highlight the influence of social environment on such motivation. Similarly, the connection between unintended pregnancy and poor social environments should be emphasized more explicitly by academic investigators, journalists and the media, politicians, and other opinion leaders interested in problems of social welfare.**

In the section on research below, the committee also notes the need to learn more about the complicated interplay of poverty, motivation, hopes for the future, and their combined effects on contraceptive use and unintended pregnancy.

· ***Campaign Goal 4:*** **Develop and scrupulously evaluate a variety of local programs to reduce unintended pregnancy.**

One aspect of the committee's work that it found most distressing was how little is known about effective programming at the local level to reduce unintended pregnancy. Given all of the public concern about teenage pregnancy, nonmarital childbearing, AIDS, and high-risk sexual behavior, it is quite remarkable that, even using fairly flexible inclusion criteria, the committee was able to identify fewer than 25 programs whose effects on unintended pregnancy, broadly defined, had been carefully evaluated. This lack of program information indicates that there is great need for research to determine various ways to reduce unintended pregnancy. Accordingly, as the fourth element of the campaign to reduce unintended pregnancy:

· **The committee recommends that public- and private-sector funders support a series of new research and demonstration programs to reduce unintended pregnancy. These programs should be designed to answer a series of clearly articulated questions, evaluated very carefully, and replicated when promising results emerge.**

The focus and design of these new programs should be based, at a minimum, on a careful assessment of the 23 programs identified by the committee that have been well enough evaluated to provide an understanding of their effects on specific fertility measures related to unintended pregnancy. Evaluation data from these programs support several broad conclusions: (1) even those few programs showing positive effects report only modest gains, which demonstrates how difficult it can be to reduce unintended pregnancy; (2) because most evaluated programs target adolescents, especially adolescent girls, knowledge about how to reduce unintended pregnancy among adult women and their partners is exceedingly limited; (3) there is insufficient evidence to determine whether "abstinence-only" programs for young adolescents are effective, but encouraging results are being reported by programs with more complex messages stressing both abstinence and contraceptive use once sexual activity has begun; (4) few evaluated programs actually provide contraceptive supplies, which may help to explain the small effects of many programs; (5) only mixed success has been reported from programs trying to prevent rapid repeat pregnancies among adolescents and young women; and (6) virtually none of the evaluated programs attempt to influence the surrounding community environment shaping sexual activity and contraceptive use.

The design of these new research and demonstration programs should also reflect four additional themes. First, unintended pregnancies derive in roughly equal proportions from couples who report some use of contraception, however imperfect, and from couples who report no use of contraception at all at the time of conception. Although many individuals move back and forth between these two states over time, it may nonetheless be useful to develop specific strategies for each group, especially for the very high-risk group of nonusers. For example, the former group may benefit particularly from ongoing support and special attention to developing better skills in contraceptive use, whereas the latter group may require a greater focus on underlying psychodynamics and couple interaction. Second, available data suggest that multifaceted programs to reduce unintended pregnancy are particularly effective—i.e., programs that include the actual provision of contraceptive supplies, as well as information, education, case management and follow-up, ongoing support, explicit attention to underlying attitudinal and motivational issues, and specific training in contraceptive negotiation and skills.

A third theme that should shape these new programs is the need to develop and test out new ways to involve men more deeply in the issue of pregnancy prevention and contraception. Although there is ever more talk about this idea, little investment in program-based research has been made to investigate the effectiveness of various strategies. Some advocate punitive approaches in order to force boys and men to "act responsibly," whereas others are convinced that carrots, not sticks, are needed. Research can help to develop effective interventions, particularly if experimental interventions address men's different ages, life stages, and cultural and personal preferences.

A fourth theme that these programs should explore is how to build community support for contraception. Although contraceptive use is ultimately a personal matter, community values and the surrounding culture clearly shape the actions of individuals and couples. Accordingly, at least some demonstration programs should target both the community and the individual, and some might also work exclusively at the community level. This approach has been used successfully in other areas such as the development of programs to reduce cardiovascular risk factors, and it would be wise to build on this experience for the problem of unintended pregnancy (Puska et al., 1985).

Within these broad themes, several additional issues seem particularly important for attention in a new research and demonstration program directed at reducing unintended pregnancy. These include such questions as: How can women over age 35 and their partners, and especially women over age 40, be reached with information and services to reduce unintended pregnancy? Can more "non-health" settings be used to serve adults, such as places of employment or community centers? What ways are especially useful in correcting the serious misinformation that many Americans apparently hold about the risks and benefits of contraception? How can programs effectively combine messages about abstinence with encouragement to use contraception?

Designing and evaluating these programs will be assisted by better and more plentiful state and local data on unintended pregnancy. "Mini" NSFGs would help in this regard and should be included as part of the overall package of new program-based research. State and local data also help to identify areas where unintended pregnancy is especially prevalent and can be valuable supplements to federal surveys.

Without new investments in measuring the effectiveness of intervention programs, the nation risks wasting large sums of money on failed strategies. Program evaluation is often expensive and can be difficult to do, but it is essential. At the same time, not every program must be evaluated; only certain model programs need be selected for detailed evaluation, whereas replications of successful models with minor modifications may just need expanded management information systems.

Several groups could help to fund the recommended research and demonstration programs. Within the federal government, the Office of Population Affairs, the Maternal and Child Health Bureau, the Centers for Disease Control and Prevention, the Bureau of Primary Care, the Agency for Health Care Policy and Research, and the Behavioral and Demographic Research Branch of the National Institute of Child Health and Human Development all have a potential interest in these issues. State entities and private foundations could take a leadership role as well.

· ***Campaign Goal 5:*** **Stimulate research to (a) develop new contraceptive methods for both men *and* women, (b) answer important questions about how best to organize contraceptive services, and (c) understand more fully the determinants and antecedents of unintended pregnancy.**

The fifth and final prong of the recommended campaign emphasizes research. With regard to the first area, the committee, like many other groups, has concluded that currently available methods of reversible contraception are generally effective but imperfect. Even when used properly, most methods have higher than desired failure rates. Some users balk at a particular method because of its side effects, aesthetic considerations (including whether it interrupts sexual intimacy), or cost. Reliable methods that are highly effective in preventing both pregnancy and STDs are lacking, as are methods that might prevent the spread of STDs but permit pregnancy. Particularly glaring is the lack of effective male methods of reversible contraception other than the condom. Accordingly, the committee supports the recommendations of the Institute of Medicine's Committee on Contraceptive Development (1990:1–5):

> Currently available contraceptive methods are not well suited to the religious, social, economic or health circumstances of many Americans and, therefore, a wider array of safe and effective contraceptives is highly desirable. . . . New methods would help men and women meet the changing needs for contraception they face during the different stages of their reproductive lives. . . . Given the relatively small pool of scientists working in this field . . . special attention should be given to enhancing the training opportunities for young scientists interested in careers in reproduction and contraceptive development. . . . Unless steps are taken now to change public policy related to contraceptive development, contraceptive choice in the next century will not be appreciably different from what it is today.

As noted earlier, the pervasive importance of personal motivation in contraceptive use underscores the need for more long-acting, coitus-independent methods of contraception. Hormonal contraception via implants and injections has already added important options to the available mix of methods; continuing to refine and improve these methods is essential. There probably is no perfect contraceptive, given the varying needs that both men and women have at different ages and stages of reproductive life, and for the foreseeable future, new methods will be only modest additions to existing options. Nonetheless, even moderate improvements can make an important difference.

Developing new contraceptive methods is a key concern of the National Institute of Child Health and Human Development, several foundations, and the pharmaceutical industry as well (Science, 1994). Their combined leadership and funding will remain crucial for progress in this area.

The second area of research focuses on learning about how best to organize contraceptive services and highlights the role that health services research can play in reducing unintended pregnancy. Two aspects of such research have already been mentioned: the need for better research on the effectiveness of publicly-supported programs that help to finance contraceptive services and the need for new research and demonstration programs at the community level to learn more about how to reduce unintended pregnancy. Many other important questions need answers as well: How is access to contraception enhanced or restricted by various managed care arrangements in health care? In which instances is it best to offer contraceptive care as a separate, specialized service and in which cases is it preferable to combine such care with other health services (such as STD services)? Many of the same funding entities noted earlier could also take a leadership role on these and related topics in health services research.

The third area of research addresses gaps in knowledge about the complex cultural, economic, social, biological, and psychological factors that lie behind widely varying patterns of contraceptive use and therefore unintended pregnancy. There are two basic reasons for the limited state of knowledge about the determinants and antecedents of unintended pregnancy—one methodological and the other theoretical. The methodological issue centers on the serious design and measurement problems in most of the existing research on determinants and antecedents, as noted throughout this report. For example, numerous definitions of contraceptive use have been employed; studies typically have been conducted with small convenience samples composed of students or low-income clinic patients; and many studies depend on a single predictor with minimal controls for confounding factors. Even those large-scale surveys that have used representative samples and multiple indicators (such as the NSFG) are limited by their heavy emphasis on social and demographic factors to the virtual exclusion of psychosocial and cognitive factors.

The theoretical issue, perhaps even more important than the methodological one, is that there is insufficient collaboration across disciplines in research on the determinants and antecedents of unintended pregnancy. Conceptualizations are often shaped by the leanings of the researchers' own discipline. Typically, demographers and sociologists have ignored the psychological underpinnings of contraceptive use and unintended pregnancy, psychologists have overlooked the social and demographic factors at work, and economists have limited themselves to economic influences on fertility. Greater interdisciplinary collaboration will be needed to blend these many perspectives into useful predictive models.

Moreover, even though contraception occurs in the context of a social interaction between two partners, few studies have examined men's knowledge, attitudes, and perceptions about contraception and pregnancy; and fewer studies have examined gender differences on these issues. Furthermore, in the majority of studies, data on male involvement have been obtained from the women interviewed, not from men. And little research has been done on couple interaction and decision-making that, for example, explores differing power relationships between the sexes and how age, income, and other status inequities affect both sexual behavior and contraceptive use, and therefore unintended pregnancy.

Finally, a new variable has entered into the contraceptive equation: concern for the prevention of STDs, including HIV and AIDS. Although there is an obvious overlap between pregnancy prevention and STD prevention, there are also important differences. For example, the condom is very effective in preventing the transmissions of many STDs, but it is not as effective as some other methods available for pregnancy prevention. By contrast, oral contraceptives are excellent at preventing pregnancy but offer no protection against STDs. So, when only one method is used, rather than a combination that would maximize protection against both consequences, a judgment of some sort is being made between the relative risk and importance of STDs versus the relative risk and importance of pregnancy. Research on the determinants of contraceptive behavior has yet to integrate this new dynamic into existing theories used to explain varying patterns of contraceptive use or method selection.

Although it is unreasonable to think that it is possible to achieve perfect understanding of all the predictors of unintended pregnancy or the relative importance of each, the scientific community could clearly be farther down the road than it is now. There are abundant clues and some important leads, but more research is needed to understand fully why more than half of all pregnancies in the United States are unintended at the time of conception and, in particular, why it is that half of these pregnancies occur among women who did not desire to become pregnant, but were nonetheless using no method of contraception when they conceived. The committee suspects that the effectiveness of intervention programs to reduce unintended pregnancy will remain modest until the knowledge base in this area is strengthened.

The material on personal feelings and beliefs summarized in Chapter 6 (especially the ethnographic information on motivation) and the many issues covered in Chapter 7 (particularly as regards the conflicting views and attitudes in American toward sexual behavior, which in turn may impede candid discussion about contraception, among other things) offer intriguing and very appealing explanations for the observed phenomena. Careful multidisciplinary work is needed to elaborate these inquiries and to integrate them with the more traditional explanations of unintended pregnancy, such as inaccessible contraception or insufficient knowledge about contraception and reproductive health. Research is also needed on factors outside of individuals (such as the impact of media messages on the contraceptive behavior of individuals), on factors within couples (such as the relative power and influence of women and men in decisions to use or not use particular methods of contraception), and on the combination of individual, couple, and environmental factors considered together. In all such multivariate research, it will be important to study the determinants of sexual behavior as well as contraceptive use, inasmuch as the two are often intimately connected and may jointly influence the risk of unintended pregnancy.

Research in these areas will be enhanced by more refined and differentiated tools to measure the intention status of a given pregnancy. As this report has repeatedly noted, the concept of an "unintended pregnancy" may be too simplistic to capture what is often a complicated set of feelings, frequently involving ambivalence, denial, and confusion. Moreover, the two partners involved may have quite different views regarding the intendedness of a particular conception—a consideration rarely reflected in existing research on unintended pregnancy. The new questions being used in the 1995 NSFG to probe intendedness represent an important step forward (Appendix C), as does the work of Miller (1992) and other investigators. Additional work along these general lines merits support.

Many players can help to lead and finance research on the determinants and antecedents of unintended pregnancy. Within the federal government, various agencies of the U.S. Public Health Service will be key (such as the Behavioral and Demographic Research Branch of the National Institute of Child Health and Human Development and the Centers for Disease Control and Prevention), as will the private foundation community.

CAMPAIGN LEADERSHIP

Progress toward achieving the five campaign goals outlined above would be enhanced by the existence of a readily identifiable group whose mission is to lead the suggested campaign.

- **The committee recommends that an independent, public-private consortium be formed at the national level to lead the campaign to reduce unintended pregnancy.**

Funding and leadership of this consortium should be provided by private foundations, given their proven capacity to draw many disparate groups together around a shared concern. Members of this consortium should be recruited from the health and education sectors, from private businesses and institutions, and from religious bodies and the media. Researchers and program administrators in reproductive health should be included along with government leaders (federal, state, and local) from both the executive and legislative branches. Experts in community development, employment training, and related fields of social service will be central to the effort as well. Similar groups that have been formed to address equally complex problems include, for example, the Partnership for a Drug-Free America and the National Commission to Prevent Infant Mortality, both of which were constituted with broad representation and, in particular, were successful in stimulating the development of parallel groups at the state and local levels.

One sector that could be especially effective in this consortium is the "children's lobby," that is, the many groups that speak on behalf of children and their needs. As this report has documented, unintended pregnancy has far-reaching consequences for children, affecting their health and development in numerous ways. Although groups representing women's issues—reproductive health in particular—have long been vocal in their support of contraception and pregnancy planning, the groups focused on children's issues have been far less visible, especially the maternal and child health community. The national campaign to reduce unintended pregnancy will need their voices as well, not only because of the substance of this issue but also because children's groups have great political appeal and credibility.

* * * * *

This report concludes where it began: unintended pregnancy is frequent and widespread, has significant negative consequences, and is poorly understood as a major public health and social challenge. Reasonable remedies are within reach, and they merit widespread support. All pregnancies should be intended—consciously and clearly desired at conception—and it is our shared responsibility to create a climate that helps the nation achieve this clear goal.

REFERENCES

Bumpass L, Sweet J, Cherlin A. The role of cohabitation in declining rates of marriage. J Marriage Fam. 1991;53:913–927.

Centers for Disease Control and Prevention. Abortion Surveillance: Preliminary Data—United States, 1992. MMWR. 1994;33:930–932.

Henshaw SK, Van Vort J. Abortion services in the United States, 1991 and 1992. Fam Plann Perspect. 1994;26:100–112.

Institute of Medicine and Commission on Behavioral and Social Sciences and Education. Developing New Contraceptives: Obstacles and Opportunities. Washington, DC: National Academy Press; 1990.

Institute of Medicine. Prenatal Care: Reaching Mothers, Reaching Infants. Washington, DC: National Academy Press; 1988.

Institute of Medicine. Legalized Abortion and the Public Health. Washington, DC: National Academy Press; 1975.

The Lancet. Editorial. Abortion: One Romania is enough. Lancet. 1995;345:137–138.

Miller WB. An empirical study of the psychological antecendents and consequences of induced abortion. J Soc Issues. 1992;48:67–93.

Puska P, Nissisen A, Tuomilehto J, et al. The community-based strategy to prevent coronary heart disease: Conclusions from the ten years of the North Karelia project. Ann Rev Public Health. 1985;6:147–193.

Science. Special section. Reproduction: New developments. 1994;266:1484–1527.

U.S. Department of Health and Human Services. Healthy People 2000: National Health Promotion and Disease Prevention Objectives. Washington, DC; 1990.

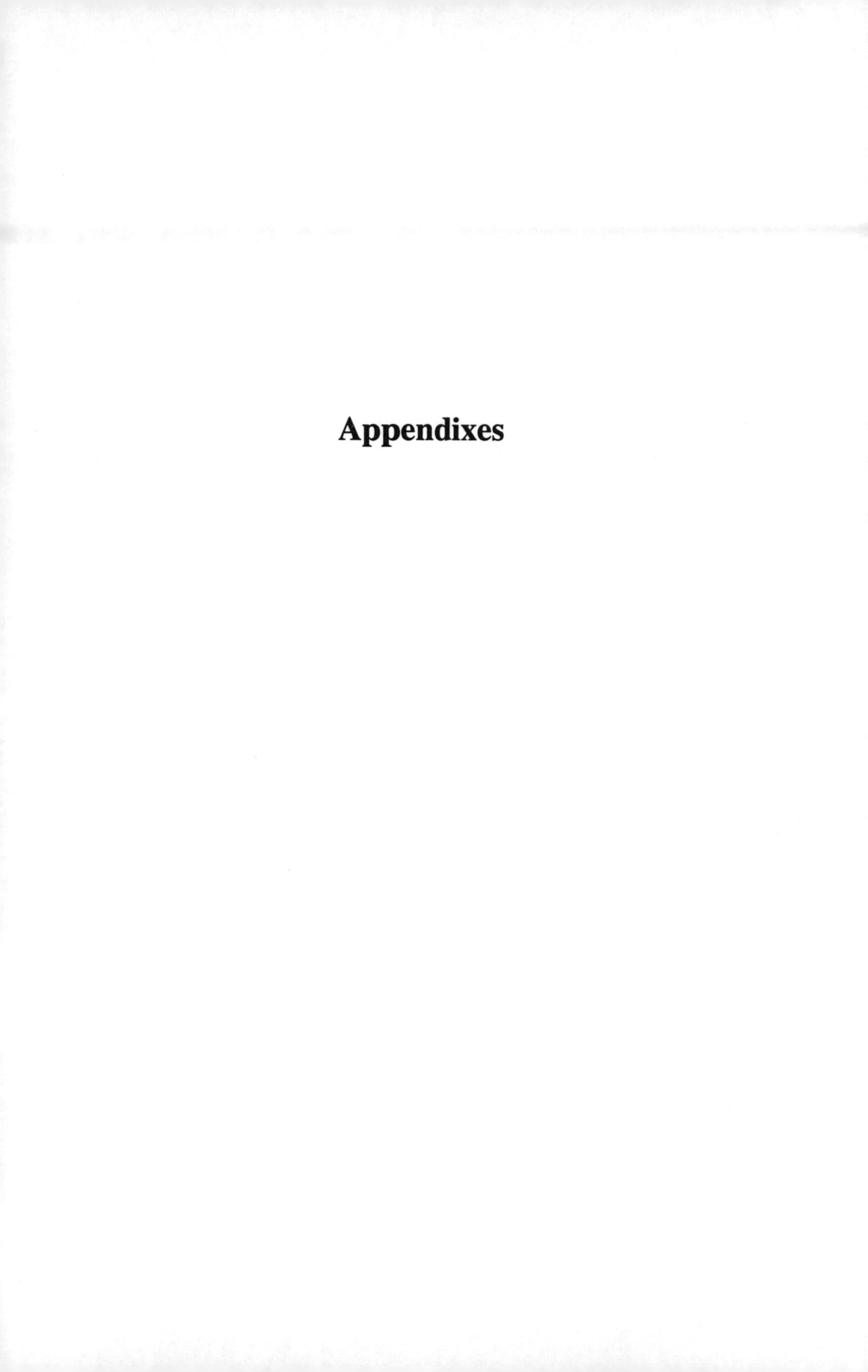

Appendixes

A

Commissioned and Contributed Papers

Nancy Adler, Ph.D., Professor of Medical Psychology, University of California, San Francisco, CA, and Warren Miller, M.D., Director, Transnational Family Research Institute, Palo Alto, CA. "Individual-Level Variables: The Reasons Behind the Rates"

Jane Delano Brown, Ph.D., Professor of Journalism and Mass Communications, and Jeanne Steele, M.S., Docotoral Candidate, School of Journalism and Mass Communications, University of North Carolina, Chapel Hill, NC. "Sex, Pregnancy and the Mass Media"

Allan Carlson, Ph.D., President, The Rockford Institute, Rockford, IL. "The Views of Theologically and Socially Conservative American Groups on Contraception, Family Planning and Related Issues"

Betty Connell, M.D., Professor of Obstetrics and Gynecology, Emory University School of Medicine, Atlanta, GA. "Contraception"

William D'Antonio, Ph.D., retired Executive Officer of the American Sociological Association. "Human Sexuality, Contraception, and Abortion: Policies, Attitudes and Practices Among America's Major Religious Groups"

Jacqueline Darroch Forrest, Ph.D., Vice President for Research, Katherine Kost, Ph.D., Senior Research Associate, and Susheelah Singh, Ph.D., Associate Director of Research, The Alan Guttmacher Institute, New York, NY. "Investigation of the Impact of Pregnancy Intention Status on Women's Behavior During Pregnancy and Birth Outcomes"

Vanessa Gamble, M.D., Ph.D., Assistant Professor, and Judith Houck, M.A., Graduate Student, Department of the History of Medicine, University of Wisconsin School of Medicine, Madison, WI. "'A High Voltage Sensitivity': A History of African Americans and Birth Control"

Shelly Gehshan, M.A., Deputy Director, Southern Regional Project on Infant Mortality, Washington, DC. "The Provision of Family Planning Services in Substance Abuse Treatment Programs"

Debra Haffner, M.P.H., Executive Director, Sex Information and Education Council of the United States, New York, NY. "Sexuality Issues and Contraceptive Use" and "Sexuality Education and Contraceptive Instruction in U.S. Schools"

Lisa Kaeser, J.D., Senior Public Policy Associate, and Cory L. Richards, Vice President for Public Policy, The Alan Guttmacher Institute, Washington, DC. "Barriers to Access to Reproductive Health Services"

Frances Kissling, President, Catholics for Free Choice, Washington, DC. "Roman Catholic Perspectives and Policy Initiatives on Sexuality and Reproduction"

Jacob Klerman, Ph.D., Economist, Rand Corporation, Santa Monica, CA. "Economic Perspectives on Fertility and Unintended Pregnancy"

Mort Lebow, M.A., Consultant, American College of Obstetricians and Gynecologists, Washington, DC. "Contraceptive Advertising in the United States"

Kathryn London, Ph.D., Linda Peterson, M.A., and Linda Piccinino, M.P.S., Family Growth Survey Branch, National Center for Health Statistics, Washington, D.C. "The National Survey of Family Growth: Principal Source of Statistics on Unintended Pregnancy"

James Marks, M.D., M.P.H., Director, Division of Reproductive Health, Centers for Disease Control and Prevention, Atlanta, GA. "Health Effects of Induced Abortion" and "Spontaneous and Induced Abortions and the Risk of Breast Cancer"

Rebecca Maynard, Ph.D., Trustee Professor of Education, Social Policy and Communication, University of Pennsylvania, Philadelphia, PA. "The Effectiveness of Interventions on Repeated Pregnancy and Childbearing"

Kristin Moore, Ph.D., Executive Director, and Dana Glei, M.A., Child Trends, Inc., Washington, DC. "The Consequences of Teenage Childbearing" and "The Demography of Unintended Pregnancy"

Kathleen Morton, M.S., Graduate Research Assistant, Center for Population and Family Health, Columbia University, New York, NY. "Effects of Pregnancy Planning on Women's Health and Well-Being"

Jeannie Rosoff, J.D., President, The Alan Guttmacher Institute, New York, NY. "The Political Storms Over Family Planning"

Freya Sonenstein, Ph.D., Director, Population Studies Center, The Urban Institute, Washington, DC, and Joseph Pleck, Ph.D., Senior Research Associate, Wellesley College, Wellesley, MA. "The Male Role in Family Planning: What Do We Know?"

Koray Tanfer, Ph.D., Senior Research Scientist, Centers for Public Health Research and Evaluation, Battelle Memorial Institute, Seattle, WA. "Determinants of Contraceptive Use: A Review"

* * * * *

Many of these papers have been submitted to journals for publication. Individuals wishing to receive copies of selected papers may contact the Institute of Medicine to request single copies, to be put in touch with the primary authors, and/or to locate the journal(s) in which selected papers have been published.

B

The Political Storms over Family Planning: Supplement to Chapters 1 and 7

Jeannie I. Rosoff
President, The Alan Guttmacher Institute

One of the more surprising political developments of the past decade has been the resurgence of political and legislative controversy over family planning, an issue that most thought had been settled some 25 years ago by the overwhelming congressional approval of the Family Planning and Population Research Act of 1970—Title X of the Public Health Service Act. This, however, was not to be.

The year 1994 marked the ninth consecutive year that this federal program, intended to equalize opportunity of access to family planning services, proved unable to secure a formal congressional authorization. This is not to suggest that public and congressional support for family planning or the provision of family planning services to the needy (however defined) had in any way lessened. On the contrary, the program continued to be supported by federal appropriations year after year even in the absence of a legislative authorization (although at increasingly lower levels because of the small but steady erosion due to inflation). In the mind of its champions on Capitol Hill, however, it was clear that the consideration of any family planning legislation was bound to bring forth a raft of hostile amendments (some of which might have survived the legislative process), making it hazardous to bring up the subject altogether. However, the November 1994 election of a new, more conservative U.S. Congress makes the prospects for the continuance of the Title X program, at least in its current form, dim at best. If it is retained at all as a federally administered program, it is likely to be further weakened, if not eviscerated, by amendments from its handful of opponents unlikely to be checked by the new Republican leadership. On the other hand, it may be caught in a wave of consolidation of federal programs into block grants, thereby losing its national identity and character (and most of its funding). Nevertheless, it can now be seen, at least in retrospect, that under the apparent early consensus about family planning, there lurked a number of either unanticipated or unresolved issues that were to fester over a period of years and that are still, in part, unresolved.

The first unresolved issue is that the term *family planning* itself lacked and, to a lesser extent, still lacks a clear, commonly agreed on definition. As representatives of the Roman Catholic Church stated repeatedly during the congressional hearings that preceded the passage of Title X, the postponement of childbearing, the spacing of children, and the limitation of family size—what most people viewed as "family planning"—could be achieved in many ways: by periodic sexual abstinence (the only method approved by the Roman Catholic Church), by contraception, by contraceptive sterilization, by abortion, or by all four means of fertility regulation at different times or under different circumstances in anyone's life.

At the time, the fact that there were numerous ways to achieve one's desired family size may have appeared irrelevant to Congress: in the mid- or late 1960s, abortion was illegal in nearly all states and the use of contraceptive sterilization among the general population was low. The Title X legislation included "comprehensive, voluntary" family planning services, but without specification. It did contain a provision, adopted at the request of the U.S. Catholic Conference, prohibiting the use of Title X funds "in programs where abortion is a method of family planning." The Conference Report that accompanied the legislation further specified that the funds could be used "only to support preventive family planning services, population research, infertility services, and other related medical, informational, and educational activities." Thus, although the prohibition on the use of family planning funds for abortion was clear, the inclusion of contraceptive sterilization could only be inferred by a careful interpretation of the phrasing "preventive family planning." The only unambiguously endorsed means of family planning (beyond periodic abstinence) was contraception, as defined and understood at the time, but this was no small achievement given a century or more of religious and public controversy and the continuing opposition of some religious organizations.

HISTORICAL BACKGROUND

Until the middle of the twentieth century, all religious denominations had condemned contraception as immoral. Largely because of the crusading activity of Anthony Comstock, the U.S. Congress in 1873 enacted a statute prohibiting the shipping of contraceptives (and of information about contraception) through the mail on the grounds of obscenity. Numerous states followed suit, passing laws banning the display, advertising, sale, and distribution of contraceptives. (Condoms, however, were exempted from the general ban because of their essential prophylactic role in the protection of men against "venereal" infection.) Although partially invalidated by court decisions or largely ignored in practice, these laws were to remain on the books until the middle 1960s, when they were declared unconstitutional by the U.S. Supreme Court. The federal statute itself, although not in force, was not officially repealed until 1972, 2 years after the passage of Title X.

The first major religious endorsement of contraception in the United States took place in 1931, when the Federal Council of Churches of Christ in America declared:

> As to the necessity for some form of effective control of the size of the family and spacing of children, and consequently of the control of conception, there can be no question. It is recognized by all churches and physicians. There is general agreement that sex union between *husbands* and *wives* as an expression of mutual affection without relation to procreation is right [italics added].

A consensus among Protestant denominations and Jewish religious groups grew rapidly in the following decades. The consensus was that the use of contraception was necessary to achieve "responsible parenthood" and that the responsibility for family limitation and child spacing had been delegated by God to the parents to be exercised in the light of their individual circumstances and informed consciences.

This consensus among some religious denominations failed, however, to bring about any changes in the position of the Roman Catholic Church, in spite of intensive ecumenical efforts to bring about a rapprochement about doctrinal and other matters among major Christian faiths. Although the Roman Catholic Church did endorse the concept of responsible parenthood, it insisted that every act of sexual intercourse between *husband and wife* be "open" to the possibility of conception and to oppose all methods of "artificial" contraception. In 1964, Pope Pius XII appointed the Commission on the Study of Population, the Family, and Births to review the position of the Catholic Church on contraception. The commission, with representatives of the laity, the scientific and medical communities, and theologians and members of the top hierarchy of the Catholic Church, did eventually recommend, after a 2-year period of deliberation and by a sizable majority, the approval of all medically appropriate methods of fertility regulation with the exception of abortion and contraceptive sterilization. Contrary to the commission's recommendations, however, the Pope reaffirmed, via the 1967 Encyclical Humanae Vitae, the Catholic Church's ban on sterilization and abortion and also on all forms of contraception, as distinct from periodic sexual abstinence, which is considered a licit method of family planning.

During these years, the legitimacy of the use of fertility regulation methods was discussed in the public arena only in the context of marriage. Indeed, in an attempt to avert the specter of sexual license, the terminology used by advocates attempted to stress this point. Even Margaret Sanger, the editor of the *Woman Rebel* and the founder of the American Birth Control League, renamed her organization the Planned Parenthood Federation of America, and in some common parlance, *family planning* and *planned parenthood* became terms often used interchangeably. Both terms, by inference at least, assumed sexual activity to occur only between married monogamous persons jointly establishing a family and planning the birth and spacing of their children.

At the same time, however, sexual and family mores were undergoing fundamental change with the gradual postponement of the age of marriage, the increased incidence of cohabitation outside of marriage, as well as steep increases in rates of marital disruption and divorce. The corollaries of these trends were substantial increases in the length of the interval between the initiation of sexual activity and marriage (now an average of 10 years among young men and 7 years for young women) as well as more sexual activity occurring outside of marriage. Under these circumstances, the use of family planning methods to prevent unwanted conceptions acquired a euphemistic connotation, when the purpose of using contraception was far removed from the desire to plan one's family but rather the purpose was to avoid starting a family at all. These developments were accompanied in many of the mainline Protestant and Reform Jewish organizations by an examination or re-examination of the essential nature of relationships—marital or otherwise—with the emphasis on the morality of sexual relationships shifting somewhat from a strict prohibition of all intercourse outside of a religiously sanctioned marriage, to the importance of such relationships being non-exploitative and being based on a commitment between equal partners to mutual support and growth.

The Catholic Church and a number of fundamentalist Protestant churches continue to maintain that any sexual activity outside the bounds of a properly sanctified marriage is by definition impermissible and sinful. Moreover, as the involvement of fundamentalist churches in the political process has grown over the last two decades, their views on sexual morality have come to exert a potent influence on the direction of public policy. It is important to note, however, that their members are not normally opposed, in principle, to the use of contraception or contraceptive sterilization within the confines of marriage; however, their opposition to the provision of contraceptive services to unmarried individuals (particularly teenagers), to school-based sex education including instruction on contraception, and to abortion has been strenuous. Although many Catholics ignore their church's admonitions regarding sexual morality, including the use of contraception, sterilization, and abortion, many members of Protestant fundamentalist groups are likely to organize and campaign militantly for the supremacy of their positions.

Religious and moral considerations aside, policymakers have been faced with very concrete issues demanding immediate and practical decisions. For example, under Medicaid (Title XIX of the Social Security Act [SSA]) the federal government reimburses the states for a portion of their expenditures for "necessary medical services" on behalf of the eligible population. Abortions and sterilizations, if they are deemed necessary by the attending physician, could therefore be paid for routinely by the states and reimbursement could be claimed from the federal government. As the use of contraceptive sterilization increased among the general population, its popularity also rose among Medicaid recipients, and demand for the procedure grew.[1] Abortions began to be reimbursed after a dozen states legalized abortion or reformed their abortion laws between 1967 and 1973; claims also increased after the U.S. Supreme Court decision of 1973. At the same time, Congress adopted amendments to the SSA in 1972 that specifically required the states to provide "family planning services and supplies" to all Medicaid recipients desiring these services, including "minors who can be considered sexually active." To encourage the states to do so, Congress also provided a preferential federal matching rate to the states of 90 percent. In June 1973, a few months after the landmark Supreme Court decision legalizing abortion throughout the United States, the U.S. Department of Health, Education and Welfare (now the U.S. Department of Health and Human Services) published a set of regulations intended to implement the 1972 SSA amendments. These regulations described the purpose of family

---

[1]The debate over sterilization that took place in the 1970s did not focus on its legitimacy as a method of birth control, but rather on its potential for coercion and its actual coercive use among minority or low-income women. Although the overall rate of contraceptive sterilization is not substantially different among the poor than among the more affluent population, it is heavily skewed by age and sex. Among the poor and minorities, among whom the use of vasectomy is minimal, virtually all contraceptive sterilizations are undergone by women. Also, sterilizations tend to take place at relatively young ages among women who start childbearing early and often experience repeated unintended pregnancies. Thus, thorough counseling as to the permanent nature of the procedure is particularly important for this group of women who may come to regret their decision if they experience a change in circumstances later in life or a change of heart. However, in some instances, counseling has clearly been perfunctory, offered, for example, during the throes of childbirth. There have even been reported instances of operations performed without the consent or knowledge of the patient. In 1978, to prevent such abuses, federal regulations were promulgated that require documentation of full informed consent and a waiting period of 30 days between the time that the patient's consent is obtained and the surgery is actually performed.

planning as the ability of individuals to freely "determine the number and spacing of their children" and the family planning services themselves as "any medically approved means" to achieve that end. By inference, at least, this definition would have included not only all of the contraceptive modalities approved by the U.S. Food and Drug Administration but contraceptive sterilization and abortion as well. An immediate controversy ensued, with some groups demanding positive assurance that sterilization and abortion be covered unambiguously and others objecting vehemently to the apparent inclusion of abortion. The final regulations were never promulgated, essentially leaving the states free to provide their own definitions. By 1976, the year of the first Hyde amendment, named after Representative Henry Hyde of Illinois, which prohibited the use of Medicaid funds for abortion, roughly one-third of the states were claiming federal reimbursements for Medicaid abortions under the family planning rubric.

After 1973, the controversy over abortion proceeded along two separate and parallel paths: (1) attempts to reverse the Supreme Court's decision on abortion through the adoption of a constitutional amendment (a prospect that has been dormant since 1983) and (2) a successful ban on the use of federal funds for abortions, first and foremost for Medicaid-eligible women. A by-product of these debates was the intrusion of the abortion issue into what most people viewed as "family planning" or, more narrowly, contraception. In the early legislative proposals to ban the use of federal monies to reimburse the states' expenditures for abortion under their Medicaid programs, the ban would have extended to the use of "abortifacient" drugs and devices. Although the specific drugs and devices were never precisely defined, they were widely claimed to include such artificial methods as oral contraceptives and intrauterine devices (although their modes of action do not normally interfere with the fertilized ovum). In rallying opposition to the proposed ban, pro-choice groups seized on this potential threat to methods of birth control used by millions of American women to help defeat the proposals in their entirety. This issue resurfaced many years later during deliberations of the Supreme Court in the *Webster* case concerning the continuing legality of abortion. At that time, the pro-choice attorney argued before the Supreme Court that the "bright line, if there ever was one (between contraception and abortion), has been extinguished" by the newer birth control methods. Justice Scalia concurred that it is indeed "impossible to distinguish between abortion and contraception when (abortion is defined) as the destruction of the *first* join of the ovum and the sperm."

Indirectly, these various maneuvers served to blur what many people and policymakers had heretofore believed to be clear lines of demarcation between contraception, the purpose of which is to prevent pregnancy, and abortion, which is intended to terminate a pregnancy that has already occurred. Underlying the ambiguity of the modes of action of certain types of fertility control is that the definition of what constitutes "pregnancy" is itself contested. Given the fact that the fertilized ovum in its early stages of division is both an unstable and a fragile entity, the medical and scientific definition of pregnancy is generally defined to be the time at which the process of the implantation of the blastocyst in the uterine wall has been completed, approximately 14 days after fertilization has taken place. On the other hand, some contend that the defining event is the moment of fertilization or conception. The use of "morning after" drugs and the development of RU-486 further confound the debate as to what properly marks the beginning of individual human life, what defines the state of pregnancy, and the possible "abortifacient" effect (depending on one's definitions) of certain means of fertility control techniques heretofore popularly believed to belong to the realm of contraception.

The desire of many politicians and much of the public at large was to (in the words of Senator Orrin Hatch of Utah) "erect a wall of separation" between contraception and abortion. This approach was tested on yet another front in 1988 when the Reagan administration promulgated regulations that prohibited federally funded family planning clinics from making referrals for abortion even at the request of women themselves. This ignored the fact that women facing an unintended pregnancy may be contraceptive users whose method failed or who had failed to use the method properly or consistently. These women as well as women who were not using contraception at all at the time that they became pregnant accidentally were likely to turn for help to the agencies or facilities whose business is the prevention of unintended pregnancies. The desire to, in effect, pigeonhole women into two categories, responsible contraceptors and wanton individuals without regard for human life, proved ultimately to be neither realistic nor politic. Even in the face of repeated veto threats on the part of President Bush, Congress came closer year by year (and, in 1992, within a few votes) to overriding this policy by the necessary two-thirds majority. However, this issue may well be rekindled in the present Congress as part of the House Republicans' "Contract with America," which seeks to prohibit the provision of information about abortion to welfare recipients.

CONCLUSION

Review of these developments leads to several conclusions. The first is that the development of public policy is both slow and deeply conservative in nature, particularly when it comes to matters within the rightful province of religious and personal morality. The second is that euphemisms, although they may help gain the superficial acceptance of new and potentially threatening concepts and values, also bring their own built-in backlash when the magnitude of their implications becomes better understood. The third is that, although largely ignored by its own communicants and perhaps because of dwindling political significance, the position of the Catholic Church continues to affect the behavior of significant community and quasi-public institutions. Although they may be supported in large part by tax monies, Catholic hospitals and the equally extensive Catholic social services network are bound, by the very nature of their affiliation, to refuse to provide services deemed "illicit" or even to refer their quasi-public clients to other facilities, assuming that they are available elsewhere in the community. Finally, although it is probably true that most Americans do not view abortion "as a method of family planning" in the sense that they would make a deliberate decision to use it as such, it is also clear that neither in science, in practice, nor in law is there a "bright line" to be drawn or a "wall of separation" to be erected in "matters so fundamentally affecting a person as the decision whether to bear or beget a child," in the words of the U.S. Supreme Court.

C

The National Survey of Family Growth: Principal Source of Statistics on Unintended Pregnancy: Supplement to Chapter 2

Kathryn London, Ph.D., Linda Peterson, M.A., and Linda Piccinino, M.P.S.
National Center for Health Statistics

The National Survey of Family Growth (NSFG) is the most comprehensive source of information available on pregnancy and contraceptive use among reproductive-age women (15–44 years) in the United States. The greatest strengths of the NSFG as a source of data on unintended pregnancy are (1) the wealth of information that it contains on pregnancy, contraceptive use, and related topics and (2) the repetition of the questions on unintended pregnancy in each round of the NSFG, permitting analysis of long-term trends. Besides detailed questions on the intendedness of each of a woman's pregnancies, the NSFG collects information on contraceptive use and method choice, infertility, use of family planning services, birth expectations, and marriage and cohabitation. The survey also collects information on other social and demographic characteristics that have been found to influence reproductive behaviors, such as family background, income, education, and labor-force participation.

The NSFG is federally funded and is conducted by the National Center for Health Statistics (NCHS). Surveys have been conducted in 1973, 1976, 1982, and 1988. In 1973 and 1976 the samples were restricted to ever-married women, among whom most childbearing in the country had occurred. In 1982 and 1988, women of all marital statuses were included. In 1990, respondents from the 1988 survey were briefly reinterviewed by telephone. The next round of the NSFG is being conducted in 1995, and with a brief telephone reinterview planned for 1997.

DEFINITIONS AND MEASUREMENT ISSUES

Since the first NSFG in 1973 (and also in four national fertility surveys that were precursors to the NSFG, conducted in 1955, 1960, 1965, and 1970), married women have been asked whether they and their husbands wanted each of their pregnancies. The questions were extended to unmarried women and their partners in 1982. The series of questions on unintended pregnancy has remained essentially unchanged, preserving the comparability of the data over time and permitting trend analysis. Women's responses to the following questions are used to code pregnancies as intended (wanted) or unintended (mistimed or unwanted):

Question C-1. Before you became pregnant . . . , had you stopped using all methods of birth control?

Yes	1 (If the answer is yes, go to question C-2)
No	2 (If the answer is no, go to question C-3)

Question C-2. Was the reason you had stopped using any methods because you yourself wanted to become pregnant?

Yes	1 (go to question C-5)
No	2 (go to question C-3)

Question C-3. At the time you became pregnant . . . , did you yourself, actually want to have a(nother) baby at *some* time?

Yes	1 (go to question C-5)
No	2 (go to question C-6)
Don't know	3 (go to question C-4)

Question C-4. It is sometimes difficult to recall these things but, just before that pregnancy began, would you say you probably wanted a(nother) baby at *some* time or probably not?

Probably yes	1 (go to question C-5)
Probably no	2 (go to question C-6)
Didn't care	3 (go to question C-6)

Question C-5. Did you become pregnant sooner than you wanted, later than you wanted, or at about the right time?

Sooner	1
Later	2
Right time	3
Didn't care	4

Question C-6. And what about your partner at the time you became pregnant . . . , did he want you to have a(nother) baby at *some* time?

Yes	1 (go to question C-7)
No	2 (skip out)
Don't know	3 (skip out)

Question C-7. Did you become pregnant sooner than he wanted, later than he wanted, or at about the right time?

Sooner	1
Later	2
Right time	3
Didn't care	4

Pregnancies are classified as "wanted" if the answer to question C-5 was "later" or "right time." Pregnancies for which the answer to question C-5 was "didn't care" are also commonly classified as "wanted." Pregnancies are classified as "mistimed" if the answer to question C-5 was "sooner." Finally, pregnancies for which the answer to question C-3 was "no" or the answer to question C-4 was "probably no" are classified as "unwanted."

Although the NSFG has effectively measured trends in unintended pregnancy, there are some limitations to the kinds of analysis that can be done. First, as with most fertility surveys, the NSFG suffers from underreporting of abortion. An estimated 35 percent of the actual abortions in the 4-year period prior to the 1988 survey were reported in the survey (Jones and Forrest, 1992). Because not all women surveyed report all of the abortions that they have had, most studies of unintendedness have minimized bias by restricting the sample to live births. Many analysts also adjust for underreported abortions by assuming that 100 percent of unreported abortions were unintended pregnancies.

A second limitation of the data is that the wantedness questions are misunderstood by some respondents. Teenagers seem particularly vulnerable to misunderstanding, as indicated by the large proportion of recent births to teens that were reported unwanted—22 percent of births to women ages 15–19 in the 5 years before the 1988 interview date (Piccinino, forthcoming). Testing of a follow-up clarifying question in the NCHS Questionnaire Design Research Laboratory found evidence that although some women accurately reported a pregnancy as unwanted (they did not want to get pregnant then or at any time in the future), other women who reported pregnancies as unwanted corrected their answers to say that they had become pregnant sooner than they had wanted, that is, the pregnancy was mistimed, but not unwanted. Two often-mentioned circumstances that apparently led women to mistakenly answer that they "did not want to have a(nother) baby at some time" were (1) the pregnancy occurred much earlier than desired, possibly by many years, and (2) they had no desire to have a baby with that particular partner, even though they wanted to have a baby at some time.

Third, respondents are asked to classify pregnancies in a fairly rigid way—either they wanted to get pregnant or they did not. Feelings of ambivalence are not measured. Understanding of unintended pregnancy would no doubt be advanced by measuring ambivalence in men's and women's attitudes toward becoming pregnant, the determinants and magnitude of the ambivalence, and its relation to contraceptive practices.

Fourth, the role of ineffective contraceptive use has not been well measured. The NSFG consistently finds that most women at risk of unintended pregnancy use contraception, yet a large percentage of births are unintended. Several studies have looked at the planning status of pregnancies to try to better understand the role of contraception in unintended pregnancy. In such studies pregnancies are classified as "planned" or "unplanned" rather than "intended" or "unintended" (Pratt et al., 1992; Williams and London, 1992). The NSFG collects information on the planning status of every pregnancy, that is, whether the woman was using birth control at the time of conception (question C-1 above) and, if not, whether her purpose was to become pregnant (question C-2 above). Pregnancies are considered unplanned if they were conceived while a woman was using birth control or while she was using no birth control but not because she desired pregnancy. Thus, whereas "unplanned" has been used to emphasize the behavioral aspects of wantedness, "unintended" reflects attitudes toward a pregnancy.

From questions C-1 and C-2 listed above, one can classify women's unplanned pregnancies by type, that is, method or user failures versus failures to use contraception at all. Yet further information is needed. From the current questions, one cannot discern whether women who reported using contraception during the month that they became pregnant actually used a method at the time that they conceived. Method users do not necessarily use their method correctly or every time that they have sexual intercourse. The NSFG lacks measures of the extent to which unplanned pregnancies result after the incorrect use of methods, from methods that are faulty themselves, and from failure to use a method at all.

NSFG PLANS FOR THE FUTURE

The revised 1995 NSFG questionnaire may produce better data on unintended pregnancy. Four goals have been identified: (1) to improve abortion reporting (and therefore permit unbiased analysis of all pregnancies, not just live births), (2) to clarify questions on unwanted and mistimed pregnancies, (3) to measure women's ambivalent feelings about becoming pregnant, and (4) to improve understanding of unplanned pregnancies through better measures of contraceptive use.

Improving Abortion Reporting

Two new techniques seek to improve abortion reporting: (1) allowing respondents to record their abortion histories in private via audio computer-assisted self-interviewing (A-CASI), and (2) paying respondents an incentive so that they will participate in the survey (which apparently has the additional benefit of eliciting more honest answers). NCHS and their data collection contractor, Research Triangle Institute (RTI), tested both techniques in the NSFG pretest in 1993 with encouraging results. Using A-CASI, a subset of NSFG pretest respondents listened via headphones to recorded questions asking whether and when they had had abortions. Women typed their answers directly into the computer; the interviewer did not see their answers. Some NSFG pretest respondents received a $20 or a $40 incentive to participate whereas other respondents received no incentive.

NSFG pretest results showed that both A-CASI and monetary incentives significantly increased abortion reporting. About 14 percent of respondents who received no incentive and no A-CASI interview reported ever having had an abortion, whereas 30 percent of respondents who received both an incentive and an A-CASI interview reported ever having had an abortion (Research Triangle Institute, 1994). According to an independent estimate, 29 percent of women aged 15–35 in 1992 have had one or more abortions (Baldwin et al., forthcoming). The NSFG pretest sample was small (500 respondents) and not nationally representative, so one must view its findings with some caution. Yet the findings raise the hope that through these new techniques abortion reporting in the 1995 NSFG will improve significantly, and perhaps even approach complete reporting.

Clarifying Questions on Unwanted and Mistimed Pregnancies

NSFG staff have redesigned some of the questions used to measure unwanted and mistimed pregnancies. First, the 1995 NSFG has added the following preamble stressing the importance of the wantedness series, in the hope of improving the quality of reporting: "The next few questions are important. They are about how you felt when you became pregnant." In the NSFG pretest, similar preambles improved the quality of reporting on other topics (Research Triangle Institute, 1994).

Second, two questions were added to the wantedness series itself. The goal was to make the questions clearer but to preserve the ability to measure changes in unintended pregnancy over time. The 1995 NSFG asks the standard version of wantedness questions, but this is followed by a new question that confirms that respondents who report an unwanted pregnancy mean that they did not want to become pregnant then or at any time in the future:

> So when you became pregnant, you thought you did not want to have any children *at any time in your life*, is that correct?

The 1995 NSFG also includes a new question to clarify the meaning of a "mistimed" pregnancy:

> How much sooner than you wanted did you become pregnant? (Record answer in months or years.)

Measuring Ambivalence about Pregnancy

NSFG and RTI staff designed a series of questions to measure ambivalence about pregnancy. They patterned questions after an instrument developed and used by Irene M. Rich. Rich's questionnaire measured ambivalent feelings during pregnancy (Rich, 1993). The NSFG and RTI staff designed similar questions to measure ambivalence about becoming pregnant, that is, to measure ambivalent feelings at the time of conception. The questions, which follow, were tested in the NSFG pretest in 1993 and will be asked in the 1995 NSFG of women under 25 years of age.

> Question E-9. Please look at the scale on Card E-3 and tell me which number on the card best describes how you felt when you found out you were pregnant. On this scale, a one means that you were very unhappy to be pregnant and a ten means that you were very happy to be pregnant.

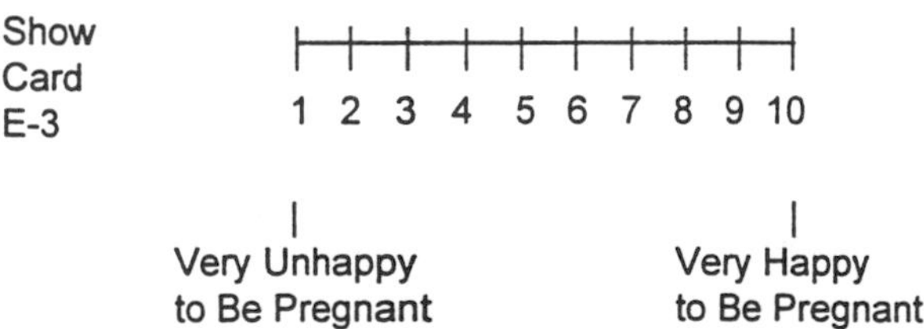

> Next, I am going to read a list of feelings and concerns women sometimes have about becoming pregnant. Please look at the scale on Card E-4.

Question E-10. For each statement I read, please tell me which number on the card best describes your opinion about becoming pregnant. On this scale, a one means that you strongly disagree with the statement and a ten means you strongly agree with the statement.

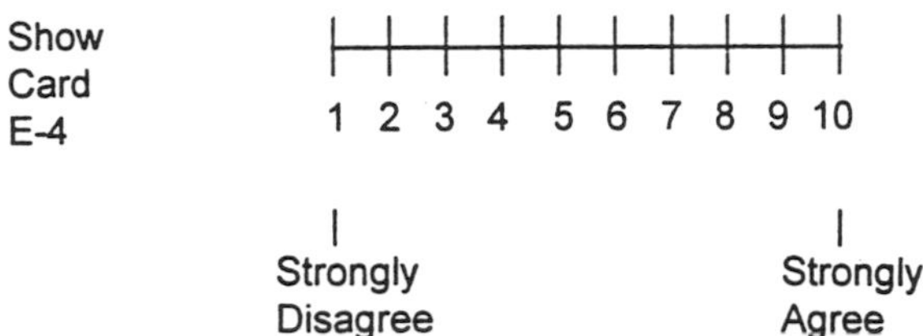

You were worried that you did not know enough about how to take care of a baby.

You thought that a new baby would keep you from doing the things that you were used to doing like working, going to school, going out and so on.

You looked forward to teaching and caring for a new baby.

You looked forward to the new experiences that having a baby would bring.

You looked forward to experiencing the changes in your body that come with carrying a baby.

You looked forward to telling your friends that you were pregnant.

You were worried about what being pregnant would do to your body.

You were worried that you did not have enough money to take care of a baby.

You dreaded telling your friends that you were pregnant.

You looked forward to buying things for a new baby.

Improving Questions on Unplanned Pregnancies and Use of Contraception

NSFG staff have added method-specific questions about how consistently women used contraception before becoming pregnant. The goal is to get a better sense of how many unplanned pregnancies occurred while methods were being used consistently and correctly and how many stemmed from incorrect or irregular use of contraception. The new questions follow.

For users of birth control pills:

Question E-11. In the month before you became pregnant, how many pills that you were *supposed* to take did you miss? Would you say you . . .

Never missed a pill,	1
Missed only one pill, or	2
Missed two or more pills?	3

For users of rhythm or natural family planning:

Question E-12. In the month before you became pregnant, did you have intercourse during your "safe time only," during your "safe time" and at other times, or during other times only?

Safe time only	1
Safe time and other times	2
Other times only	3

For users of other (coitus-dependent) methods:

Question E-13. Although you were still using a method in the month before you became pregnant, how often did you and your partner *usually* use a method of birth control for any reason? Would you say you used a method . . .

Less than half the time,	1
About half the time,	2
More than half the time, or	3
Every time you had intercourse?	4

The A-CASI section of the questionnaire may also improve data on unplanned pregnancy by giving respondents a second chance to accurately report their contraceptive use. During the in-person part of the interview, respondents who fail to report abortions may also fail to report their contraceptive use accurately. For example, a woman who used a contraceptive method inconsistently and who as a result had an unplanned pregnancy and an abortion may be reluctant to report this information to the interviewer and may instead report a period of successful contraceptive use. To address this possibility, the A-CASI section of the 1995 NSFG follows up any new reports of abortions with a set of questions about the contraceptive method the woman used before she became pregnant:

> So that we can understand how well birth control methods work, we would like you to list the methods of birth control you were using—if you used any—during the month you became pregnant.

Question J-1. In (month and year of conception), the month you became pregnant, were you using any birth control methods?

Yes	1 (go to question J-2)
No	2 (flow check question J-7)

Question J-2. Which methods did you use in (month and year of conception), the month you became pregnant? Did you use . . .

	Yes	No
Birth control pills?	1	2
Condoms?	1	2
A vasectomy?	1	2
A diaphragm?	1	2
Foam?	1	2
Jelly or cream?	1	2
A cervical cap?	1	2
A suppository or insert?	1	2
The Today sponge?	1	2
A female condom?	1	2
An intrauterine device?	1	2
Norplant?	1	2
Depo-provera injectables?	1	2
Rhythm or safe period by calendar?	1	2
Safe period by temperature or cervical mucus test or natural family planning?	1	2
Withdrawal?	1	2
Some other method?	1	2

Flow check question J-6: If more than one method reported in question J-2, ask question J-3. Else, go to question J-4.

Question J-3. Did you use those methods together, that is, at the same time, or did you use them at different times during the month?

Same time	1 (go to question J-4)
Different times	2 (go to question J-4)

Question J-4. How many months in a row had you been using that method when you became pregnant?

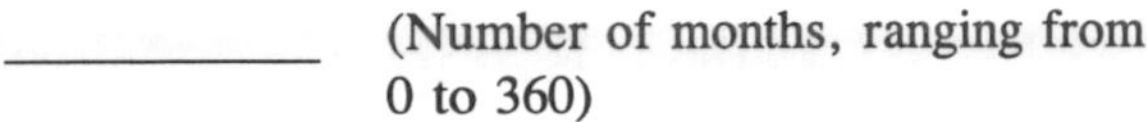

(Number of months, ranging from 0 to 360)

Finally, the 1995 NSFG uses a memory aid that may, among other benefits, improve data on contraception. NSFG staff have designed a calendar for respondents to refer to throughout the interview to help them remember the dates of the events that they report. A respondent writes important events on the calendar as she proceeds through the interview, such as her date of marriage, the dates of birth of her children, and dates when she was not having sexual intercourse for an extended time. The hope is that giving the woman a context in which to remember her contraceptive use will produce more accurate data.

The trends in unintended pregnancy seem clear and their measurement fairly straightforward. The NSFG is striving to improve the measurement of the more elusive concepts related to unintended pregnancy. It is hoped that the NSFG will continue to take the lead in producing the data needed to understand the causes of unintended pregnancy.

REFERENCES

Baldwin AK, Jobe JB, London KA, Rasinski KA, Pratt WF, Tourangeau R. Answering sensitive questions in a health survey. Forthcoming.

Jones E, Forrest J. Underreporting of abortion in surveys of U.S. women: 1976–1988. Demography. 1992;29:113–126.

Piccinino, LJ. Unintended pregnancy and childbearing. In From Data to Action. Wilcox L, Marks J, eds. Washington, DC: U.S. Department of Health and Human Services and Centers for Disease Control and Prevention; Forthcoming.

Pratt WF, Peterson LS, Piccinino LJ. Trends in Contraceptive Practice and Contraceptive Choice, United States: 1965–1990. Paper presented at the NIH Conference on Opportunities in Contraception: Research and Development. Bethesda, MD: National Institutes of Health; 1992.

Research Triangle Institute. National Survey of Family Growth, Cycle V, Pretest Report. Research Triangle Park: Research Triangle Institute; 1994.

Rich IM. General Pregnancy Attitudes, Ambivalence, and Psychological Symptom Distress During Pregnancy. Ph.D.dissertation. Catholic University of America; 1993.

Williams LB, London KA. The planning status of births to ever-married women in the United States: 1982-1988. Fam Plann Perspect. 1992;26:121–124.

D

Tables of Odds Ratios: Supplement to Chapter 3

Carol J.R. Hogue
Member, Committee on Unintended Pregnancy

Chapter 3 includes an assessment of the literature published within the last 30 years that addresses various health and health-related consequences of unintended pregnancy. The literature base for most consequences studied does not permit a numerical survey. However, some effects, particularly ones related to pregnancy and pregnancy outcome, have been studied sufficiently to permit a structured assessment. These consequences include timing of the initiation of prenatal care, an estimate of the adequacy of prenatal care based on both timing and the number of visits, exposure of the fetus to smoking and alcohol, and the incidence of low birthweight (<2,500 grams) among live-born infants. A graphical presentation of studies on these issues is provided in Chapter 3.

This appendix provides more detail regarding those studies. To be included in this structured assessment, an investigation had to compare outcomes between women reporting intended conceptions and women reporting unintended conceptions, variously defined. When unintended was subdivided into mistimed and unwanted, estimates of effects (usually odds ratios) are included for both categories of unintended conception. An odds ratio is an estimate of the relative risk, that is, the risk of a poor outcome among the "exposed" group (unintended conception) relative to the risk of a poor outcome among the "unexposed" group (intended conceptions). These results, with 95 percent confidence intervals, are shown in column 5 of the tables in this appendix. The results in Figures 3-3 through 3-5 of Chapter 3 were selected from these results. If a study calculated both a crude and an adjusted odds ratio, only the adjusted one was included in the figure. When the results were available for both mistimed and unwanted conceptions, they were included in the figures. The references for this appendix are provided in Chapter 3.

TABLE D-1 Studies of Prenatal Care Attainment Associated with Pregnancy Intention

Definition of Intention	Population/ Sample	Retrospective/ Prospective	Control Factors	Results	Reference/ Comments
		Initiation of Prenatal Care (PNC) after the First Trimester			
Unwanted: (a) at conception, (b) at fourth month, (c) in last trimester	120 black women, Boston City Hospital, married with at least one living child, 1964	Prospective at three points during gestation	None	Late PNC, (a) OR[a] = 2.89 (0.96,9.02)[c], (b) OR= 3.57 (1.38,9.36)[c], (c) OR= 2.42 (0.65,9.31)[c]	Watkins, 1968; (a) 77.5%, (b) 27.9%, (c) 11.7%
(a) Mistimed, (b) unwanted	NSFG, 1982 (random sample of U.S. women 15–44, with live births 1979–1982)	Retrospective (≤3 yrs. postpartum)	Race	(a) RR[b], all = 1.6[c]; RR, white = 1.6[c]; RR, black = 1.4[c] (b) RR, all = 1.8[c]; RR, white = 1.7[c]; RR, black = 1.75[c]	Pamuk and Mosher, 1988
"Intended" vs. "unintended"	NNS, 1980 (random sample of U.S., married)	Retrospective (>6 mo postpartum)	Race, residence, education, birth order	Crude OR = 1.25[c] Adjusted OR = -1.19[c]	Wells et al., 1987
Planned vs. unplanned	416, central Harlem residents in PNC, 1982–1983	Retrospective (at first PNC visit)	None	OR = 1.31[c]	McCormick et al., 1987;73% were unplanned

Continued

TABLE D-1 Continued

Definition of Intention	Population/ Sample	Retrospective/ Prospective	Control Factors	Results	Reference/ Comments
Intended (stopped using contraception because of pregnancy desire or just before pregnancy, wanted to become pregnant) vs. unintended	NLSY, 1984, women 18–26, nationally representative sample of 6,015	Retrospective (78%), prospective (22% during pregnancy)	Race, economically disadvantaged (white), southern or urban resident at age 14, grandmother's education, maternal age	For unintended, crude RR = 1.14[c]; adjusted OR = 1.6[c]	Marsiglio and Mott, 1988; they used the term "wanted" but the questions more closely reflect intended
"Intended" vs. "unintended"	Random sample, 1,490; births in England, 1,984	Retrospective (≥4 mo postpartum)	None	Risk of entry after first trimester; OR = 1.9 (1.33,2.17)[c]	Cartwright, 1988; interview asked pregnancy intention
(a) Mistimed, (b) unwanted	NMIHS, 1988 nationally representative sample of 9,953	Retrospective (at least 1 yr postpartum)	None	(a) RR = 2.88[c] (b) RR = 2.62[c]	Kost et al., 1994
(a) Mistimed, (b) unwanted	Oklahoma PRAMS, 1988–1993, (a) N = 2,329 (b) N = 933	Retrospective (4–12 mo postpartum)	Age, education, source of family income, timing of pregnancy recognition, parity	(a) Crude OR = 2.7 (2.1,3.4); adjusted OR = 1.4 (1.04,1.9) (b) crude OR = 4.6 (1.3,6.1); adjusted OR = 1.7 (1.1,2.5)	DePersio et al., 1994

Planned vs. "surprise"	Hispanic, Houston, TX, public hospital patients, 100 each entered PNC in 1st, 2nd, 3rd trimester or none	Retrospective (at delivery)	None	Risk of entry after first trimester OR = 2.64 (1.50,4.66)[c]	Byrd, 1994; early PNC associated with hospital access card, fewer perceived barriers, more benefits to baby
			Inadequate Prenatal Care (PNC)		
See Results column	Random sample in Oklahoma, births, 1985	Retrospective (at delivery)	Multiple	Receipt of inadequate care, mistimed, family support OR = 1.15[c] (NS); mistimed, pregnancy discussed OR = 1.09[c] (NS); unwanted, family support, OR = 1.15[c] (NS); unwanted, pregnancy discussed, OR = 1.36 ($p < 0.05$)	St. John and Winston, 1989; see text
Unwanted	Case–control study, three sites in Missouri; adequate, N=720; inadequate, N=764	Retrospective (at delivery)	Multiple	Receipt of inadequate care; OR = 1.39 (1.11, 1.67)	Sable, 1992;74% of women with inadequate care had not wanted the pregnancy

Continued

TABLE D-1 Continued

Definition of Intention	Population/ Sample	Retrospective/ Prospective	Control Factors	Results	Reference/ Comments
Initial attitude: negative, mixed, or positive	200 poor, mainly black women, Detroit, MI	Retrospective (at delivery)	Attitudinal	Zero-order correlation = 0.39 (p <0.05)	Poland et al., 1990
Planned vs. unplanned; somewhat/very unhappy vs. neutral/happy	Case–control, 400 inadequate care,100 adequate care,Mecklenburg, NC, 1990– 991	Retrospective (at delivery)	None	For unplanned, OR = 1.86 (1.10,3.18)[c] for unhappy, OR = 2.2 (0.96,3.70)[c]	Boggs and Miles, 1991; among cases with inadequate care, 81% unplanned and 21.2% unhappy
(a) Mistimed, (b) unwanted	Oklahoma PRAMS, 1988–1993 (a) N = 2,092 (b) N = 810	Retrospective (4–12 mo postpartum)	Education, marital status, source of family income, timing of pregnancy initiation, parity	(a) crude OR = 2.7 (1.9,3. 7); adjusted OR = 1.3 (0.8,1.9) (b) crude OR = 5.5 (3.8,8.0); adjusted OR = 1.9 (1.2,3.1)	DePersio et al., 1994

NOTE: NSFG (National Survey of Family Growth); NNS (National Natality Survey); NLSY (National Longitudinal Survey of Youth); NMIHS (National Maternal and Infant Health Survey); PRAMS (Pregnancy Risk Assessment Monitoring System); NS (not significant).
[a]The OR (odds ratio) is the odds of adverse outcome among exposed persons relative to the odds among unexposed persons.
[b]The RR (relative risk) is the risk of the adverse outcome among exposed persons relative to the risk among unexposed persons. Relative risk and odds ratios are similar when adverse outcome is rare.
[c]Calculated for this report.

TABLE D-2 Studies of Behavioral Risk Factors for Low Birthweight or Preterm Delivery Associated with Pregnancy Intention

Definition of Intention	Population/Sample	Retrospective/ Prospective	Control Factors	Results	Reference/ Comments
			Smoking		
"Intended" vs. "unintended"	NNS, 1980 (random sample of U.S. married women)	Retrospective (>6 mo postpartum)	Race, residence, education, birth order, early PNC	Whether didn't stop smoking: crude OR[a] = 1.13[c]; adjusted OR = 1.07[c]	Wells et al., 1987; early PNC had similar but independent impact on smoking cessation, as planning the pregnancy did
Planned vs. unplanned	416, central Harlem residents in PNC, 1982–1983	Retrospective (at first PNC visit)	None	OR = 1.08[c]	McCormick et al., 1987; 41% smoked during pregnancy
(a) Mistimed, (b) unwanted	NSFG, 1982 (random sample of U.S. women ages 15–44, with live births 1979–1982)	Retrospective (≤3 yr postpartum)	Race	(a) RR[b], all = 1.3[c] RR, white = 1.25[c] RR, black = 1.05[c] (b) RR, all = 1.3[c] RR, white = 1.4[c] RR, black = 1.2[c]	Pamuk and Mosher, 1988

Continued

TABLE D-2 Continued

Definition of Intention	Population/ Sample	Retrospective/ Prospective	Control Factors	Results	Reference/ Comments
"Intended" vs. "unintended"	Random sample, 1,490; births in England, 1,984	retrospective (≥4 mo postpartum)	Social class	Smoking OR = 1.66 (1.25,2.22)[c]	Cartwright, 1988; interview asked pregnancy intention
Intended (stopped using contraception because of pregnancy desire or just before pregnancy, wanted to become pregnant) vs. unintended	NLSY, 1984, women 18–26, nationally representative sample of 6,015	Retrospective (78%) and prospective (22% during pregnancy)	Race, economically disadvantaged (white), southern or urban resident at age 14, grandmother's education, maternal age	For unintended, crude RR = 1.04[c]; adjusted OR = 0.97[c]	Marsiglio and Mott, 1988; they used the term "wanted" but the questions more closely reflect intended
(a) Mistimed, (b) unwanted	NMIHS, 1988, nationally representative sample of 9,953	Retrospective (at least 1 yr postpartum)	Marital status	(a) Crude RR = 1.71[c] (b) crude RR = 1.47[c]	Kost et al., 1994; smoked during pregnancy; married women with wanted conception smoked much less than other subgroups

(a) Mistimed, (b) unwanted	Oklahoma PRAMS, 1988–1993 (a) N = 2,267 (b) N = 900	Retrospective (4–12 mo postpartum)	Age, education, race, martial status, source of family income	(a) Crude OR = 1.3 (1.02, 1.6); adjusted OR = 1.0 (0.8,1.3) (b) crude OR = 2.4 (1.9, 3.1); adjusted OR = 1.8 (1.3,2.4)	DePersio et al., 1994; smoking 3 mo before delivery
			Alcohol		
Planned vs. unplanned	416, central Harlem residents in PNC, 1982–1983	Retrospective (at first PNC visit)	None	OR = 2.67[c]	McCormick et al., 1987; 9.2% drank during pregnancy

Continued

TABLE D-2 Continued

Definition of Intention	Population/ Sample	Retrospective/ Prospective	Control Factors	Results	Reference/ Comments
Intended (stopped using contraception because of pregnancy desire or just before pregnancy, wanted to become pregnant) vs. unintended	NLSY, 1984, women aged 18-26, nationally representative sample of 6,015	Retrospective (78%), prospective (22% during pregnancy)	Race, economically disadvantaged (white), southern or urban residents at age 14, grandmother's education, maternal age	For unintended, crude RR = 1.05[c]; adjusted OR = 1.25[c]	Marsiglio and Mott, 1988; they used the term "wanted," but the questions more closely reflect intended
(a) Mistimed, (b) unwanted	NMIHS, 1988, nationally representative sample of 9,953	Retrospective (at least 1 yr postpartum)	None	(a) RR = 1.11[c] (b) RR = 1.77[c]	Kost et al., 1994; drank one or more times per week

NOTE: NNS (National Natality Survey); NSFG (National Survey of Family Growth); NLSY (National Longitudinal Survey of Youth); PRAMS (Pregnancy Risk Assessment Monitoring System); NMIHS (National Maternal and Infant Health Survey).

[a]The OR (odds ratio) is the odds of adverse outcome among exposed persons relative to the odds among unexposed persons.

[b]The RR (relative risk) is the risk of the adverse outcome among exposed persons relative to the risk among unexposed persons. Relative risk and odds ratios are similar when adverse outcome is rare.

[c]Calculated for this report.

TABLE D-3 Studies of Low Birth Weight (LBW) (<2,500 grams) Associated with Pregnancy Intention

Definition of Intention	Population/Sample	Retrospective/ Prospective	Control Factors	Results	Reference/ Comments
Wanted vs. unwanted	17 selected U.S. sites, 1971–1972; 4,891 white and 3,030 black women	Retrospective (at delivery)	Race	Crude OR[a] = 1.2[c] OR for whites = 1.36[c] OR for blacks = 0.94[c]	Morris et al., 1973; women with high education and unwanted conceptions had babies with significantly higher LBW rates
Intended (stopped using contraception because of pregnancy desire or just before pregnancy, wanted to become pregnant) vs. unintended	NLSY, 1984, women ages 18–26, nationally representative sample of 6,015	Retrospective (78%) and prospective (22% during pregnancy)	Race, economically disadvantaged (white), southern or urban resident at age 14, grandmother's education, maternal age	For unintended, crude RR[b] = 1.3[c]; adjusted OR = 0.92[c] adjusted OR = 0.88[c] (including behavioral risk factors)	Marsiglio and Mott, 1988
(a) Mistimed, (b) unwanted	NSFG, 1982 (random sample of U.S. women aged 15–44, with live births 1979–1982)	Retrospective ($\leq$3 yr postpartum)	Race	(a) RR, all = 1.4[c] RR, white = 1.2[c] RR, black = 1.3[c]	Pamuk and Mosher, 1988

Continued

TABLE D-3 Continued

Definition of Intention	Population/ Sample	Retrospective/ Prospective	Control Factors	Results	Reference/ Comments
Unintended vs. intended	Case–control study, 1984; 83 LBW cases, 1,392 NBW controls	Retrospective (at delivery)	Smoking	Crude OR = 1.28[c] adjusted OR = 1.17[c] (0.70,1.95)[c]	Cartwright, 1988
Wanted vs. unwanted	1,518 multiparous, indigent women in Birmingham, AL, 1985–1988, with risk of IUGR	Prospective (at PNC visit)	None	OR = 1.3[c]	Goldenberg et al., 1991; sample was limited to women receiving early PNC
Mistimed, unwanted	1988 NSFG, most recent singleton birth	Retrospective (<5 yr postpartum)	Smoking, race	Reduction in LBW if all unwanted conceptions had been avoided No. / % change Black 69,000 7 White 67,000 4 Smoker 70,000 6 Non-smoker 66,000 7	Kendrick et al., 1990; mistimed not associated with LBW
(a) Mistimed, (b) unwanted	NMIHS, 1988, nationally representative sample of 9,953	Retrospective (at least 1 yr postpartum)	None	(a) Crude RR = 1.21[c] (b) crude RR = 1.80[c]	Kost et al., 1994

(a) Mistimed, (b) unwanted	Oklahoma PRAMS, 1988–1993 (a) $N = 2,215$ (b) $N = 888$	Retrospective (4–12 mo postpartum)	Education, black race, marital status at delivery, smoking three months before delivery, trimester that PNC began, infant gender, parity, plurality	(a) Crude OR = 1.2 (1.1,1.4); adjusted OR = 1.0 (0.8,1.1) (b) crude OR = 1.4 (1.2,1.6); adjusted OR = 0.9 (0.7,1.1)	DePersio et al., 1994
(a) Mistimed, (b) unwanted	1990 NICHD/MOMIH survey	Retrospective (>6 mo postpartum)	Multiple	(a) No increased risk (b) crude OR = 1.44 for LBW adjusted or NS VLBW not associated	Sable, 1992

NOTE: NLSY (National Longitudinal Survey of Youth); NBW (Normal birthweight is over 2,500 grams); IUGR (intrauterine growth retardation); NSFG (National Survey of Family Growth); NMIHS (National Maternal and Infant Health Survey); PRAMS (Pregnancy Risk Assessment Monitoring System); NICHD/MOMIH (National Institute of Child Health and Development/Missouri Mothers and Infant Health); VLBW (very low birthweight is under 1,500 grams)

[a]The OR (odds ratio) is the odds of adverse outcome among exposed persons relative to the odds among unexposed persons.

[b]The RR (relative risk) is the risk of the adverse outcome among exposed persons relative to the risk among unexposed persons. Relative risk and odds ratios are similar when adverse outcome is rare.

[c]Calculated for this report.

E

Technical Notes on the Recalculation Exercise: Supplement to Chapter 3

Larry Bumpass
Member, Committee on Unintended Pregnancy

How much change in children's family contexts could potentially be achieved if there were no childbearing derived from unintended pregnancy? Unwanted and mistimed pregnancies figure differently in this estimation. Births unwanted at conception* would, by definition, simply not occur, whereas births that were mistimed at conception would occur later—some to parents who are married and some to parents who are unmarried.

BIRTHS UNWANTED AT CONCEPTION

Births that are unwanted at conception are those that occur to women who say, prior to pregnancy, that they did not want to have any more children. The avoidance of such births would have a surprisingly large effect on the proportion of children born to unmarried mothers. It is little appreciated how large a proportion of childbearing among unmarried women is to women of higher parity, to women over age 25, and to women who want no more children.

It is necessary to adjust for some possible misreporting of mistimed births as unwanted births. Although the estimation of "unwantedness" is quite good in the aggregate, this is a category of births for which misclassification seems to

*In this appendix only, births resulting from unwanted pregnancies are referred to as unwanted births, and births resulting from mistimed pregnancies are referred to as mistimed births.

result in some bias. For example, it seems unlikely that many women who had their first child when unmarried and at a young age and who reported a birth as unwanted actually intended to remain childless in the future. In this exercise, first births to women under age 25 that were reported as unwanted at conception were recoded as mistimed. Although the resulting difference in estimated reduction of unwanted births is small (approximately 2 percent), it seems the most appropriate way to proceed.

For this exercise, it is necessary to begin with estimates based on births in 1986–1988, the most recent years for which there is complete information from the National Survey of Family Growth (NSFG). With these data and the above procedures, it is estimated that 28 percent of all births in 1986–1988 were either unwanted births (10.6 percent) or wanted births to unmarried women (17.6 percent). When the unwanted births are removed from the denominator (as would be the case in the absence of childbearing derived from unwanted pregnancy), 19.9 percent of the wanted births are to unmarried women. Hence, the avoidance of unwanted births in 1986–1988 would have resulted in a reduction in the percentage of all births that were either unwanted or to an unmarried mother, from 28 to 20 percent.

One further step is necessary, however, given the continued increase in the proportion of births that are to unmarried women. About one-quarter of all births in the 1986–1988 period were to unmarried women and the proportion is at present more likely one-third. In the recalculation, the relationships observed in the 1986–1988 data are applied to the current level, although this is a somewhat conservative procedure since levels of unwanted fertility also appear to have increased since that time. Under these assumptions, it is estimated that currently 27.2 percent of all births are wanted births to unmarried women, and (again) 10.6 percent are unwanted births. Removing unwanted births from both the numerator and the denominator implies a change from 38 to 30 percent of all births being either unwanted births or wanted births to unmarried women.

BIRTHS MISTIMED AT CONCEPTION

Births that are mistimed are those births that were wanted at some time in the future but that occurred sooner than they were wanted as a result of contraceptive misuse, nonuse, or failure. The effect of mistimed fertility cannot be properly estimated by simply observing the distribution of births intended at conception, since this would incorrectly reallocate births away from groups with higher proportions of unintended births, such as women with less education. For this reason, a logit regression is used in the recalculation to estimate the potential reduction from the elimination of mistimed fertility, since this procedure allows the distribution of births on other variables to be kept constant. Whether wanted births occurred outside of marriage (for births occurring 1986–1988 as reported in the NSFG) was predicted in a logit equation that included the mother's race, education, and parity, as well as whether the birth resulted from an unintended pregnancy. The resulting coefficients were then used to estimate the proportion of wanted births that occurred outside of marriage, first with all variables set at their observed means and then with all other variables set at their means and the "unintended" variable set to zero. The first simulation closely replicates the observed proportion of births to unmarried women; the second simulation is 24 percent lower than the observed proportion of births to unmarried women. Hence, this analysis implies that, in addition to the reduction in the number of children born to unmarried women through the avoidance of unwanted births noted above, about a quarter of the wanted births that occurred to unmarried women would be delayed until after marriage. This would reduce the proportion of births estimated to be wanted births to unmarried women from 27.2 to 20.7 percent of births.

In sum, then, instead of the likely current level of 38 percent of all births that are either unwanted births (10.6 percent) or are wanted births to unmarried women (27.2 percent), the avoidance of unintended fertility could potentially reduce this proportion to the 21 percent that are intended births to unmarried mothers—a 45 percent reduction overall. Of course, the complete elimination of unintended fertility is an unrealistic goal, but the experience of other countries makes it likely that a serious effort could move the United States substantially in that direction—with proportional improvements in the well-being of future generations.

F

Summaries of Evaluated Programs: Supplement to Chapter 8

Dana Hotra
Staff, Committee on Unintended Pregnancy

This appendix presents detailed information on the 23 programs profiled in Chapter 8.

COMMUNITY OF CARING

Summary: Several sites around the country providing prenatal care for pregnant adolescents, with an emphasis on planning for future goals, including prevention of repeated pregnancy.

Program: The Community of Caring program operated at 16 sites nationwide and targeted pregnant and parenting adolescents between the ages of 13 and 19. It was designed to help the teenager to have a healthy pregnancy, learn how to care for the baby, complete her education, and/or become employed. The program highlighted five themes (family, personal responsibility, sexual maturity and commitment, planning for future goals, and commitment to parenthood), although each site implemented the curriculum slightly differently.

Evaluation: Two of the sites were evaluated between 1985 and 1988: a hospital-based program in Boston, MA and a community-based program in Las Cruces, NM. Participants were not randomly assigned; instead, a quasi-experimental design was developed in which individuals with similar background demographics made up the comparison group. This design was complicated when some young women in the comparison group switched to the intervention group. The researchers designated three groups at each site: high treatment, low treatment, and a comparison group. A baseline pretest was given, as was a posttest following delivery. A third survey was administered at 1 year posttest (79 percent response rate). The two sites had different results at the 1-year follow-up. At the Las Cruces site, contraceptive knowledge had increased among the high-treatment group, but there was no significant difference in sexual behavior. At the Boston site, the low-treatment group scored consistently lower in knowledge, attitudes, and behavior than either the high treatment or comparison groups. The high-treatment group showed no statistically significant differences in behavior from the comparison group.

Primary Reference:

Miller BC, Dyk PH. Community of Caring effects on adolescent mothers: A program evaluation case study. Fam Relat. 1991;40:386–395.

CONDOM MAILING PROGRAM

Summary: Direct mail program for adolescent men designed to increase their knowledge about and access to condoms.

Program: The Condom Mailing Program was a direct mail program initiated in 1987 that was designed to increase knowledge about condoms through an informational packet called *The Man's World* and to increase access to contraception through an order form for free condoms. The target population was low-income adolescent men aged 16–17. The actual population reached was primarily middle-income rather than low-income men.

Evaluation: The experimental design was developed by randomly dividing a list of names purchased from a list broker into an intervention group (n = 985) and a control group (n = 1,033). The direct mail packet was sent to the intervention group. Both groups were interviewed by telephone 5 weeks after the mailing to elicit information on their knowledge, attitudes, and behavior. The researchers reached 86 percent of the sample by telephone. The experiment was double-blind, in that the interviewer did not know which group the respondent was in, nor did the respondent probably realize that he was part of an experiment. At follow-up, 72 percent of the intervention group recalled receiving the materials; 91 percent of that group read the pamphlet, 36 percent discussed the pamphlet with their parents, and 44 percent discussed it with their friends. As compared to the control group, men in the intervention group were more likely to be knowledgeable about contraception, sexually transmitted diseases, and pregnancy, although there were no differences in use of contraception. Receiving the materials and order form did not have a significant effect on whether the respondent had ever had intercourse, but those respondents who had read the materials reported fewer acts of intercourse ($p < 0.05$). Also, 9 percent of those men who had read the pamphlet ordered the free condoms, a response rate much higher than typical direct mail response rates.

Primary Reference:

Kirby D, Harvey PD, Claussenius D, Novar M. A direct mailing to teenage males about condom use: Its impact on knowledge, attitudes and sexual behavior. Fam Plann Perspect. 1989;21:12–18.

ELMIRA NURSE HOME VISITING PROGRAM

Summary: Comprehensive program of prenatal and postpartum infancy nurse home visitation for low-income women bearing their first child.

Program: Located in New York State during the early 1980s, this was a comprehensive program of prenatal and postpartum nurse home visitation for socially disadvantaged white women (47 percent of whom were adolescents) bearing their first child. Registered nurses who had participated in a 3-month training program helped women improve their prenatal health-related behaviors and infant caregiving skills, and encouraged the women to clarify their future plans. The advantages of various types of contraception were discussed with the women and their partners. Nurses visited one group of pregnant women in their homes during the pregnancy and another group during the pregnancy and through the following 2 years. Program objectives included encouraging the women to complete their education, identify vocational interests, and increase their interpregnancy interval.

Evaluation: An evaluation was conducted with an experimental design. The researchers followed women in the two intervention groups and a control group for 4 years following the birth of their first child. (The results reported here contrast the women who were nurse-visited during pregnancy and infancy with women who were not nurse-visited at all.) During the first 22 months after delivery, low-income unmarried women visited during pregnancy and infancy ($n = 72$) had 33 percent fewer subsequent pregnancies than did their counterparts in the control group ($n = 124$). By 48 months postpartum, these women experienced 43 percent fewer subsequent pregnancies, and they postponed the birth of a second child an average of 12 months longer than did women in the control group. Among women in the intervention groups there was an 83 percent increase in the number of months that women participated in the workforce. The researchers argue that the reduction in subsequent pregnancy enabled the nurse-visited women to participate in the workforce to a greater extent than their counterparts in the control group. Moreover, the intervention also reduced the rates of child maltreatment by 80 percent (19 percent in the comparison group compared with 4 percent in the nurse-visited group) among low-income, unmarried adolescents during the first 2 years postpartum. Although the program was designed to directly improve qualities of infant caregiving and reduce child abuse and neglect, the researchers attribute part of the positive effect of the program to the reduction in subsequent pregnancies, many of which would probably have been unintended.

Primary References:

Olds D, Henderson C, Tatelbaum R, Chamberlin R. Preventing child abuse and neglect: A randomized trial of nurse home visitation. Pediatrics. 1986;78: 65–78.

Olds DL, Henderson CR, Phelps C, Kitzman H, Hanks C. Effects of prenatal and infancy nurse home visitation on government spending. Med Care. 1993;31:155–174.

Olds DL, Henderson CR, Tatelbaum R, Chamberlin R. Improving the life-course development of socially disadvantaged mothers: A randomized trial of nurse home visitation. Am J Public Health. 1988;78:1436–1455.

FACTS AND FEELINGS

Summary: Home-based abstinence program using sex education videotapes to encourage discussion between parents and early adolescents about sexual issues.

Program: In the mid-1980s, families of seventh and eighth grade adolescents in northern Utah were asked to participate in a home-based program in which they received a series of sex education videotapes called "Facts and Feelings." The objective of the program was to encourage discussion about sexual issues between the parents and the adolescent, and the long-term goal was to reduce early adolescent sexual behavior. The videotape did not include contraceptive information. This program was initiated in several communities in Utah among young adolescents who were not likely to have already initiated sexual intercourse.

Evaluation: Using an experimental design, 548 families were randomly assigned to receive either the videotapes and a newsletter, the videotapes alone, or no videotapes or newsletter. A pretest, posttest, and delayed posttest (at 1 year) were administered by program staff in the home. The questionnaire focused on parent–child communication, knowledge, values, and sexual activity. Although intervention groups did experience significantly increased communication between parents and adolescents, similar rates of adolescent sexual activity (3 to 5 percent had begun having intercourse) were found across the three groups at 1-year follow-up.

Primary Reference:

Miller BC, Norton MC, Jenson GO, Lee TR, Christopherson C, King PK. Impact evaluation of Facts and Feelings: A home-based video sex education curriculum. Fam Relat. 1993;42:392–400.

GIRLS INCORPORATED PREVENTING ADOLESCENT PREGNANCY

Summary: Nationwide sexuality education program divided into four age-appropriate components.

Program: Preventing Adolescent Pregnancy is a sexuality education program developed in the 1980s by Girls Incorporated, a national organization serving girls and young women. The program is divided into four age-appropriate components. The first component, Growing Together, focuses on parent–daughter communication for young girls and encourages delaying sexual initiation. The second component, Will Power/Won't Power, targets 12- to 14-year-olds, using a series of fun, skill-building exercises focused on assertiveness training, again encouraging postponement of sexual intercourse. Taking Care of Business, the third component, uses the life options model to target adolescents ages 15–17 and focuses both on the delay of sexual intercourse and on contraceptive use. The fourth component, Health Bridge, is patterned on the school-linked health clinic model, including access to reproductive health services and contraceptives. Some young women participated in more than one program component, and the Will Power/Won't Power component had the highest enrollment.

Evaluation: Two evaluations are summarized here: one evaluates Growing Together and Will Power/Won't Power together; the other compares the impact of participating in one or more program components with no program participation.

Growing Together and Will Power/Won't Power were evaluated by using a quasi-experimental design. The sample consisted of girls ages 12 to 14 who had participated in the programs for at least 1 year and had never had sexual intercourse ($n = 295$). The control group consisted of eligible girls who did not enroll in either program ($n = 117$). Background characteristics of the Growing

Together group differed from the background characteristics of the control group in that on the basis of sociodemographic characteristics, intervention participants appeared to be less likely than control participants to have begun having sexual intercourse. Background characteristics of Will Power/Won't Power participants appeared similar to those of the control group. Evaluation results indicated that significantly fewer Growing Together participants began sexual intercourse during the follow-up period. There was no difference in rates of initiation of sexual intercourse among Will Power/Won't Power participants and controls. Additional analysis suggests that those girls who participated in Will Power/Won't Power for a longer period were significantly less likely to initiate sexual intercourse than were those who participated for a shorter period or those in the control group.

Another evaluation used a quasi-experimental design to establish three groups: adolescents who had participated in two or more components, adolescents who had participated in only one component, and the control group. As in the other evaluation, members of the control group were young women eligible for the program but who did not enroll. The intervention group totaled 237, and the control group totaled 106. Demographic characteristics were similar for the three groups. Evaluation results were mixed. For example, adolescents who participated in one program component were more likely to have had sexual intercourse without contraception than were adolescents who had participated in two or more components or in no components (i.e., the control group). There was no difference in the rate of unprotected intercourse between participants in two or more components and adolescents in the control group. Young women who participated in one or more program components were less likely to report becoming pregnant than those in the control group. This finding was marginally significant.

Primary References:

Girls Incorporated. Truth, trust and technology: New research on preventing adolescent pregnancy. Indianapolis, IN; Girls Incorporated; October 1991.

Nicholson HJ, Postrado LT. A comprehensive age-phased approach: Girls Incorporated. In Preventing Adolescent Pregnancy: Model Programs and Evaluations. Miller BC, Card JJ, Paikoff RL, Peterson JL, eds. Newbury Park, CA: Sage Publications; 1992.

Postrado LT, Nicholson HJ. Effectiveness in delaying the initiation of sexual intercourse of girls aged 12–14: Two components of the Girls Incorporated Preventing Adolescent Pregnancy Program. Youth Soc. 1992;23:356–379.

GROUP COGNITIVE BEHAVIOR CURRICULUM

Summary: School-based sexuality curriculum using group cognitive behavior theory to personalize accurate information about sexuality and contraception.

Program: This curriculum used group cognitive behavior theory to implement an adolescent pregnancy prevention program in 1979. Trained college staff helped adolescents to personalize and act on accurate information about sexuality and contraception. The program used a four-step process: (1) accurate information about reproductive health, contraceptive methods, and sexuality in adolescent development was made available; (2) program staff ensured that information had been accurately perceived by using small groups to test and reinforce students' knowledge; (3) information was personalized so that the transition was made from knowledge to decision-making; and (4) behavioral skills necessary to implement decisions made on the basis of the new information were practiced.

Evaluation: Using a small sample size of 36 students, the researchers made random assignments to intervention and control groups. The intervention group received the program outlined above. Questionnaires were completed at baseline, immediately postintervention and 6 months postintervention. At the 6-month follow-up, intervention group participants were practicing more effective contraception than controls. A second evaluation with a larger sample size (N = 107) did not show any significant difference between the intervention and control groups, although intervention group participants were better able to raise and discuss contraceptive issues.

Primary References:

Gilchrist LD, Schinke SP. Coping with contraception: Cognitive and behavioral methods with adolescents. Cognit Ther Res. 1983;7:379–388.

Schinke SP, Blythe BJ, Gilchrist LD. Cognitive-behavioral prevention of adolescent pregnancy. J Couns Psychol. 1981;28:451–454.

Schinke SP, Gilchrist LD, Small RW. Preventing unwanted adolescent pregnancy: A cognitive-behavioral approach. Amer J Orthopsychiatry. 1979; 49:81–88.

McCABE CENTER

Summary: Alternative public school for pregnant students providing prenatal and postnatal education, with an emphasis on delaying rapid repeat pregnancy.

Program: The Polly T. McCabe Center in New Haven, CT, was an alternative public school for pregnant students, one objective of which was to delay subsequent childbearing. The center stressed intensive, health-focused prenatal and postnatal education by nurse practitioners and counseling services for pregnant and recently delivering adolescents. The program provided case management by nurses and social workers for up to 4 months after delivery. Such care included follow-up counseling about contraceptive choices made at the hospital in order to be confident that the young mothers felt comfortable with their contraceptive choices and knew how to use their methods most effectively. Approximately 120 young women were served each year in the 1980s.

Evaluation: The demonstration project was evaluated by examining the 1979–1980 birth cohort using a quasi-experimental, longitudinal design. The evaluation did not compare pregnant adolescents who attended the school with those who did not, but compared adolescents who spent different lengths of time at the school. Students who were permitted to remain at the school for more than 7 weeks postpartum were compared with those who returned more quickly to their regular school (this was due to administrative procedures and was not by the student's choice, and essentially randomized the students). A total of 102 women participated in the 18-month follow-up, and 99 participated in the 5-year follow-up. Students who were permitted to remain at the school for more than 7 weeks postpartum were significantly less likely to have another child within 2 years ($p < 0.005$) and within 5 years ($p < 0.015$). The researchers note that "the most surprising finding in this study was that relatively brief postnatal intervention with new adolescent mothers significantly reduced their likelihood of subsequent childbearing over the next five years." They suggest that the critical period is the second month following the birth of the child, in that this typically marks the end of the postnatal recovery period and sexual activity often then resumes.

Primary References:

O'Sullivan A, Jacobson B. A randomized trial of a health care program for first-time adolescent mothers and their infants. Nurs Res. 1992;41:210–215.

Seitz V, Apfel N. Effects of a school for pregnant students on the incidence of low-birthweight deliveries. Child Develop. 1994;65:666–676.

Seitz V, Apfel NH. Adolescent mothers and repeated childbearing: Effects of a school-based intervention program. Amer J Orthopsychiatry. 1993;63:572–581.

NEW CHANCE

Summary: National demonstration program offering comprehensive services for low-income parenting adolescents and young adults.

Program: New Chance was a national demonstration program that tested a model offering young parents intensive and comprehensive services including education, training, personal development counseling, parenting support, and case management. Intended to improve the employment prospects of participants, to improve their parenting skills, and to enhance the development of their children, it also sought to delay repeat pregnancies. Those eligible to participate were mothers ages 16–22 who were high school dropouts, received Aid to Families with Dependent Children (AFDC), and gave birth to their first child before age 20. The demonstration project began in 1989 and ended in 1992. The model was put in place in 16 local sites, of which 12 are still in existence; sites operated on a small scale to create a warm and supportive environment. The intervention was divided into two phases. Phase I focused on education, career exploration and pre-employment skills, parenting, life skills, and family planning (including arranging visits to family planning providers), and phase II centered on skills training, work experience, and job placement assistance.

Evaluation: The evaluation involved the random assignment of young women meeting the eligibility criteria either to an intervention group, whose members were eligible to received the treatment described above, or to a control group, whose members could not participate in New Chance, but could have received other services available in their communities. An evaluation (published in 1994) was based on follow-up interviews with 2,088 members of both groups conducted 18 months after random assignment; a subsequent round of follow-up is being conducted at 42 months after random assignment. At the 18-month point, comparable rates of repeat childbearing were found in both intervention and control groups (approximately 25 percent). Participants in the intervention group reported a higher rate of pregnancy (57 versus 53 percent) as well as a higher rate of abortion (15 versus 11 percent).

Primary References:

Manpower Demonstration Research Corporation. New Chance: A New Initiative for Adolescent Mothers and Their Children. New York, NY: Manpower Demonstration Research Corporation; April 1993.

Quint J, Musick J, Ladner J. Lives of Promise, Lives of Pain. New York, NY: Manpower Demonstration Research Corporation; January 1994.

Quint JC, Fink BL, Rowser SL. Implementing a Comprehensive Program for Disadvantaged Young Mothers and Their Children. New York, NY: Manpower Demonstration Research Corporation; December 1991.

Quint JC, Polit DF, Bos H, Cave G. New Chance: Interim Findings on a Comprehensive Program for Disadvantaged Young Mothers and Their Children. New York, NY: Manpower Demonstration Research Corporation; September 1994.

THE OUNCE OF PREVENTION FUND'S PARENTS TOO SOON PROGRAM

Summary: Statewide program for pregnant and parenting adolescents using home visiting and parent groups.

Program: The Ounce of Prevention Fund's Parents Too Soon Program is a state-wide network of 27 community programs for pregnant and parenting adolescents to encourage young women to complete their education, increase their employability, improve their parenting skills, and reduce their rates of repeat childbearing. The programs serve adolescents for 2 years and provide different types of support according to individual needs. The two primary services are home visiting (to reduce isolation) and parent groups (a peer-support model). These programs are currently ongoing, and are supported by the Illinois Department of Children and Family Services.

Evaluation: A sample of 1,004 young women who entered the program between June 1985 and July 1987 was compared with a sample (n = 790) from the National Longitudinal Survey of Youth (NLSY). Program participants who were under age 20 at program entry and had participated in the program for at least 12 months were matched with a sample of NLSY women who were also adolescent parents. The baseline point was considered to be date of program entry for the Parents Too Soon participants and date of birth of the first child for the NLSY comparison group. Follow-up data were measured at 12 months post–baseline for both groups. When age at first birth, ethnic background, living arrangements, level of education, school enrollment, and employment status at baseline were controlled, participants in the NLSY comparison group were 1.4 times more likely to experience a subsequent pregnancy than the intervention group. Although the use of national data is an innovative way to address the problem of identifying a comparison group, there was a serious inadequacy in using the NLSY group because the NLSY survey had not always asked about subsequent pregnancies. Therefore, the number of subsequent pregnancies was determined by noting subsequent births, leaving a wide margin for undercounting of subsequent pregnancies in the NLSY group.

Primary Reference:

Ruch-Ross HS, Jones ED, Musick JS. Comparing outcomes in a statewide program for adolescent mothers with outcomes in a national sample. Fam Plann Perspect. 1992;24:66–71, 96.

POSTPONING SEXUAL INVOLVEMENT

Summary: School-based curriculum encouraging middle school students to delay initiation of sexual intercourse in combination with a human sexuality and contraception component.

Program: Postponing Sexual Involvement: An Education Series for Young Teens began in 1983 as one of two components of a hospital-based outreach program. It is given in combination with a component on Human Sexuality that provides students with basic health and reproductive information, including contraceptive use. The Postponing Sexual Involvement component was developed in response to an early evaluation of the human sexuality component, which indicated that this unit alone was not effective in reducing the rate of sexual activity or adolescent pregnancy. Based on the social influence model, Postponing Sexual Involvement uses older adolescent leaders to teach young adolescents to practice specific attitudes and skills related to decision-making about their sexual behavior. The Postponing Sexual Involvement component emphasizes that abstinence is the best choice for young adolescents. The Postponing Sexual Involvement Educational Series is being used in multiple sites throughout the United States, Canada, and England. The Human Sexuality component is used elsewhere but not as widely.

Evaluation: A quasi-experimental design was used to evaluate the program. The intervention group consisted of low-income eighth-grade students from one school district, and the control group consisted of low-income students from three adjacent school districts who did not participate in the experimental program ($N = 536$). Data were collected by telephone interviews at baseline and postintervention, at the end of the eighth grade. Longer-term follow-up data were collected by telephone interviews at the end of the ninth and twelfth grades. The following findings in the intervention group were significant at the $p < 0.05$ level: less initiation of intercourse at postintervention and at the end of ninth grade follow-up; less frequency of intercourse among those who were sexually inexperienced at pretest but initiated sex by the end of ninth-grade follow-up; more contraceptive use among those who were sexually inexperienced at pretest but initiated sex by end of ninth-grade follow-up. The significance of the intervention was most apparent at the end of eighth-grade posttest and the end of ninth-grade follow-up; by the twelfth-grade follow-up, the difference between groups was not significant. The combined two-component program demonstrates, among other things, that the two messages—abstinence and use of contraception—are not incompatible.

Primary References:

Howard M, McCabe JB. An information and skills approach for younger teens. In Preventing Adolescent Pregnancy: Model Programs and Evaluations. Miller BC, Card JJ, Paikoff RL, Peterson JL, eds. Newbury Park, CA: Sage Publications; 1992.

Howard M, McCabe JB. Helping teenagers postpone sexual involvement. Fam Plann Perspect. 1990;22:21–26.

PROJECT REDIRECTION

Summary: Comprehensive demonstration program targeting pregnant and parenting adolescents age 17 or younger, including an employment-orientation component.

Program: Project Redirection was a comprehensive demonstration program targeting pregnant and parenting adolescent girls age 17 or younger. This was the first major demonstration to include employment issues in a model for school-age women. The adolescents were supported by community women acting as mentors, peer groups, and the development of individualized participant plans. Four sites were maintained in New York, Boston, Phoenix, and Riverside, CA. The program served 805 young women between 1980 and 1982, and the average enrollment was 1 year. Program objectives included continuation of education, delay of subsequent pregnancies, acquisition of employability and job skills, improved maternal and child health, and acquisition of life management skills.

Evaluation: The evaluation used a comparison site design. The intervention group included 305 young women, and the comparison group (n = 370) was developed from those adolescents who met the program eligibility criteria but lived in communities that did not offer the program. Nevertheless, many types of services were available in these other communitites , and young women in the comparison group were likely to have received some types of support. Thus, the evaluation became a comparison of Project Redirection with other types of services. Interviews were done at baseline, and at 1, 2, and (for a subgroup of adolescents) 5 years after the program. One-year evaluation results indicated that young women in the intervention group were significantly less likely to have a repeat pregnancy ($p < 0.01$), but 5-year evaluation results indicated that although the intervention group had the same number of pregnancies as the comparison group, they had fewer abortions and thus more births (the difference between the groups was significant at $p < 0.01$). The intervention group also had improved employment outcomes and greater self-sufficiency, and their children were better off than the children of the comparison group on a number of cognitive, social, and emotional indicators.

Primary References:

Polit DF. Effects of a comprehensive program for teenage parents: Five years after Project Redirection. Fam Plann Perspect. 1989;21:164–187.

Polit DF, Kahn JR. Project Redirection: Evaluation of a comprehensive program for disadvantaged teenage mothers. Fam Plann Perspect. 1985;17:150–155.

Polit DF, Quint JC, Riccio JA. The Challenge of Serving Teenage Mothers: Lessons from Project Redirection. New York, NY: Manpower Demonstration Research Corporation; October 1988.

PROJECT TAKING CHARGE

Summary: School-based program combining abstinence-only sexuality education and vocational education.

Program: This school-based program combined sexuality education and vocational education, targeting low-income seventh-grade students and their parents at three sites around the country (Wilmington, DE; West Point, MS; and Ironton, OH), during the fall of 1989. The curriculum length was 6 weeks. The program was designed to promote abstinence from sexual activity through promotion of communication between adolescents and their parents and planning for their future lives in the world of work. The curriculum focused on occupational goals and community support, self-development, and parental involvement. Basic sexual anatomy and development were taught, but contraception was not a part of the curriculum. Nearly one-quarter of the students reported that they were sexually active at the pretest.

Evaluation: A quasi-experimental design was used in which control groups were developed from students and parents from the same school as the intervention groups. A total sample of 136 adolescents and 126 parents were involved; however, the sample size at each separate site was small, not allowing for intersite comparisons. Pretest and posttest questionnaires were used for both students and parents at 6 weeks postintervention and again at 6 months postintervention. Results from the 6-week posttest indicated that adolescents in the intervention group were somewhat less likely than the students in the control group to have initiated sexual intercourse, but the difference was not statistically significant. This trend was also seen in the 6-month posttest, but again it was not significant.

Primary References:

Jorgensen SR. Project Taking Charge: An evaluation of an adolescent pregnancy prevention program. Fam Relat. 1991;40:373–380.

Jorgensen SR, Potts V, Camp B. Project Taking Charge: Six-month follow-up of a pregnancy prevention program for early adolescents. Fam Relat. 1993; 42:401–406.

REDUCING THE RISK

Summary: School-based curriculum, based on several interrelated theoretical approaches, encouraging avoidance of unprotected intercourse through abstinence or contraceptive use.

Program: The Reducing the Risk curriculum was based on three interrelated theoretical approaches: social learning theory, social inoculation theory, and cognitive behavior theory. The curriculum explicitly emphasized the idea that adolescents should avoid unprotected intercourse, either through abstinence or by using contraception. The curriculum was taught in such a way as to personalize sexuality, reproductive, and contraceptive information, and students were trained in decisionmaking and assertive communication skills. Personal communication skills were practiced through role-playing as well as real-life situations such as finding and obtaining information about nonprescription contraceptives at local stores and clinics. Adolescents were also encouraged to initiate parent–child discussions. The curriculum was implemented in 13 high schools in urban and rural areas of California during the late 1980s.

Evaluation: A quasi-experimental design was developed in which classrooms of students were designated as either intervention ($n = 586$) or comparison ($n = 447$) groups. Comparison groups received the typical sex education course; thus, students in the Reducing the Risk curriculum were compared with students in a general sex education course, rather than with students receiving no information at all. The students completed questionnaires at baseline, immediately following the program, and at 6 and 18 months postintervention. Results indicated that increases in knowledge were significantly greater among the intervention group ($p < 0.001$) at both 6 and 18 months of follow-up. Significantly fewer intervention students had initiated sexual intercourse by the 18-month follow-up ($p < 0.05$). Among those students who had not initiated sexual intercourse before the program, significantly fewer intervention students practiced unprotected sex at the 18-month follow-up ($p < 0.05$), either by delaying the onset of intercourse or increasing the use of contraceptives. Female students and students who were at lower risk for engaging in risk-taking behavior (based on background characteristics) appeared to be more likely to use contraception ($p < 0.05$), although the sample size for these subgroups was small.

Primary References:

Barth RP, Leland N, Kirby D, Fetro JV. Enhancing social and cognitive skills. In Preventing Adolescent Pregnancy: Model Programs and Evaluations. Miller BC, Card JJ, Paikoff RL, Peterson JL, eds. Newbury Park, CA: Sage Publications; 1992.

Kirby D, Barth RP, Leland N, Fetro JV. Reducing the risk: Impact of a new curriculum on sexual risk-taking. Fam Plann Perspect. 1991;23:253–263.

REPRODUCTIVE HEALTH SCREENING OF MALE ADOLESCENTS

Summary: Hospital-based reproductive health counseling for adolescent boys, aged 15–18.

Program: The Reproductive Health Screening of Male Adolescents program at Northwest Kaiser Permanente was designed to measure the effects of reproductive health counseling on young men (ages 15–18). Nearly 1,200 adolescent men were recruited by phone between June 1985 and November 1986 to participate in the study. Study participants received a 1-hour reproductive health consultation, during which they viewed a slide-tape program (which focused on explicit photographs of and information on reproductive anatomy, fertility, hernia, testicular self-examination, abstinence, contraception, sexually transmitted diseases, couples communication, and access to health services) and met with a health care practitioner to discuss sexuality, fertility goals, reproductive health, interpersonal skills in a sexual context, and contraception.

Evaluation: Subjects were randomly distributed to intervention and control groups ($N = 1{,}200$). All subjects completed a pretest questionnaire. Those in the intervention group received the intervention described above, and the control group received no special information. Knowledge, attitudes, and behavior were tested in a follow-up questionnaire 1 year later. There was little difference in sexual activity between the groups, although sexually inexperienced young men in the intervention group were significantly less likely ($p < 0.01$) to be sexually impatient (i.e., negative feelings about having never engaged in sexual intercourse). Sexually active participants were more likely to be using contraception at follow-up ($p < 0.05$), particularly those who had not been sexually active at the baseline ($p < 0.01$). Those participants who were sexually inexperienced at pretest and who became sexually active in the interim were most likely to use effective contraception. Participants in the intervention were more likely to be protected from unintended pregnancy by their partners' use of oral contraceptives ($p < 0.05$). The researchers hypothesize that the intervention increased knowledge about the safety of oral contraceptives: among those who were sexually active at baseline, participants were significantly more likely to believe that "birth control pills are a very safe method" ($p < 0.05$).

Primary References:

The Center for Health Training. Male involvement in family planning: A bibliography of project descriptions and resources. Seattle, WA: The Center for Health Training; February 1988.

Danielson R, Marcy S, Plunkett A, Wiest W, Greenlick MR. Reproductive health counseling for young men: What does it do? Fam Plann Perspect. 1990;22:115–121.

SCHOOL/COMMUNITY PROGRAM FOR SEXUAL RISK REDUCTION AMONG TEENS

Summary: Community-based program to delay initiation of sexual intercourse and improve use of contraceptives by sexually active adolescents.

Program: Located in western South Carolina, this rural community- and school-based program used a variety of coordinated approaches to reduce high rates of adolescent pregnancy. Its objectives were to promote postponement of sexual intercourse and the use of contraception by adolescents who were sexually active. The educational component included educating teachers, clergy, parents, and community leaders to improve their understanding of human sexuality and adolescent pregnancy and to enhance their skills in helping youth to avoid pregnancy. The program offered public school teachers tuition-free university-level graduate courses that dealt with these issues and that resulted in the development of a sex education curriculum that was integrated into the teachers' various subject areas. Program staff recruited parents and church and community leaders to participate in workshops that addressed these issues. Staff also trained students to serve as peer counselors. In addition, the program conducted a public media campaign to highlight the objectives of the program, its special activities, and achievements. Finally, a school nurse provided contraceptive counseling and services. She counseled students to abstain from sexual intercourse, and to those who did not do so, she provided contraceptive methods. She supplied condoms to male students and took female students to the county family planning clinic. Later, for a short period, contraceptives were provided in a school-based clinic; still later, they stopped being provided in any way at the school. Although the school nurse and school-based clinic were funded by sources different from those that funded the education–media program, the contraceptive services were an integral part of the total intervention.

Evaluation: Two evaluations of this program have been made. The first evaluation used a quasi-experimental design and compared pregnancy rates for women aged 14–17 in the intervention area with adolescent pregnancy rates in a nonintervention portion of the same county as well as in three other demographically similar counties. In the 2 years following the intervention, adolescent pregnancy rates in the intervention area dropped significantly ($p < 0.05$) as compared to the nonintervention areas. A later reanalysis of the data selected comparison areas by matching preprogram adolescent pregnancy rates in addition to socioeconomic variables, and extended the time period during which adolescent pregnancy rates were examined. The reanalysis confirmed that the adolescent pregnancy rate in the intervention area dropped during the early intervention years (1984–1986). However, it found that the rate rose during the later intervention years (1987–1988) to levels that were not significantly different from the preprogram rates. The reanalysis differed from the original evaluation in that it included an examination of the provision of contraceptive counseling and services as part of the total intervention. The authors of the reanalysis suggest that the educational program combined with the provision of contraceptive counseling and services accounted for the initial decrease in adolescent pregnancy rates. They also suggest that the cessation of the contraceptive counseling and services in the school, together with a loss of momentum of the educational program, explained the subsequent rise in adolescent pregnancy rates to preprogram levels.

Primary References:

Koo HP, Dunteman GH, George C, Green Y, Vincent M. Reducing adolescent pregnancy through a school- and community-based intervention: Denmark, South Carolina, revisited. Fam Plann Perspect. 1994;26:206–211, 217.

Vincent ML, Clearie AF, Schluchter MD. Reducing adolescent pregnancy through school and community-based education. JAMA. 1987;257:3382–3386.

SELF CENTER

Summary: Full reproductive health services as well as health education and counseling services provided through a school-linked clinic.

Program: The Self Center program in Baltimore, MD, combined school and clinic operations and provided full reproductive health services as well as health education and counseling services; some of these services were offered through the Self Center clinic, and others through counselors and educators sent in to the school. The pregnancy prevention program began in November 1981, and the clinic opened in January 1982; services were provided through June 1984. The target population included all students in the two local junior and senior high schools in an urban, low-income neighborhood. Most services were offered in a school-linked clinic located close to both schools. Educational and counseling services were provided by health and social work professionals through in-class presentations, small group and individual counseling in schools, formal and informal after-school discussions, peer groups, and group and individual counseling in the clinic. Activities were designed to widen access to information about sexuality and contraception. Contraceptive services and other reproductive health services (such as pregnancy testing and treatment for sexually transmitted diseases) were provided in the clinic and were free of charge.

Evaluation: The program was evaluated using both pretest/posttest and experimental control methodologies that allowed the researchers to assess changes in knowledge, attitudes, and sexual behavior over time. The control groups consisted of students at similar junior and senior high schools that were not associated with the special health clinics. Questionnaires were administered at pretest and annually for 3 years. The analysis was done as a multiwave study, and the sample size ranged from 3,646 students completing baseline questionnaires to 2,950 students completing the final survey 3 years later. Methodological problems unique to a school-based sample, such as no two schools being truly comparable and the use of the entire school as the relevant sample, were addressed. At follow-up, significantly more students in the intervention schools attended a clinic before the initiation of sexual activity; significantly more students in the intervention schools also attended a clinic during the first months of sexual activity. Young men in the intervention junior high school were as likely to attend a clinic as were the young women. A significant delay in the initiation of sexual intercourse for young women in the intervention schools ($p < 0.01$) was noted; the median delay was 7 months. In addition, a significant increase in the use of contraceptives at last intercourse was noted among both adolescent women and men. For example, after exposure to the intervention, the percentage of young women using oral contraceptives increased significantly among all grade levels, particularly among the younger girls. Follow-up showed a significant reduction of pregnancy rates among the older adolescents relative to those in the control schools (a decrease of 30 percent and an increase of 58 percent, respectively). A small decrease in the pregnancy rates among younger adolescents was found, although the pregnancy rates in the control school increased dramatically. The researchers note that a longer follow-up period to the program would be useful in monitoring pregnancy rates.

Primary References:

Zabin LS, Hirsch MB. Evaluation of Pregnancy Prevention Programs in the School Context. Lexington, MA: Lexington Books; 1987.

Zabin LS, Hirsch MB, Smith EA, Streett R, Hardy JB. Evaluation of a pregnancy prevention program for urban teenagers. Fam Plann Perspect. 1986;18:119–126.

Zabin LS, Hirsch MB, Streett R, Emerson MR, Smith M, King TM. The Baltimore Pregnancy Prevention Program for Teenagers. I. How did it work? Fam Plann Perspect. 1988;20:182–192.

SIX SCHOOL-BASED CLINICS

Summary: School-based clinics providing comprehensive health care to students located in six sites around the country.

Program: A group of six school-based clinics that provided comprehensive health care to students in the mid-1980s framed the basis of a program analysis. Although the sites were located all around the country (Gary, IN; San Francisco, CA; Muskegon, MI; Jackson, MS; Quincy, FL; and Dallas; TX), all six served low-income populations. The services and supplementary education offered at each site differed substantially. For example, the Gary site placed a strong emphasis on treating medical problems but did not consider preventing pregnancy a major goal, and therefore did not prescribe or dispense contraceptives; the San Francisco site emphasized pregnancy prevention as well as preventing AIDS and other sexually transmitted diseases, although contraceptives, including condoms, were not prescribed or distributed; the Muskegon site emphasized pregnancy prevention in the classroom as well as the clinic and provided vouchers for contraceptive pills; the Jackson site focused on risk-taking behaviors (including unprotected intercourse), encouraged abstinence, and dispensed contraceptives; the Quincy site emphasized sexuality and reproductive health education, including the benefits of abstinence, and dispensed contraceptives; and the Dallas site focused on health care, including reproductive health care, and provided contraceptives.

Evaluation: Program implementation at four of the six sites was already under way by the time that evaluation began, so closely located comparison groups with similar social and demographic characteristics were identified for each of the four sites. The other two sites had not yet begun their programs, so it was possible to collect preclinic and postclinic data from the populations served. Data collection consisted of administering surveys to the entire student body or, in some cases, large samples. The surveys measured social and demographic characteristics, clinic use, general use of medical services, risk-taking behavior, sexual activity, contraceptive use, and pregnancy. Some evaluation results varied among sites. Among males, there was no significant relationship between clinic presence and the initiation of intercourse at five of the sites; at one site, clinic presence was associated with a lower proportion of male students having initiated sexual intercourse. Among females, there was no relationship at four sites, a positive relationship at one site, and a negative relationship at one site. At all sites, clinic presence was not significantly related to frequency of intercourse either among males or females. Overall, substantial proportions of students who were at sites that dispensed contraceptives used the clinics to obtain contraceptives. Among males, clinic presence was not significantly related to condom use at four sites; it was positively related to condom use at two sites. Among females, clinic presence was not significantly related to contraceptive use at five sites; it was positively related to contraceptive use at one site. Clinic presence was not significantly related to pregnancy rates at any of the sites. The researchers note that although sites that dispensed contraceptives obviously increased access to contraceptives for far more students than the other sites, providing contraceptives alone may not have been enough to increase contraceptive use. However, school and community programs and a combination of education, counseling, contraceptive provision, and careful follow-up may have increased contraceptive use.

Primary Reference:

Kirby D, Waszak C, Ziegler J. Six school-based clinics: Their reproductive health services and impact on sexual behavior. Fam Plann Perspect. 1991; 23:6–16.

ST. PAUL SCHOOL-BASED HEALTH CLINICS

Summary: One of the first school-based health clinic systems in the country providing comprehensive health care, including reproductive health care.

Program: One of the first school-based health clinic systems in the country, the clinics in St. Paul, MN, have been in operation since 1973. Comprehensive health care that included reproductive health care was provided at six sites. Such services included education, counseling about how to make decisions about sexual behavior, physical examinations, contraceptive prescriptions, and pregnancy testing. A nearby hospital agreed to fill the contraceptive prescriptions for free. Nearly three-quarters of the students used the clinics for health services such as sports physicals, care for minor injuries, immunizations, personal counseling, nutrition counseling, and testing and treatment for sexually transmitted diseases. The clinics were easily accessible to the students. The clinics were staffed by nurse practitioners, social workers, medical assistants, health educators, and part-time physicians.

Evaluation: This program has been evaluated twice, in the late 1970s and the late 1980s. The earlier evaluation found higher contraceptive use and lower birth rates among the students attending the schools with school-based clinics. This evaluation has been criticized for making comparisons over time based on a single baseline year rather than multiple baseline years, for computing birth rates on estimates made by clinic staff, and for not calculating tests of significance. The later evaluation calculated annual birth rates at each school separately (sample size ranged from 1,838 to 2,988 depending on the year). To do so, the total number of female students in each school was used as the denominator, and only those female students whose names could be matched with birth certificates were used in the numerator. The data indicated that birth rates fluctuated between individual schools and at each school for different years. The researchers could not find any evidence that the school-based clinics reduced birth rates. Contraceptive use was not addressed in the second evaluation.

Primary References:

Edwards L, Steinmann M, Hakanson E. Adolescent pregnancy prevention services in high school clinics. Fam Plann Perspect. 1980;12:6–15.

Kirby D, Resnick MD, Downes B, et al. The effects of school-based health clinics in St. Paul on school-wide birthrates. Fam Plann Perspect. 1993;25: 12–16.

SUCCESS EXPRESS

Summary: School- and community-based program emphasizing abstinence for middle school students.

Program: Funded through the Adolescent Family Life Act, Success Express was an abstinence-only school-based program for sixth through eighth graders who were from primarily low-income and minority families. The curriculum was implemented across 20 sites (in schools and community centers) and emphasized attitudes, skills, and behaviors consistent with premarital abstinence. The curriculum focused on family values and self-esteem, pubertal development and reproduction, communication strategies and interpersonal skills about "how to say no," examination of future goals, the effects of peer and media pressures, and complications of premarital sexual activity, adolescent pregnancy, and sexually transmitted diseases.

Evaluation: Two evaluations were made of Success Express, both of quasi-experimental design (the first evaluation sample size was 320 students and the replication was 528 students), in the mid- to late 1980s. In both evaluations, the intervention sample consisted of five health education classes that received the Success Express curriculum; the comparison groups were students in health education classes with traditional curricula. Matched questionnaire data were collected at the baseline and after the 6-week intervention. Separate analyses were made for students who were sexually experienced at pretest and those who were not. In the first evaluation there was an increase in precoital sexual behavior among intervention participants, especially among male participants. The second evaluation found a similar trend among those male participants who had not initiated sexual intercourse.

Primary References:

Christopher FS, Roosa MW. An evaluation of an adolescent pregnancy prevention program: Is "just say no" enough? Fam Relat. 1990;39:68–72.

Roosa MW, Christopher FS. A response to Thiel and McBride: Scientific criticism or obscurantism? Fam Relat. 1992;41:468–469.

Roosa MW, Christopher FS. Evaluation of an abstinence-only adolescent pregnancy prevention program: A replication. Fam Relat. 1990;39:363–367.

Thiel KS, McBride D. Comments on an evaluation of an abstinence-only adolescent pregnancy prevention program. Fam Relat. 1992;41:465–467.

SUMMER TRAINING AND EDUCATION PROGRAM

Summary: Summer school program combining work experience with educational skills and information about responsible sexual decision-making.

Program: The Summer Training and Education Program (STEP) combined work experience with educational skills and information about responsible sexual decision-making. Its target audience was young adolescents (ages 14–15) from economically and educationally disadvantaged backgrounds. Students spent classroom time on mathematics and reading skills. They also received instruction that emphasized the value of planning life goals and delaying early parenthood and included information about contraception. Part-time employment was provided as part of the federal summer jobs program. The summer program was supplemented by adult mentors who met with the students bimonthly during the academic year. The program began in 1984 with five demonstration sites and 1,500 participants. It has been replicated throughout the country at 150 sites across 19 states and has served more than 40,000 adolescents.

Evaluation: The evaluation at the demonstration sites used an experimental design. Adolescents were assigned to an intervention group or a control group (N = 4,800). A baseline questionnaire and follow-up questionnaires (annually for 5 years) were administered. Although students in STEP gained significant life skills knowledge, no significant differences were noted in the sexual behaviors between the two groups during longitudinal follow-up. The researchers hypothesize that once the involvement ended "there was no vehicle to reinforce and continue STEP's positive impacts . . . and a brief, modest intervention is no match for life and school performance problems that were already well-formed." To address the need for multiyear program involvement, Public/Private Ventures has designed developmentally appropriate options for STEP graduates.

Primary Reference:

Walker G, Vilella-Velez F. Anatomy of a Demonstration: The Summer Training and Education Program (STEP) from Pilot through Replication and Postprogram Impacts. Philadelphia, PA: Public/Private Ventures; 1992.

TEENAGE PARENT DEMONSTRATION

Summary: Large-scale field test of a change in welfare rules and services, increasing self-sufficiency through enhanced services.

Program: The Teenage Parent Demonstration was a large-scale field test of a change in welfare rules and services, similar to changes made by a provision of the Family Support Act of 1988 that mandated work-oriented activities for recipients of AFDC. The three demonstration sites instituted new eligibility requirements for low-income parenting adolescent women and included Project Advance in Illinois (Chicago) and Teen Progress in New Jersey (Newark and Camden). Approximately 5,300 young women participated in a demonstration of the new welfare policies between 1987 and early 1991. To be eligible to receive the maximum AFDC grant, the adolescents were required to participate in the demonstration project: half were randomly assigned to the regular social and support services associated with AFDC benefits, and the other half were assigned to receive enhanced services. Enhanced services included special activities oriented toward self-sufficiency, such as completing education or becoming employed, and were based on a case management system. All three sites required participants in the enhanced services group to attend workshops on personal and parenting skills, on reproductive health (including information about contraceptive methods), and on preparation for continued education and job training. The demonstration projects were held accountable for keeping the participants engaged in some useful activity such as school, work, or job training. If the participant chronically failed to engage in such activities, program staff were required to issue a request for the participant's AFDC grant to be reduced by approximately $160 a month. The primary objective of the program was to promote self-sufficiency, but one of the secondary goals was to delay subsequent pregnancy directly through knowledge acquired at the workshops and indirectly through expected increases in school enrollment, job training, and employment.

Evaluation: An evaluation using an experimental design was conducted to measure a wide range of outcomes. The focus of one evaluation track was on factors that contribute to contraceptive use and repeat pregnancy. In this component, the sample consisted of the 3,400 adolescents who completed the follow-up survey at least 23 months after intake; 1,721 of these young women received the enhanced services described above, and 1,691 of them received regular AFDC benefits. Contraceptive use among participants in both the enhanced and regular services groups increased during the program: at baseline, 54 percent of the participants did not use contraception; this dropped to 17 percent by follow-up. Use of oral contraceptives increased from 29 to 49 percent, and condom use increased from 11 to 24 percent. However, as a consequence of method misuse and failure as well as substantial nonuse, 64 percent of participants had at least one repeat pregnancy within 29 months; 21 percent had two or more repeat pregnancies. Women receiving enhanced services were no more or less likely to use contraception than women receiving regular services. The likelihood of repeat pregnancy varied across the sites. For example, young women receiving enhanced services in Camden were significantly less likely to have a repeat pregnancy than those receiving regular services; young women in Newark and Chicago were significantly more likely to have a repeat pregnancy. The researchers suggest that the current strategy of offering reproductive health workshops and ensuring access to family planning services is not powerful enough to reduce the incidence of repeat pregnancies.

Primary References:

Hershey A, Rangarajan A. Implementing employment and training services for teenage parents. Princeton, NJ: Mathematica Policy Research, Inc.; 1993.

Maynard R, ed. Building self-sufficiency among welfare-dependent teenage parents: Lessons for the Teenage Parent Demonstration. Princeton, NJ: Mathematica Policy Research; June 1993.

Maynard R, Rangarajan A. Contraceptive use and repeat pregnancies among welfare-dependent teenage mothers. Fam Plann Perspect. 1994;26:198–205.

TEEN OUTREACH PROGRAM

Summary: School-based program involving students in community volunteer service, designed to reduce adolescent problem behaviors.

Program: The Teen Outreach Program is a school-based program involving students in community volunteer service and is designed to reduce problem behaviors such as school suspension, failure of courses in school, dropping out of school, and adolescent pregnancy. The program, which began in St. Louis, MO, in 1978, is implemented by local junior leagues or other community groups, and has served more than 4,000 students ages 11–19 at more than 130 sites nationally. The program consists of two major components: student volunteer involvement in the community and facilitator-led small group discussions. It has been suggested that the program's emphasis on volunteerism applies the "helper-therapy" principle and also increases the identification of adolescents with adults in the larger community, thus fulfilling the social development needs of the adolescent. The curriculum component of the program focuses on life options and includes topics on life planning, communication skills, family relationships, and community responsibilities. Although the curriculum contains some traditional sex education information, such information is not its primary emphasis.

Evaluation: A national evaluation system has been maintained since 1984. Evaluations of 5 academic years (1984–1985 to 1988–1989) suggest positive results for intervention students. For example, when the five academic years are analyzed together, program students had significantly lower pregnancy rates than the comparison students (3.2 versus 5.4 percent, respectively). These results remain after analyses have controlled for grade level, gender, racial/ethnic status, parents' level of education, household composition, and problem behaviors at the start of the program. (Although the overall evaluation is quasi-experimental, an experimental study within the larger evaluation indicates that the program results for the students who were randomized did not differ from program results obtained from those who were not randomized.) Over time, the evaluation emphasis has moved beyond the traditional focus of program outcomes by attempting to link specific program components with various effects for students at different ages. For example, sites that most fully implement the volunteer service component are more successful in decreasing problem behaviors than those sites that do not. The program also appears to be more effective for older students. Most recently, another small study was again embedded in the larger evaluation; data were collected from 66 sites and more than 2,000 students. In this study, promotion of student autonomy and feelings of relatedness were predictive of reduced levels of problem behaviors in the younger students. A self-reported high quality, although not quantity, of volunteer work was also related to positive results in the younger students.

Primary References:

Allen JP, Kupermine GP, Philliber S, Herre K. Programmatic prevention of adolescent problem behaviors: The role of autonomy, relatedness, and volunteer service in the Teen Outreach Program. Am J Commun Psychol. Forthcoming.

Allen JP, Philliber S, Hoggson N. School-based prevention of teen-age pregnancy and school dropout: Process evaluation of the national replication of the Teen Outreach Program. Am J Commun Psychol. 1990;18:505–524.

Philliber S, Allen JP. Life options and community service. In Preventing Adolescent Pregnancy: Model Programs and Evaluations. Miller BC, Card JJ, Paikoff RL, Peterson JL, eds. Newbury Park, CA: Sage Publications; 1992.

TEEN TALK

Summary: Sexuality education program based on the health belief model and social learning theory.

Program: The Teen Talk sexuality education program was based on the health belief model and social learning theory. The target population was adolescents (ages 13–19), 80 percent of whom were low income or from inner-city families in California and Texas. The 12- to 15-hour curriculum was designed to make adolescents aware of the seriousness of adolescent pregnancy and the probabilities of such a pregnancy happening to them, as well as the benefits of and barriers to abstinence and contraceptive use. Content areas included discussion about reproductive and contraceptive information, values, feelings and emotions, decisionmaking, and personal responsibility. Small group discussion format was a key feature, and lectures, leader-guided discussions, role-playing, refusal skills, script-writing, and guided practice were used to implement the program. The program was staffed by trained family planning educators and school staff.

Evaluation: Between June 1986 and September 1988, the evaluation compared the program with several publicly funded community-based and school-based interventions. Using an experimental design, the researchers randomly assigned either individuals or classroom units (N = 1,444) to intervention and control groups. The intervention and control groups completed questionnaires at baseline, postintervention, and 1 year after the end of the program. Some 62 percent of the original sample completed the 1-year follow-up questionnaire. Investigators measured a variety of personal factors and attitudes (such as perceived probability of pregnancy occurring, feelings about the seriousness of a pregnancy, etc.) and then related these factors to the outcome measures. Males in the intervention group were significantly more likely to remain abstinent than males in the control group ($p < 0.05$) at the 1-year follow-up. There did not appear to be a similar program effect on women. Among participants who became sexually active following the program, women in the control group were significantly more likely to have used contraception at last intercourse ($p < 0.01$). Among participants who were sexually active before the program, all groups showed significantly more contraceptive use at the 1-year follow-up; however, men in the intervention group were significantly more likely to use contraception than men in the control group ($p <$ p.05). The researchers suggest that the program appeared to have the most positive effect on high-risk young men, but was less useful for young women in general and for young women making the transition to sexual intercourse in particular.

Primary References:

Eisen M, Zellman GL. A health beliefs field experiment. In Preventing Adolescent Pregnancy: Model Programs and Evaluations. Miller BC, Card JJ, Paikoff RL, Peterson JL, eds. Newbury Park, CA: Sage Publications; 1992.

Eisen M, Zellman GL, McAlister AL. Evaluating the impact of a theory-based sexuality and contraceptive education program. Fam Plann Perspect. 1990; 22: 261–271.

G

Assessing Program Effectiveness and Cost-Effectiveness: Supplement to Chapter 8

Mark R. Montgomery
Member, Committee on Unintended Pregnancy

This appendix discusses several principles of evaluation that can be applied to family planning programs. As the body of Chapter 8 makes clear, the formal tools of program evaluation have only occasionally been brought to bear on U.S. family planning programs. This is surprising, especially as there exists a lively literature on family planning programs in developing countries, and many of the issues are precisely the same, although the contexts in which these issues emerge are, of course, quite different.

The evaluation concepts discussed in this appendix can be distinguished according to the objectives of the evaluation and the specific tools that are applied in the course of the evaluation. Although other forms of evaluation exist, this appendix concentrates on the evaluation of program outcomes. A fundamental objective is to determine whether a given program is effective, that is, whether it exerts a measurable influence on the outcome or outcomes of interest. A program's effectiveness can be determined through the use of experimental methods where these are feasible, but more commonly, effectiveness must be assessed by an application of statistical methods to non-experimental data. The first main section below describes what is involved in establishing program effectiveness with such non-experimental data. In this area, a good deal can be learned from the literature on family planning programs in developing countries.

Once given a set of programs whose effectiveness has been demonstrated, a second evaluation objective then comes into play: to determine their cost-effectiveness. Cost-effectiveness is a difficult and much-misunderstood concept in program evaluation. It is a relative concept, in that it involves a comparison between at least two programs that achieve the same level of effectiveness or "output." To assess cost-effectiveness, one asks which of the two programs achieves this output at lower total social cost; it is this program that can be described as "cost-effective." In practice, formidable conceptual and empirical issues confront even the simplest of cost-effectiveness analyses, particularly when unit costs vary with the level of output or when outcomes have multiple dimensions that must be considered. These issues are discussed in the second main section below. Only the most rudimentary forms of cost-effectiveness analysis have been applied to family planning programs, whether in the United States or in developing countries. As is made clear in what follows, perhaps the most informative literature on these issues is that concerned with health care costs in the United States, also reviewed in the second main section.

Finally, it is important to mention yet an additional objective of evaluation that arises in some circumstances: to determine the net social benefits generated by a particular program. This is termed a cost-benefit analysis. Cost-benefit analysis requires a means of translating outcome measures—such as pregnancies averted—into a single metric or standard that permits comparisons among quite different programs operating, perhaps, in quite different sectors. Even if attention is confined to the health sector, controversy must inevitably accompany any effort to force very dissimilar outcomes into a common metric or index for evaluation. A well-known recent attempt is that of the World Bank (1993), which sought in the concept of DALYS (disability-adjusted life-years saved) an index for assessing a great range of programs in developing-country health care.[1] Such approaches are commented on only briefly below.[2]

---

[1]The DALYS index relies on a combination of subjective rankings and empirical data to represent the degree of health disability associated with various illnesses and conditions. If these rankings are accepted one has a means of comparing the benefits from investing in (for example) family planning programs with those derived from investments in malaria control.

[2]As discussed in the body of Chapter 8, the term cost-benefit analysis is sometimes misapplied in reference to the net effects of public investments in family planning service delivery for public budgets in health and social service sectors in general. Levey et al., (1988) term this a "taxpayer's benefit-cost" perspective. A taxpayer's benefit-cost analysis asks whether public expenditures are likely to be reduced, on net, by public funding of family planning services. This perspective frames the evaluation issue very narrowly, being concerned only with the impact of one form of public expenditure on another form. There is no clear or necessary relationship between the claims that programs make on government budgets and their cost-effectiveness or social desirability. Thus, the terms "benefit" and "cost" that appear in a taxpayer's benefit-cost analysis bear no obvious correspondence to social benefits and costs.

ASSESSING PROGRAM EFFECTIVENESS

This section discusses some of the issues regarding evaluation of program outcomes when no randomized, experimental data are available. It is assumed that individuals have access, to a greater or lesser degree, to a variety of contraceptive methods supplied by the private market as well as by various programs. The focus of evaluation is on the net contribution made by one or perhaps a set of these programs. The outcome of principal interest is the degree of protection against unintended pregnancy. This analysis begins by considering the issues from the viewpoint of a representative woman.

Figure G-1 depicts the environment in which her decisions regarding contraception are made, and shows the potential ramifications of these decisions over the near term. (The highlighted boxes represent features of particular interest to this report.) The figure is meant to represent one period in the sequence of decision periods that make up a woman's reproductive life cycle. One may think of this decision period as being as short as a month, although the consequences of decisions made within that period are played out over the ensuing nine months and beyond (the later events are not shown). The individual woman entering this decision period is assumed not to be pregnant; she may or may not be sexually active, and may or may not believe herself to be capable of conceiving.

The information and constraints bearing on her contraceptive choices encompass a range of factors that have been discussed in several chapters of this report. Here only a few of the major dimensions are indicated. The woman's age (a), her current marital status, and her level of current income or poverty status (as denoted by y) are important, not only because of the obvious connections to contraceptive motivation, but also because of the fact that in the United States, access to service subsidies is conditioned on income. Under the current system of public funding, a woman's income relative to the poverty line determines the fee schedule that she faces for services in Title X clinics and establishes her rights to free services through Medicaid.[3]

In choosing among alternative providers, a woman will rely on the information available to her regarding the characteristics X_{priv} of private physicians or other non-program sources of contraceptive methods and the out-of-pocket prices of these methods $p_{priv}(y)$, the latter of which will vary according to her current income; likewise, she will take into account the characteristics X_{clinic} and prices $p_{clinic}(y)$ of clinic or program sources. Included in X_{priv} and X_{clinic}

[3]See Ku (1993) and Levine and Tsoflias (1993:50–54) for reviews of Title X and Medicaid funding and a discussion of typical fee schedules for women at various percentiles above and below the federal poverty line.

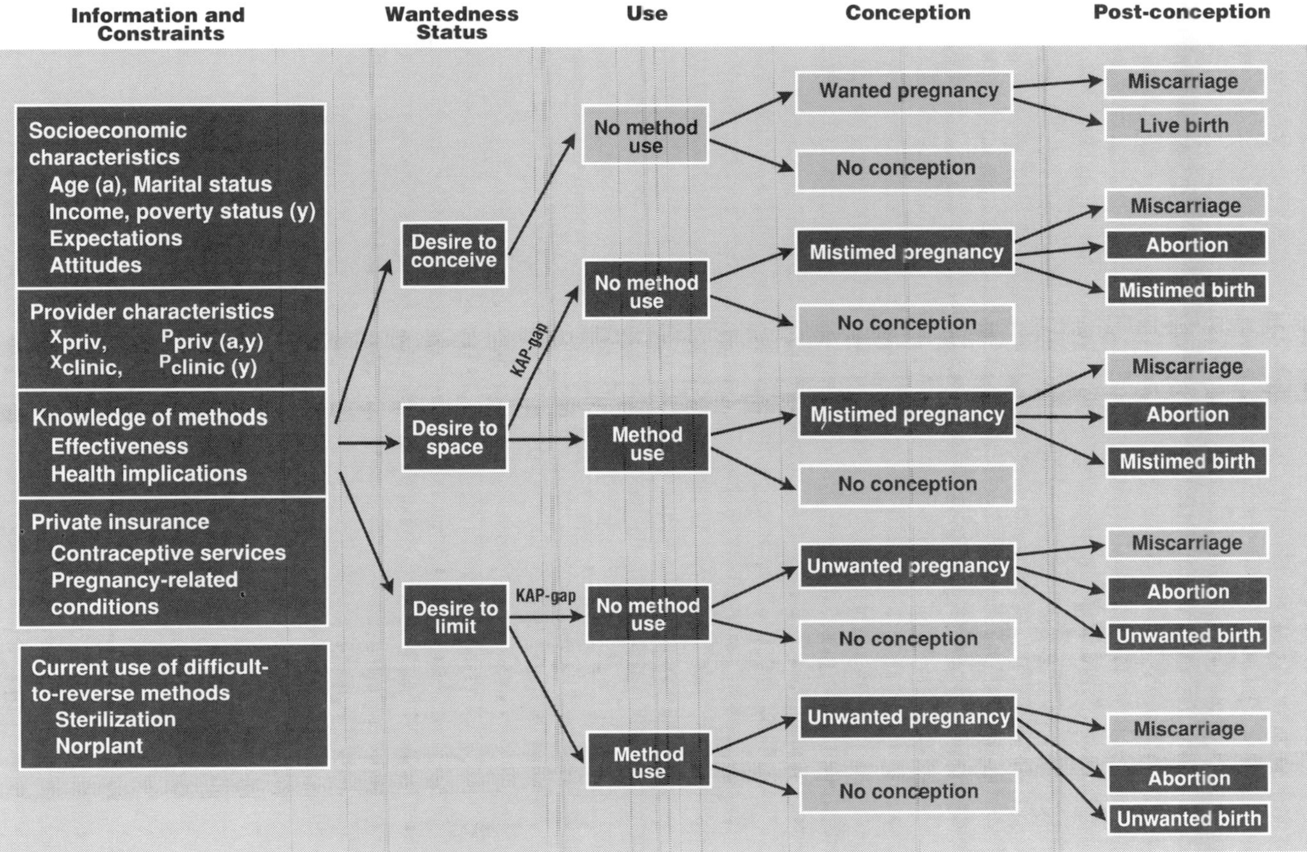
Information and Constraints
Wantedness Status
Use
Conception
Post-conception
Socioeconomic characteristics
Age (a), Marital status
Income, poverty status (y)
Expectations
Attitudes
Provider characteristics
X_{priv}, P_{priv} (a,y)
X_{clinic}, P_{clinic} (y)
Knowledge of methods
Effectiveness
Health implications
Private insurance
Contraceptive services
Pregnancy-related conditions
Current use of difficult-to-reverse methods
Sterilization
Norplant
Desire to conceive
Desire to space
Desire to limit
KAP-gap
KAP-gap
No method use
No method use
Method use
No method use
Method use
Wanted pregnancy
No conception
Mistimed pregnancy
No conception
Mistimed pregnancy
No conception
Unwanted pregnancy
No conception
Unwanted pregnancy
No conception
Miscarriage
Live birth
Miscarriage
Abortion
Mistimed birth
Miscarriage
Abortion
Mistimed birth
Miscarriage
Abortion
Unwanted birth
Miscarriage
Abortion
Unwanted birth

are the time and money costs that a woman faces to gain access to services.[4] Another factor of potential significance is whether private insurance is available to the woman and, if so, whether it covers contraceptive and pregnancy-related services.[5] The woman's current knowledge about methods, which may have been derived from previous method use on her part and from program and non-program counseling, will certainly affect her choices among methods and may also influence her propensity to use any method. Finally, various features of the woman's attitudes and preferences are important, including her subjective expectations about future income opportunities, the likelihood, as she perceives it, of sexual activity in the decision period, her perceived abilities to conceive, her skill and self-confidence in negotiations with sexual partners, and (especially for teens) her attitudes in respect to risk-taking.

Although the woman may have been informed by previous decisions she has made about contraception, she may also find herself constrained by these decisions. A constraint may arise if the woman has adopted methods such as sterilization, Norplant, or the IUD, which are either very difficult to reverse or costly (in money terms or otherwise) to remove.

All these factors, when taken in combination, express themselves in a woman's current wantedness status, that is, in her desire either to conceive within the decision period, or to defer conception to some later date, or to avert conception altogether.[6] The wantedness categories are, in fact, little more than markers of the current intensity with which a woman wishes to avoid conception; no doubt there is great variability in desires within as well as between categories. The categories are nevertheless convenient in that they correspond to the data gathered in fertility surveys such as the NSFG.[7]

---

[4]The *X* variables should also include indices of perceived quality of care; see Levine and Tsoflias (1993: 33–34). Confidentiality of care is one aspect of quality that appears to be particularly important for adolescents; see National Research Counci (1987:164–165). Note that access to care may be determined by the age and marital status of the woman, in that some private physicians will not accept unmarried teenage clients without parental consent (National Research Council, 1987:155–159). Nor will all private physicians accept Medicaid clients. See Ku (1993: 32ff) for further discussion of Medicaid eligibility criteria in the context of family planning.

[5]See Ku (1993:4–9).

[6]Women who currently wish to conceive, but are prevented from doing so by an earlier sterilization or the costs of removing a method, face a somewhat different set of decisions and consequences; these are not shown in Figure G-1.

[7]Although the desire to avoid conception is something that is expressed in the current decision period, a woman's expectations about future events figure into this desire. Consider a woman who, at present, wishes to avert conception altogether. She envisions the remainder of her reproductive career and can imagine no realistic scenario in which she would desire to conceive. A woman who simply wishes to defer pregnancy, on the

The desire to avoid conception is acted upon through adoption or continued use[8] of a contraceptive method. For reasons that remain poorly understood (see Chapter 4), not all women who wish to delay or avert pregnancy make use of a contraceptive method.[9] This disjuncture between expressed preferences and behavior has been termed a "KAP-gap." Women who act on their stated preferences may obtain contraceptive methods either from program sources—these are mainly family planning clinics—or from non-program sources—these are mainly private physicians—in the case of prescription methods, and pharmacies for the non-prescription methods such as condoms and foam.

Users of contraception face some risk of conception, as do non-users, although of course method users enjoy a greater degree of protection. A woman in either category is at risk of unintended pregnancy, whether mistimed or unwanted, and this may result in a miscarriage, an abortion, or an unintended birth.

A reproductive career may be viewed as a sequence of decision periods like the one sketched in Figure G-1, in which the decisions and outcomes in one period contribute to the information, and add to the set of constraints, that form the basis for decisions in the next period. For the purposes of program evaluation, it is important to realize that many elements in the figure are variable—and some of these are highly variable—over a reproductive career. Income y may fluctuate above and below the poverty line, so that the expected length of a spell in poverty and other aspects of poverty dynamics must be taken into consideration.[10] Other elements, including marital status and expectations about future income, also vary over the life cycle. This variation in what is termed information and constraints may then influence wantedness status. Depending on circumstances, a woman may switch among categories of

---

other hand, has in mind some future decision period in which she is likely to want to conceive. These different expectations regarding the future affect the intensity of current desires to avoid conception. See Montgomery (1989) for further discussion of such dynamic and life-cycle issues.

[8]The informational costs, and perhaps the money costs, associated with a woman's first use of a given method will differ from the costs of continued use of the method. The costs of adoption, continuation, and method switching are undoubtably important in contraceptive use dynamics. See the issue of the *Journal of Biosocial Sciences* edited by A. Tsui and M. Herbertson (1989) for further discussion.

[9]According to Levine and Tsoflias (1993:ii,22), some 37 percent of poor women (with income below 150 percent of the poverty line) who were sexually active believed themselves to be fertile, were not pregnant and did not want to become pregnant nevertheless used no contraceptive method. Even among better-off women (with incomes above 150 percent of the poverty line) in these circumstances, 22 percent did not use a method.

[10]See Levine and Tsoflias (1993:15).

wantedness over time. Hence, her wantedness status at a point in time cannot be taken as a constant or be interpreted as fully predictive of her status in the future.

The individual perspective adopted above is useful in clarifying the net effects of family planning programs on individual contraceptive use. Consider the following hypothetical but instructive situations. A user of a given program might, in its absence, have obtained her information and methods elsewhere, without there being any net impact on her contraceptive use. Conversely, a well-run program might attract a woman who had formerly relied upon other programs or on private sources, again with no net change in use. An increase in one program's out-of-pocket fees for methods or services might either reduce overall contraceptive method use, or induce substitution among methods, or encourage substitution of non-program sources for program sources. The information and counseling provided by a family planning clinic at one point in time might influence a woman's contraceptive choices at some later date; but the change in her behavior, although stimulated by the program, might not ever be expressed in the choice of a method supplied by that program. All this suggests the difficulty of determining the net effectiveness of any given program in an environment where a number of program and non-program sources are operating.

Consider now the upper part of Figure G-2, which depicts the reproductive career of an individual woman. In the course of this reproductive career, she might have come into contact with a number of different program and non-program sources. As of a given point in time (say, at the time of a demographic survey), the woman will have accumulated information about contraceptive methods and related aspects of reproductive health, will have enjoyed a certain amount of cumulative protection from unintended pregnancy, and will currently use or not use a method. Each of the programs will have made some contribution to her accumulated knowledge, contraceptive protection, and current use. To isolate the net contribution of any given program, however, is clearly a difficult task, one that calls for retrospective or prospective data on program contacts and careful statistical modelling. The evaluation task is further complicated because of the aspect of self-selection in program contacts. For a general review of the statistical issues and a comparison of statistical approaches to alternatives using experimental or quasi-experimental designs, see Maddala (1985), Foster (1989), Heckman and Hotz (1989), and Hausman and Wise (1985).

The fundamental problem in establishing program effectiveness is to predict what the program clients might have done, had that program not existed, or had its characteristics been different from what they are. Such "what if?" or "counter-factual" questions can only be rigorously addressed through a statistical model of the factors that induce individual women to participate in the program. As Huntington and Connell (no date) have pointed out in another context, the

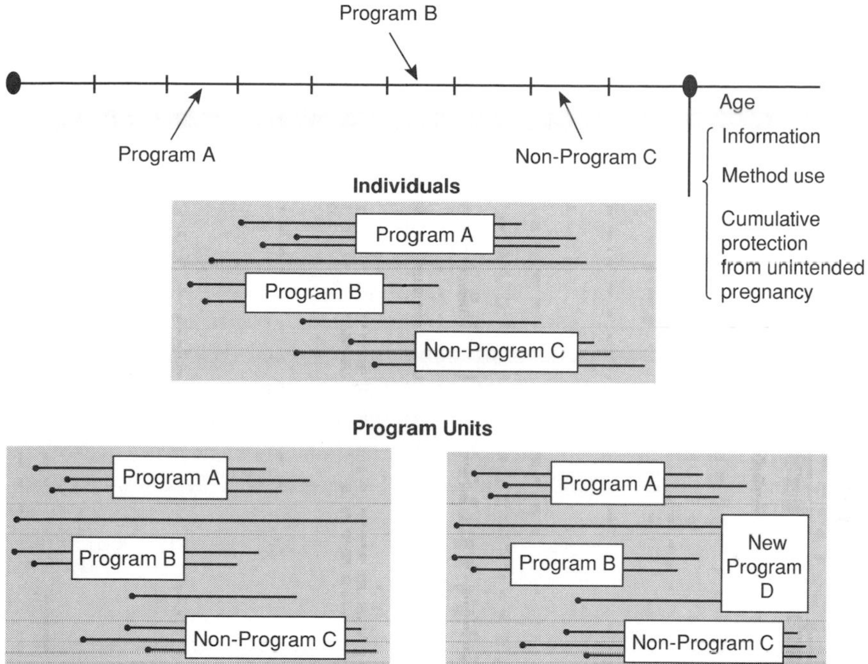

detail available in the empirical data and the statistical model brought to bear on these data are critical elements in producing defensible estimates of net effectiveness.

The ideal data include information on the nature of both program and non-program sources in the areas in which these women live. Note that when access and fees for service are income-conditioned, as they are for Title X clinics and Medicaid services, predictions about net program effects depend on the price-responsiveness of demands for contraception among women of differing income levels.[11] The committee is not aware of any detailed data concerning such issues for the United States, although there are data available for developing countries.

To understand some of the issues, consider the following equations (G.1 and G.2), which represent, respectively, the motivation to use contraception and the choice of program versus non-program method sources. The first equation represents the woman's "wantedness" status, that is, the intensity of her motivation to use contraception:

---

[11]See Foster (1989) for an illustrative analysis dealing with the introduction of a new form of health clinic in a low income neighborhood.

$$Y^*_{i,j} = Z_{i,j}\beta + X_{priv,j}\gamma_1 + P_{priv,j}\gamma_2 + X_{clinic,j}\gamma_3 + P_{clinic,j}\gamma_4 + \nu_i + \epsilon_{i,j} \quad (G.1)$$

Here $Y_{i,j}^*$ represents the intensity of motivation on the part of woman i living in area j. The $Z_{i,j}$ are her own individual characteristics (age, income and the like). Program (X_{clinic}, P_{clinic}) and non-program (here denoted by X_{priv} and P_{priv}) characteristics, or more precisely, the woman's knowledge of these program characteristics, also affect her motivation to use. For simplicity, assume that there is only 1 program and 1 non-program source in area j. There is also a place in the equation for certain unmeasured traits or constraints ν_i of the woman's that may affect her level of motivation.

Provided that motivation exceeds a certain threshold, say $Y_{i,j}^* > 0$, the woman will seek out the source of contraceptive supply that, on the basis of her own knowledge, level of income and the like, best meets her needs. This source may or may not be the program in question. The probability that she makes use of the program can be represented as

$$Prob(program)_{i,j} = \rho(Z_{i,j}, X_{clinic,j}, P_{clinic,j}, X_{priv,j}, P_{priv,j}, \nu_i) \quad (G.2)$$

which is a general function of the same set of variables as in the motivation equation. The program's own service statistics can be viewed as the summation of such probabilities across all women i in its geographic catchment area j.

From the viewpoint of evaluation, there are at least three difficulties brought to the fore by these equations. First, it is unusual for the evaluator to have any listing of all program and non-program sources in a given area, to say nothing of womens' subjective knowledge about such sources. Second, it is equally unusual for the evaluator to know which program or programs the woman chose, unless it happens to have been the program under evaluation. Third, there is the problem of self-selection, by which is meant that there will always exist unmeasured variables, represented here by ν_i, which affect both individual motivations to use and their program choices. If a particular program is eliminated, or if its characteristics are altered, one must trace the net impact first on motivation (equation G.1), and then on the probability that the program is accessed (equation G.2). A proper assessment requires data on all potential sources of supply, and also requires a means of controlling statistically for unmeasured but confounding variables such as ν_i.

To sum up this much-abbreviated discussion, it is no simple matter to document program effectiveness in a context of multiple programs and individual self-selection among programs. The evaluation literature can provide some guidance on these issues, but much depends on the availability of data at both the individual and the areal level. In view of these difficulties, some progress can be made with aggregated areal-level data. For attempts at evaluation using aggregated areal data (in this case, data on large U.S. counties), see Joyce, Corman, and Grossman (1988); Corman, Joyce, and Grossman (1987); and Frank, Strobino, Salkever, and Jackson (1992). The recent Title X evaluation of Meier and McFarlane (1994) is of this type. These authors are frank about the limitations of aggregated data and the possibility of mistaken inference owing to ecological fallacies.

ASSESSING COST-EFFECTIVENESS

The principles of cost-effectiveness come into play when one wishes to establish a ranking among alternative means of mobilizing resources to achieve a given objective x. Here x is defined principally in terms of protection from unintended pregnancy, but other dimensions will also prove to be of interest. The ranking is expressed in terms of the full social costs $C(x)$ of the resources used to produce x, with these costs being denominated in money terms. "Social costs," in this context, means the value of these resources when they are put to their best alternative use.

To engage in a cost-effectiveness analysis, one must first define the objective x in some quantifiable and measurable way, consider at least two alternative programs or ways of achieving the objective, make an accounting of the associated social costs $C_1(x)$ and $C_2(x)$ of the two programs, and assign a higher ranking to the program having lower total social costs. Often the comparison between programs is implicit, with Program 1 representing the status quo and Program 2 a newly initiated alternative.

Cost-effectiveness analysis should be carefully distinguished from cost-benefit analysis. In the latter, a social value $V(x)$ is attached to the objective x. As with the social costs, $V(x)$ is expressed in money terms, and this makes possible a direct comparison of social costs to benefits. The level of x is said to be socially optimal at the point when marginal social costs equal marginal social benefits, or $C'(x) = V'(x)$. The ideal cost-benefit analysis aims to identify the optimum level of x, or at the least, to establish whether the current level of x should be increased or reduced. A cost-effectiveness analysis, by contrast, makes no effort to assign a social value to x, and is therefore silent on its socially appropriate level. The cost-effectiveness approach leaves these larger issues to be decided by other criteria.

In spite of its limitations, cost-effectiveness is more suitable than cost-benefit analysis for the evaluation of family planning programs. These programs are necessarily concerned with the prevention of unintended pregnancies and births. To assign a social value to the prevention of an unwanted birth, in particular, is to engage in an ethical and religious debate about the valuation of life in general.[12] These are not scientific matters, nor are they matters about which economic analysis is especially informative. Thus, for the purpose at hand, the limited aims of a cost-effectiveness approach are entirely appropriate.

As it has been described to this point, cost-effectiveness analysis may seem to be little more than an exercise in accounting. Quite to the contrary: it is a difficult endeavor, requiring a blend of economic theory, expert judgment, and statistical sophistication. Consider these complications, which arise even in the most mundane of program evaluations: If two programs produce different levels of the output x, say x_1 and x_2, they are not directly comparable. That is, a comparison of total costs $C_1(x_1)$ to $C_2(x_2)$ is not informative, in itself, about cost-effectiveness. (The exception is when one of the projects can produce higher levels of x with the same or lower total costs.) It has been common practice to use average costs, $C(x)/x$, to make comparisons between programs, but this too is misleading if the average costs of a program are not constant with respect to the level of x. Furthermore, if x is defined in terms of multiple dimensions or joint outputs, then the total costs of a program with output mix x_1 are not directly comparable to the total costs of a program having output mix x_2. Programs differing in scale or output mix can only be compared indirectly through the device of cost functions, which provide a statistical means of predicting what social costs would be if the programs generated the same level of output or had the same output mix. Thus, the estimation of cost functions—a difficult task—is central to an evaluation of program cost-effectiveness.

There is also the question of units of analysis: whether these should be *individuals* within a set of well-defined geographic areas, program units such as the clinics that operate within these areas, or the reproductive health system through which individuals pass and within which a variety of programs are situated. As argued above, the effectiveness of programs is perhaps most easily established at the individual level, with data on the reproductive careers of individual women. Accurate measurement of costs, however, requires both individual-level data and data on program units. The individual data are required because important components of total social costs are borne by individuals, most notably the value of their travel time, their waiting time, and if referred elsewhere for additional services, the time that they spend in locating the next service point (Jonsson, 1985; Warner and Luce, 1982). From a broad conceptual

---

[12]Although such valuations have certainly been made (Enke, 1960), they are inherently controversial. The debate about valuation is not further clarified by the need, in a cost-benefit calculus, to summarize all values in money terms. The use of money indices of benefits and costs, while perhaps suitable for quantifying an individual's balance of production net of consumption over a life span, tends to direct attention to the measurable economic benefits and to divert attention from the non-economic or non-quantifiable dimensions of the problem.

point of view, it is the reproductive health system, taken as a whole, whose organization should be subjected to cost-effectiveness analysis.

The different units of analysis are exhibited in Figure G-2. The individual level, depicted in the upper part of the figure, has already been described. The programs themselves, each intersected by a variety of women in different stages of their reproductive careers, are shown in the middle portion of the figure. The bottom part of the figure contrasts two reproductive health systems, one having family planning programs A and B and a non-program actor or agency C (for instance, a private physician), and the other system having, in addition to these, a new program D. These two arrangments yield outputs x_1 and x_2, respectively. The full social costs $C_1(x_1)$ and $C_2(x_2)$ of the two health systems are the proper subjects of a cost-effectiveness evaluation.

The contrast between health systems need not take the form pictured in Figure G-2. For example, two organizational schemes might be envisioned, one of these being characterized by closer ties among programs units linked by a specialized referral system. Or, one can envision two health systems that differ only in respect to the organization of resources within a given program unit.

The recent history of publicly supported family planning programs shows why the appropriate comparison is between health systems rather than between lower-level program units. In the latter part of the 1980s (see Donovan 1991, and Levine and Tsoflias, 1993:42-50), family planning clinics in the United States found themselves caught between two forces: a decline in public funding, on the one side, and on the other side an increasing demand among poor clients for reproductive and other health services. The response on the part of many clinics, according to Donovan, was to increase reliance on fees for family planning and other services, and to reduce the range of services supplied in-house. The increasing use of referral by clinics, as opposed to direct service provision, has implications for the level and mix of output x, the total social costs $C(x)$ associated with this output, and the incidence of these costs among population subgroups, as between taxpayers in general and poor clients. In the late 1980s, clients were being asked, in effect, to take on a greater share of the full social costs of service provision. They were now using more of their time—a valuable resource—in order to obtain services. Clinics were directing fewer resources, on the whole, to contraceptive service delivery. The net effect on the mix of outputs x and total social costs is unknown, but it is at least conceivable that total costs $C(x)$, for any given level and mix of outputs x, were driven up. An evaluation of the reproductive health system, rather than a narrow focus on clinic costs alone, would be required to determine this.

In making the case for a comparison of health systems, the focus is on a conceptual ideal in evaluation. Many difficulties stand between this ideal and practical implementation. To begin, one must face the issue of how and where to draw the line in defining a health system. One simply cannot include all health services in a meaningful evaluation, as the range of services is too great; even within the sphere of reproductive health, it may be that attention should be concentrated on a fairly narrow range of services. The key, in the committee's view, is to restrict analysis to the set of services within which there are potential economies of scope. To understand the concept of economies of scope, let q represent the quantity of contraceptive services and let r represent the quantity of all other reproductive health services, so that the objective x is defined in two dimensions, as $x = (q,r)$. Economies of scope are said to exist if $C^*(q,r) < C_1(q,0) + C_2(0,r)$, where C^* represents total costs under an integrated service delivery scheme, and C_1 and C_2 represent costs when the services are not integrated.[13] To put it differently, economies of scope exist if there are potential cost savings to be secured by integrating service delivery in some fashion.[14] If these savings exist, or if the savings are believed to be possible under an alternative organization of the health system, then q and r should be considered jointly in a proper cost-effectiveness evaluation.

One final point should be made in respect to cost functions and evaluation of relatively new programs. In general, one expects the cost curve associated with a new program or system to be an unreliable guide to the costs that will be exhibited over the long term. New programs are unlikely to have on hand precisely the right mix of fixed inputs (such as capital) to minimize their long-run costs in the neighborhood of the output level and mix they will produce over the long run (Cowing et al., 1983). There are also learning effects to be considered, which would tend to reduce the cost curves over time, as well as differences in manager and worker motivation in pilot as compared to mature projects, which may tend either to reduce or to increase costs (Jensen 1991; Kenney and Lewis, 1991; Kristein, 1983). Thus, even if the estimated cost functions show a new program to be more costly (for given output levels) than an established program, some margin for error should be allowed.

---

[13]Another way of describing economies of scope is to say that economies of scope exist if the marginal cost of providing Q_1,

$$\frac{\partial C^*(Q_1,Q_2)}{\partial Q_1}$$

is reduced by an increase in Q_2. If the marginal cost is increased by the increase in Q_2, on the other hand, then dis-economies of scope are said to exist.

[14]By "integration," we do not mean to imply that services must necessarily be delivered within the same physical units (e.g., clinics). A referral system is one (albeit minimal) form of service integration.

Cost-effectiveness in Family Planning

The issues discussed to this point represent common themes in program evaluation in general. Family planning programs, or intervention programs having a significant family planning component, present two additional features that require special consideration.

First, they are concerned with prevention, and in this case, mainly with the prevention of unintended pregnancy. Second, family planning programs produce what should be regarded as intermediate outputs, as opposed to final outputs x, in that they provide interested clients with contraceptive methods accompanied by information on their use, the potential side-effects, and so on.

Programs aimed at prevention have impacts and benefits that take place in the future, for the most part, so that in evaluating program impact a decision must be made regarding the discounting of future benefits. Prevention programs typically cannot guarantee that a benefit will materialize or that an undesirable outcome will be avoided; rather, programs affect only the probabilities of these future events. Thus the concept of uncertainty comes into play in an evaluation of prevention programs (Warner and Luce, 1982). In some contrast to prevention programs in other areas of health, in which the illness in question can always be presumed to be unwanted, not all pregnancies are unwanted. As has been discussed above, a woman's wantedness status at a point in time—that is, whether she desires to have no more births or simply to defer pregnancy, and how intensely these desires are felt—can be expected to vary over the remainder of her reproductive life cycle. The desire to avert or delay pregnancy may change with her socioeconomic circumstances, with marital status, with stage of the life cycle, and with all manner of unforseen events. This inherent randomness in individual circumstances and desires introduces a number of subtle complications.

Consider the issues associated with discounting of future benefits. If a program supplies a woman with a 6-month allotment of oral pills, this may appear to be equivalent to 6 months of protection against unintended pregnancy, where the degree of protection is defined by the failure rate of the pill. But setting aside the possibility of method failure, do 6 months of protection necessarily result? If the woman's wantedness status remains unchanged over the 6-month period, she will make use of her full allocation of pills. But if her wantedness status happens to change, let us say after 3 months' time, she may discontinue the pill and strive to conceive. Has the program then supplied her with 6 months of protection or with only 3 months? From the woman's point of view, the program has supplied her with the means to avoid unintended pregnancy for as many as 6 months, although in the event, she chooses not to make full use of this. At the time she receives her allotment of pills, their value to her is affected by the probability, as she perceives it, that her wantedness status will change. The amount of protection supplied by the program thus depends on the expected span of time over which her wantedness status will remain unchanged.[15] In short, the service rendered by the program depends on the characteristics of the method and of the individual.

To further develop this point, consider the example of a non-reversible method. Envision a woman who, after counseling and referral from a family planning program, decides to undergo sterilization. She has all but guaranteed herself protection from unwanted pregnancy for the remainder of her reproductive career. (Evidently some risk of conception remains, see Trussell and Kost (1987), but the risk is very small.) Yet because her wantedness status may change in the future, perhaps owing to changes in marital or economic circumstances, a woman who has been sterilized may find herself later regretting the operation. She has been well-protected against unwanted conception, to be sure, but in selecting a method that is very difficult to reverse, she has also constrained her ability to have a wanted conception.

How should the contribution of the program be assessed in this instance? Wantedness status is to a great degree an individual matter, something that lies beyond the reach and the responsibilities of family planning programs. Programs play an important role, however, in providing the information on which individual decisions are based. A woman who at present wishes to have no more children, and who then makes inquiries regarding the option of sterilization, can reasonably expect to learn about all the costs and risks of the operation, the possibilities for reversal, and the characteristics of other effective methods (e.g., Norplant) which are more easily reversed. Having been fully informed as to the options facing her, she will then weigh the benefits of sterilization against the

---

[15]More formally, let the woman be in "state 1" if she is not pregnant and does not wish to conceive, in "state 2" if she is not pregnant and does wish to conceive, and in "state 3" if she is pregnant. (See Figure G-3 later in this appendix for illustration.) Let r_{12} be the instantaneous transition intensity associated with changes in wantedness status (that is, a move from state 1 to state 2), and let r_{13} represent the contraceptive failure rate for the pill, this also being expressed in instantaneous form. Assume that the period in question—6 months—is too short for more than one change in wantedness status. Then the probability that a 6-month supply of pills will yield a full 6 months of protection against unintended pregnancy is

$$e^{-\int_0^6 (r_{12}+r_{13})da}$$

a quantity that depends on both the pill failure rate, r_{13}, and the variability of conception desires, as indexed by r_{12}. Readers familiar with increment-decrement life tables or multiple-state hazard models will recognize the expression above.

strength of her desires to have no more children and the likelihood, known only to her, that these desires may someday change.[16]

Two larger points may be extracted from these examples. First, although the business of family planning programs can be defined as the prevention of unintended pregnancy, from a broader point of view their role is to assist women in the regulation of conception risks. Programs should aim to facilitate conception when conception is desired, and to help in the prevention of conception when it is not.

Second, the provision of information about methods and reproductive health has an immediate individual and social value, irrespective of whether the woman decides to use a method on the basis of what she has heard. Of course it is difficult to formulate objective and quantifiable measures of the quality of care and counseling that a program makes available, but these are fundamental outputs that must be distinguished from the provision of methods and recognized in any accounting for program cost-effectiveness.

Indeed, there is a clear link between the provision of information and the individual and social benefit attached to the supply of methods. In practice, contraceptive methods are used with greatly varying degrees of effectiveness relative to their theoretical benchmarks. The degree of use-effectiveness depends on the socioeconomic characteristics and motivations of the user, and on the information that has been made available to her. In providing contraceptive methods, a program produces an intermediate output that must be, as it were, further processed by the client to yield a final output: the level of protection against unintended pregnancy. Since different programs provide their clients with different amounts and qualities of information, they affect the way methods are used and the protection they ultimately supply against unintended pregnancy.

Dimensions of Cost-Effectiveness

Given the importance of cost functions $C(x)$ to program evaluation, and the many subtleties that arise in their specification and estimation, a brief discussion

---

[16]Let us carry forward the analysis of footnote 15 above. To understand the expected benefits and costs of sterilization, we would need to consider the expected length of time in state 1 (not pregnant but does not wish to conceive), and the expected length of time spent in state 2 (not pregnant but wishes to conceive) over the remainder of the woman's reproductive career. (The failure rates, r_{13} and r_{23}, can be set to zero in the case of sterilization, but we might want to introduce another transition intensity r_{21} to account for transitions from state 2 back to state 1.) The net benefit of sterilization *ex ante* would have to be defined in terms of the balance between these two expectations. We will return to this issue below.

of the issues is in order. Several issues merit particular attention: (1) how to account for the costs borne by individuals, these being the value of time and money expenditures they make in order to gain access to services; (2) how to deal with the multiple dimensions of services; and (3) how to make a translation from the service statistics collected by programs to measures of final outputs. These issues are seldom addressed in any rigorous manner in the literature on family planning programs.[17] For insight into the issues, one must look instead to the broader field of health economics, which in recent years has seen a profusion of cost studies. Table G-1 provides a guide to the notation used to organize this discussion.

To begin, it is important to re-emphasize here a point made earlier: family planning programs are engaged in the provision of a number of distinct services, and the supply of contraceptive methods is only one of these. Table G-1 identifies the four broad areas in which services are delivered. First, there are community outreach and informational services O, which provide information to the surrounding community and assist in bringing clients into contact with the program. These outreach services are in part responsible for the number of clients N who present themselves to the clinic or program. Second, an average amount of information I is made available per client during a typical visit. Third, contraceptive methods Q are provided to the clients who request them, either directly or through referral. Fourth, other reproductive services R are also supplied. (For notational convenience, I, Q, and R are expressed as averages per client, or in terms of proportions of clients receiving the service. Total services supplied are therefore NI, NQ, and NR.) The total social costs associated with these services may be summarized in a cost function $C_i(O,N,I,Q,R;w)$, where the i subscript is used to indicate that the program or health system is of "type i" in its organization.

The variable w appears in the cost function to denote the set of input prices facing the program, such as the prices of methods, wage and salary levels, rent, and the like. These input prices must be adjusted, if necessary, to reflect the true social costs of the resources employed. Many small or newly formed programs rely on volunteer labor or donated services. Although such resources are free in an accounting sense, they should be valued at their market-price equivalents in determining total social costs. Likewise, services made available to a program on a subsidized basis should be valued at their true social costs.

The cost function $C_i(O,N,I,Q,R;w)$ is to be viewed as a summary of all social costs associated with the delivery of the set of services (O,N,I,Q,R). These costs must include the value of travel time and waiting time on the part

---

[17]See Janowitz and Bratt (1992), and Kenney and Lewis (1991) for partial exceptions.

TABLE G-1 Dimensions of Program Output

O	$O^1, \ldots, O^K$	Information provided by community outreach efforts
N	$N^1, \ldots, N^K$	Clients, in total (N) and by age and socioeconomic type (N^k, $k = 1, \ldots, K$)
I	$I^1, \ldots, I^K$	Information provided to clients on average (I) and average by client type ($I^1, \ldots, I^K$)
$Q_1, \ldots, Q_c$	$Q_1^1, \ldots, Q_1^K$ $Q_C^1, \ldots, Q_C^K$	Contraceptive methods supplied per client, average by method ($Q_1, \ldots, Q_C$) and by method and client type
$R = (R_1, \ldots, R_S)$	$R_1^1, \ldots, R_1^K$ $R_S^1, \ldots, R_S^K$	Other reproductive health services supplied per client, average by type of service ($R_1, \ldots, R_S$) and by service and client type

of the N clients (Jonsson, 1985; Warner and Luce, 1982). Such time and travel costs must generally be imputed from information on a client's characteristics, such as her age, education, labor market experience, and the like. The distinction between the costs borne by clients and the costs tallied in program accounts is important, because different forms of program organization imply different divisions of social costs between the program and its clients. For example, a program that does little in the way of community outreach reduces its own administrative costs in comparison to more ambitious programs, but in so doing might increase total social costs. Without the guidance provided by outreach, potential clients might spend greater amounts of their time and resources in learning about and locating the program.

It is obviously misleading to compare the total costs $C_1(O_1,N_1,I_1,Q_1,R_1;w_1)$ for one program, with its own particular mix and level of services, to the total costs $C_2(O_2,N_2,I_2,Q_2,R_2;w_2)$ of another. Neither is it defensible to focus attention on only one dimension of services—say, the provision of contraceptive methods Q—and to interpret the relative costs of the two programs in light of this dimension alone. Perhaps it goes without saying that output mix and scale must matter a great deal to program costs; yet the family planning literature is full of misleading statements about costs that ignore both mix and scale.[18] Likewise, it is inappropriate to make cost comparisons without recognizing that programs face different prices w for their inputs, as would be the case when one program operates in an urban area and another in a rural area.[19] But by estimating cost functions, through which the implications of different service levels, service mixes, and input prices can be explored, one can lay down a proper foundation for meaningful cross-program comparisons.

As Table G-1 suggests, it may be useful to further disaggregate the service dimensions (O,N,I,Q,R) according to the socioeconomic characteristics of the clients being served and by type of services delivered (e.g., types of contraceptive methods) within each broad category. The various population subgroups (as indexed by the superscript k) could be defined on the basis of age and socioeconomic status, and perhaps additionally by the expressed motivation (spacing, stopping) given for family planning visit.

This disaggregation across subgroups serves several purposes. By indicating who the recipients of services are, it permits the equity dimension of service delivery to be examined. It also allows for differences in the costs of providing service to certain population subgroups, who may (for example) require greater

---

[18]The analogy would be to statements about hospital costs that ignore differences in case mix and numbers of cases in each category.

[19]Nyman and Dowd (1991) explore this issue in the context of Medicare. Note that programs operating in socioeconomically disadvantaged areas may need to pay higher wages and salaries to recruit qualified personnel.

outreach effort, counseling, or care.[20] It allows for meaningful imputation of the time and travel costs borne by clients. Disaggregation also provides the information required to convert data on the supply of contraceptives of various types into more refined measures of protection against unintended pregnancy.

Translating Service Statistics into Measures of Contraceptive Protection

A long-standing problem in the evaluation of family planning programs concerns the link between program service statistics, which are represented in this document by *(O,N,I,Q,R)*, and protection from unintended pregnancy. The essence of the problem is this: contraceptive methods are heterogeneous, so that a way must be found to aggregate across methods; and individuals themselves make use of any given method with different degrees of effectiveness, and will discontinue use as wantedness status changes. Protection from unintended pregnancy thus depends on both the method that is used and the characteristics of the individual user.

In progressing from service statistics to more refined measures of final services, two issues require discussion: (1) whether and how to adjust contraceptive failure rates for differences in program-supplied information and client characteristics; and (2) how to adjust for variations over time in wantedness status, another characteristic of clients. Curiously, the family planning literature has been more concerned with the first of these issues than with the second.[21]

To understand the difficulties, consider Figure G-3. Imagine that a woman begins in "state 1," defined as not pregnant and desiring not to conceive. In this condition, she contacts or begins her participation in a program. Upon contacting the program, she may decide to use no contraceptive method, or she may accept an allotment of s months of method type c. If the method adopted is sterilization, for instance, then s represents the length of time remaining in the woman's reproductive career. If the method is Norplant, s represents 5 years of coverage. For the pill, s corresponds to the length of the prescription issued.[22]

---

[20]See Nyman and Dowd (1991) for an exploration of the link between outpatient characteristics and program costs.

[21]For a review of some of these issues in the developing-country context, see United Nations (1979).

[22]A slightly more elaborate framework is required to deal with the possibility of unintentional expulsion of the method, or with health side effects severe enough to cause discomfort or to warrant its removal. The side effects can be considered by assigning a distinct "state" to each distinct (and measurable) degree of discomfort associated with method use. This is analogous to the method used to calculate disability-adjusted life years.

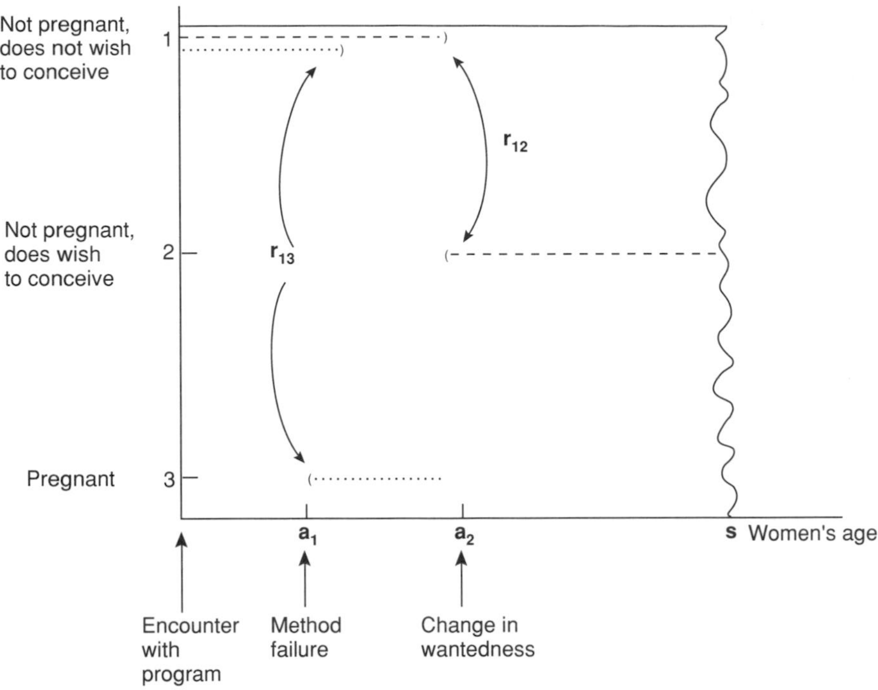

Newly armed with this length and type of contraceptive protection, the woman may then enjoy s full periods of protection from unintended pregnancy (a path represented in Figure G-3 by the long solid line) or she may experience a contraceptive failure and become pregnant (this is represented by the dashed lines showing a transition at a_1 from state 1 to state 3) or she may have a change of heart in respect to wantedness, discontinue the method, and hope to conceive (a path indicated by the dashed lines showing a transition at a_2 to state 2). Three transition rates govern the movements among states: r_{12} and r_{21} determine transitions between the wantedness statuses, and r_{13} represents the method failure rate. All three transition rates depend implicitly on the woman's characteristics (her subgroup k), and r_{13} may also depend on the contraceptive counseling that has been supplied by the program.

When a program supplies a woman with method c in allotment s, it provides her with an expected span of protection from unintended pregnancy. The *ex ante* value of the service she receives is indexed, in part, by the expected length of time $E_1(c,s;k,I_c^k)$ that the woman will spend in state 1. This quantity E_1 is, in general, less than s; how much less depends on the effectiveness of the method and the variability of conception desires. If method c is difficult to remove or reverse, then in addition to E_1 one must also consider the expected span of time $E_2(c,s;k,I_c^k)$ over which the woman finds herself in state 2, wanting to conceive but being prevented (at least temporarily) from doing so. The quantities E_1 and E_2 may be calculated by increment-decrement life tables or related methods.[23]

Given values of E_1 and E_2 for each method allotment (c,s), client type k, and program counseling strategy I_c^k, total services provided are calculated by summing E_1 and E_2 over these categories. What results is a pair of indicators of total services supplied (E_1,E_2). The E_1 dimension, representing total expected protection against unintended pregnancy, should be positively valued from a social point of view, whereas the E_2 dimension, representing total constraints on desired conception, should be negatively valued.

As the discussion suggests, rather detailed data are required to undertake calculations of E_1 and E_2. Given this, it may be useful to view E_1 and E_2 as conceptual ideals against which current standard practice can be measured.

Perhaps the most common approach now found in the family planning evaluation literature is the use of couple-years of protection, or CYP. This approach is based on two assumptions: that wantedness status is fixed (i.e., $r_{12}=0$), which removes the E_2 dimension; and that method failure rates (r_{13}) can be set equal to their theoretical values, unaffected either by client type or by the information provided by the program. Under these strong assumptions, the calculation of E_1 then becomes a trivial matter.

An alternative and better-justified measure, but one that is more demanding of data, is that of use-effectiveness. The use-effectiveness measure retains the assumption of fixed wantedness status, but allows contraceptive failure rates r_{13} to depend on the characteristics of the client served (her subgroup k, in this document) and permits the failure rates to vary (at least in principle) with the information provided by the program. Forrest and Singh (1990) give a good illustration of the use-effectiveness approach in family planning evaluation, whereas Shelton (1991) defends the CYP approach on practical grounds. As just noted, neither of these conventional approaches deals with the variability of wantedness status. Hence, neither approach can be fully justified when applied

---

[23]See earlier footnotes. E_1 and E_2 can be calculated if data are available on changes in wantedness status. Surveys such as the NSFG collect reliable data on wantedness status at survey, and the distribution of wantedness at a point in time can therefore be linked to various socioeconomic characteristics that we have subsumed under the superscript k. Reliable retrospective data on *changes* in wantedness status, however, are less common. The NSFG collects such information prior to the survey date, but only with respect to previous pregnancies. If a pregnancy took place, then its wantedness (in retrospect) can be ascertained via a standard set of survey questions. But since wantedness influences contraceptive motivation, which in turn affects the likelihood of pregnancy, these data may be subject to considerable selectivity bias.

to programs that supply irreversible methods or methods that are difficult to remove.

Predicting Net Program Effects Without Individual Data

Cost-effectiveness is inherently a relative concept: a program or health system is said to be cost-effective in relation to an alternative program or system. In practice, however, one may not have access to the cost and service level information required to compare two distinct systems or programs. Evaluation must then proceed on a hypothetical basis. The conceptual experiment is to imagine a health system much like the current system, except that the program of interest has been removed, scaled back, or otherwise altered. What would be the service level and mix x, and total social costs $C(x)$, in this hypothetical world?

It is argued above that the availability of detailed data on individuals, and an appropriate statistical model, would permit such questions to be addressed. But how should evaluation proceed if these ideal data are unavailable? The family planning literature presents no consensus, and offers surprisingly little guidance, on this central evaluation question. Essentially, one must set out different assumptions about individual choices that might be made in the absence of the program (or under an altered version of the program) and summarize these assumptions in a set of probabilities about contraceptive use and method choice.

Let p_i^k represent the probability that, in the absence of the program being evaluated, an individual woman (in socioeconomic subgroup k) would have chosen contraceptive method i. One should allow for the possibility that no method ($i=0$) might have been used. With all else held constant, her predicted E_1 becomes

$$E_1^*(k)=\sum_{i=0} p_i^k E_1(i,\bar{s}_i;k,\bar{I}_i^k)$$

where the bars over method allotments s_i and information I_i^k represent assumptions about the hypothetical values that these quantities assume in the absence of the program. An analogous expression can be specified for the expected or predicted value of E_2 in the absence of the program. Couple-years of protection (CYP) or use-effectiveness can also be predicted in this manner.

Evidently, then, the prediction issue can be reduced to the set of assumptions required to motivate a particular configuration of choice probabilities p_i^k. Some authors (e.g., Fitzgibbons, 1993) propose that information on a woman's method choices prior to her contact with the program be used to define p_i^k. The prescription is as follows. If the woman had previously used method c, then set

$p_c^k = 1$ and set the probabilities associated with all other methods to zero. If the woman had used no method, then set $p_0^k = 1$. This approach ignores the woman's level of motivation, that is, the factors that brought her to seek out the program in question. If that program had not existed, would she not have found other, non-program sources of services? Why is it reasonable to assume that the woman simply would have gone on doing what she was doing?

An attractive alternative in selecting a set of p_i^k, suggested by Forrest and Singh (1990) and used by them in an evaluation, is to employ the distribution of use and method choices that characterizes women who do not access the program in question. Forrest and Singh make a statistical adjustment to account for differences in social and economic characteristics among those who used the program (e.g., Title X clinics) as compared to the women who relied on non-program sources. The statistical adjustments described by Forrest and Singh do not take client self-selection into account, owing to a lack of data, but in other respects represent a reasonable compromise.[24]

Estimating the Cost Functions

Given all that has been said above, how can cost functions be estimated and used to establish cost-effectiveness of programs? Remarkably little guidance on this question can be found in the family planning literature. Within the broader field of health economics, however, numerous studies exist that employ cost functions, most of these studies being focused on the estimation of cost functions for hospitals. Cowing, Holtmann, and Powers (1983) provide an survey of the literature, and Cowing and Holtmann (1983), Granneman, Brown, and Pauly (1986), and Nyman and Dowd (1991) present empirical applications. Much of this literature is concerned with the cost implications associated with the delivery of a range of services. The methods are therefore of considerable relevance to the evaluation of family planning service delivery, which is also characterized by multiple service dimensions.

Cost functions are estimated from a base of cost and services data covering either a number of similar programs operating in different environments or a given program observed over time. Each data point provides information on total social costs C and the level and mix of services provided, whether these are expressed in terms of service statistics (O,N,I,Q,R) or, for the contraceptive component of services, in more refined measures of services such as $\boldsymbol{E_1}$ and $\boldsymbol{E_2}$ discussed above. Input prices w should also be available for each data point. Finally, each program under consideration should be classified according to its

[24]One questionable aspect of the Forrest-Singh analysis concerns their treatment of sterilization, which is assumed to be beyond the means of any poor or near-poor woman.

organizational type. In their studies of hospitals, for example, Cowing and Holtmann (1983), Granneman, Brown, and Pauly (1986), and Nyman and Dowd (1991) specify cost functions that incorporate shift factors representing different forms of organization, as for example, not-for-profit versus proprietary hospitals.

With such data in hand, one then selects a functional form for the cost function $C_i(O,N,I,Q,R;w)$. At this stage a decision needs to be made about how to aggregate services within the broad categories of outreach, information, provision of methods, and provision of other reproductive health services. Cowing, Holtmann, and Powers (1983) discuss the formal criteria that justify service aggregation, and of course data availability must also be taken into account. As a general rule, the less aggregation applied to the services data, the better; but some compromise is inevitable. Nyman and Dowd (1991) have estimated a cost function having as many as seven dimensions of service delivery. In principle, at least, even more dimensions could be incorporated, up to the limits imposed by the data.[25]

The estimation procedure takes the form of non-linear regression, with total costs (or the natural log of costs) being the dependent variable and with the set of explanatory variables defined in terms of levels of services and input prices. For example, suppose that a homothetic functional form is selected,

$$C_i(O,N,I,Q,R;w) = \Theta(O,N,I,Q,R)\,\Phi(w)\,e^{\beta_i D_i}$$

where D_i is a dummy variable representing program type and the sign of the coefficient β_i indicates whether, with all else constant, this type of program is associated with greater or lesser costs. A specification such as the above would typically be estimated in log form:

$$\ln C_i = \ln \Theta(O,N,I,Q,R) + \ln \Phi(w) + \beta_i D_i$$

and non-linearity arises through the functions of services Θ and input prices Φ on the right-hand side of the equation. If the estimated $\beta_i > 0$, this indicates that a program of type i is cost-inefficient relative to the benchmark program.

How can this approach be employed to assess the cost-effectiveness of a new program, on which perhaps only one data point is available? If an estimated cost function is available for a range of already established programs, then the cost-

---

[25]There are additional considerations, in particular concerning programs that provide zero levels of some service dimension (e.g., outreach). Some of the standard functional forms used in cost function estimation, such as the translog form, cannot deal with zero output levels. See Granneman, Brown, and Pauly (1986) for discussion and an alternative that can incorporate zero outputs.

effectiveness of the new program can be evaluated using the estimated function as a benchmark. In other words, by substituting into a previously estimated cost function the service levels (O,N,I,Q,R) for the new program, and the input prices w faced by that program, one can derive the predicted costs of the new program. These predicted costs can be compared to the actual costs exhibited by the new program. Although no strong conclusions about cost-effectiveness can be drawn on the basis of a single data point, a divergence of predicted costs from actual costs may nevertheless prove informative.

SUMMARY

To sum up, the assessment of program cost-effectiveness is a demanding task, particularly so in respect to the data that are required to support a rigorous analysis. If the data are not available, evaluation can proceed only on an informal basis, by invoking strong assumptions on the nature of the cost functions. Much of the cost-effectiveness literature in family planning has rested on two exceedingly strong yet rarely scrutinized assumptions: (1) that the multiple dimensions of output can somehow be collapsed into a single output indicator; and (2) that average costs, defined as total costs divided by (composite) output, are constant over the range of output. If both conditions are met, then a single observation on average costs can provide a basis for program comparisons. But in the absence of supporting evidence—the committee finds none in the literature—these strong assumptions are not well justified and may be misleading as a guide to policy.

CONCLUSIONS

This discussion and analysis has attempted to provide an introduction or guide to the evaluation literature on effectiveness and cost-effectiveness, with emphasis on those issues which are central to family planning programs. One of the more alarming facts about the state of family planning evaluation in the United States is the scarcity of research, and the degree to which techniques that have become standard practice in other fields have yet to be applied. Some of these are difficult techniques, to be sure, and results based on them lack the feel of certainty that attaches to randomized-experiments research. Nevertheless, their application to family planning evaluation is long overdue.

REFERENCES

Corman H, Joyce T, Grossman M. Birth outcome production function in the United States. J Hum Resour. 1987;22:339–360.

Cowing T, Holtmann A. Multiproduct short-run hospital cost functions: Empirical evidence and policy implications from cross-section data. Southern Econ J. 1983; 49:637–653.

Cowing T, Holtmann A, Powers S. Hospital cost analysis: A survey and evaluation of recent studies. Adv Health Econ Health Serv Res. 1983;4: 257–303.

Donovan P. Family planning clinics: Facing higher costs and sicker patients. Fam Plann Perspect. 1991;23:198–203.

Enke S. The gains to India from population control: Some money measures and incentive schemes. Rev Econ Stat. 1960;42:175–181.

Fitzgibbons E. Benefit:Cost Analysis of Family Planning in Washington State. Unpublished Master's thesis. University of Washington; 1993.

Forrest J, Singh S. Public-sector savings resulting from expenditures for contraceptive services. Fam Plann Perspect. 1990;22:6–15.

Foster R. Identifying experimental program effects with confounding price changes and selection bias. J Hum Resour. 1989;24:253–279.

Frank R, Strobino D, Salkever D, Jackson C. Updated estimates of the impact of prenatal care on birthweight outcomes by race. J Hum Resour. 1992;27:629–642.

Grannemann T, Brown R, Pauly M. Estimating hospital costs: A multiple-output analysis. J Health Econ. 1986;5:107–127.

Hausman J, Wise D. Technical problems in social experimentation: Cost versus ease of analysis. In Social Experimentation. Hausman J, Wise D, eds. Chicago, IL: The University of Chicago Press; 1985.

Heckman J, Hotz VJ, Choosing among alternative nonexperimental methods for estimating the impact of social programs: The case of manpower training. J Am Stat Assoc. 1989;84:862–880.

Huntington J, Connell F. "For every dollar spent . . ." The cost-savings argument for prenatal care. Department of Health Services, University of Washington; no date.

Janowitz B, Bratt J. Costs of family planning services: A critique of the literature. Int Fam Plann Perspect. 1992;18:137–144.

Jensen E. Cost-effectiveness and financial sustainability in family planning operations research. In Operations Research: Helping Family Planning Programs Work Better. Seidman M, Horn M, eds. New York, NY: Wiley-Liss; 1991.

Jonsson B. The value of prevention: Economic aspects. In The Value of Preventive Medicine. London, England: Pitman. (Ciba Foundation symposium 110); 1985.

Joyce T, Corman H, Grossman M. A cost-effectiveness analysis of strategies to reduce infant mortality. Med Care. 1988;26:348–360.

Kenney G, Lewis M. Cost analysis in family planning: Operations Research programs and beyond. In Operations Research: Helping Family Planning Programs Work Better. Seidman M, Horn M, eds. New York, NY: Wiley-Liss; 1991.

Kristein M. Using cost-effectiveness and cost-benefit analysis for health care policymaking. Adv in Health Econ and Health Services Res. 1983;4:199–224.

Ku L. Financing of family planning services. In Publicly Supported Family Planning in the United States. Washington, DC: The Urban Institute and Child Trends, Inc.; 1993.

Levey L, Nyman J, Haugaard J. A benefit-cost analysis of family planning services in Iowa. Eval Health Prof. 1988;11:403–424.

Levine R, Tsoflias L. Use in the 1980s. In Publicly Supported Family Planning in the United States. Washington, DC: The Urban Institute and Child Trends, Inc.; 1993.

Long D. Analyzing social program production: An assessment of Supported Work for Youths. J Hum Resour. 1988;22:551–562.

Maddala GS. A survey of the literature on selectivity bias as it pertains to health care markets. Adv Health Econ Health Serv Res. 1985;6:3–18.

Meier K, McFarlane D. State family planning and abortion expenditures: Their effect on public health. Am J Public Health. 1994;84:1468–1472.

Montgomery M. Dynamic behavioral models and contraceptive use. Dynamics of Contraceptive Use. J Biosoc Sci Suppl No. 11. 1989;17–40.

National Research Council. Risking the Future: Adolescent Sexuality, Pregnancy, and Childbearing. Vol I. Hayes C. (ed.). Washington, DC: National Academy Press; 1987.

Nyman J, Dowd B. Cost function analysis of Medicare policy: Are reimbursement limits for rural home health agencies sufficient? J Health Econ. 1991;10:313–327.

Shelton J. What's wrong with CYP? Stud Fam Plann. 1991;22:332–335.

Trussell J, Kost K. Contraceptive failure in the United States: A critical review of the literature. Stud Fam Plann. 1987;18:237–283.

Tsui A, Herbertson M, eds. Dynamics of Contraceptive Use. J Biosoc Sci Suppl No. 11. 1989.

United Nations. Manual IX: The methodology of measuring the impact of family planning programs on fertility. Popul Stud. No. 66. New York, NY: United Nations. 1979.

Vincent M, Lepro E, Baker S, Garvey D. Projected public sector savings in a teen pregnancy prevention project. J Health Educ. 1991;22:208–212.

Warner K, Luce B. Cost-Benefit and Cost-Effectiveness Analysis in Health Care. Ann Arbor, MI: Health Administration Press; 1982.

World Bank. World Development Report, 1993: Investing in Health. Washington, DC: The World Bank; 1993.

Index

B

C

D

L

M

N

S